You CAN Teach ADVANCED Med–Surg Nursing!

Mary A. Miller, RN, MSN, CCRN, is a practicing registered nurse who has worked as a medical–surgical and critical care nurse in a variety of clinical settings for over 40 years. In addition she is currently a clinical nursing instructor at Trinity University School of Nursing & Health Professions, Washington, DC. She has also served as both full-time and adjunct faculty for the past 10 years, holding positions such as lead professor in the RN to BSN program and chair of the Academic Standards Committee on Informatics. During the course of her career, she has effectively mentored many students and adjunct faculty through the challenging clinical teaching/learning experience. She has developed numerous instructional tools, interactive student exercises, and time-tested evaluation methodologies to help students excel in their clinical rotations and make a successful transition to professional practice. She received her BS degree from Shippensburg College in Maryland and her BSN and MSN degrees from University of Phoenix and is a member of the Sigma Theta Tau Honor Society of Nursing.

Deborah C. Wirwicz, BSN, MSNEd, is a practicing registered nurse and also a clinical nursing instructor at Trinity University in Washington, DC. She has held numerous clinical and leadership positions in critical care and medical–surgical nursing over the past 20 years. She received her BSN and MSN degrees from University of Phoenix and is a member of the Sigma Theta Tau Honor Society of Nursing. She has successfully developed patient educational materials for the critical care field in which she continues to work, and has initiated a progressive mobility program for the intensive care unit.

You CAN Teach ADVANCED Med–Surg Nursing!

The Authoritative Guide and Toolkit for the ADVANCED Medical–Surgical Nursing Clinical Instructor

Mary A. Miller, RN, MSN, CCRN
Deborah C. Wirwicz, BSN, MSNEd

SPRINGER PUBLISHING COMPANY
NEW YORK

Springer Publishing Company, LLC
11 West 42nd Street
New York, NY 10036
www.springerpub.com

Acquisitions Editor: Elizabeth Nieginski
Composition: diacriTech

ISBN: 978-0-8261-2666-5
e-book ISBN: 978-0-8261-1908-7
PowerPoints ISBN: 978-0-8261-2898-0
Forms ISBN: 978-0-8261-2899-7

Instructor's Materials: Qualified instructors may request supplements by emailing textbook@springerpub.com

14 15 16 17 / 5 4 3 2 1

The author and the publisher of this Work have made every effort to use sources believed to be reliable to provide information that is accurate and compatible with the standards generally accepted at the time of publication. The author and publisher shall not be liable for any special, consequential, or exemplary damages resulting, in whole or in part, from the readers' use of, or reliance on, the information contained in this book. The publisher has no responsibility for the persistence or accuracy of URLs for external or third-party Internet websites referred to in this publication and does not guarantee that any content on such websites is, or will remain, accurate or appropriate.

Library of Congress Cataloging-in-Publication Data

Miller, Mary A. (Mary Alice), author.
  You can teach advanced med–surg nursing! : the authoritative guide and toolkit for the advanced medical-surgical nursing clinical instructor / Mary A. Miller, Deborah C. Wirwicz.
    p. ; cm.
  ISBN 978-0-8261-2666-5
  I. Wirwicz, Deborah C., author. II. Title.
  [DNLM: 1. Education, Nursing. 2. Perioperative Nursing–education. 3. Clinical Competence. 4. Teaching–methods. WY 18]
  RT73
  610.73071'1–dc23
                    2014026959

Special discounts on bulk quantities of our books are available to corporations, professional associations, pharmaceutical companies, health care organizations, and other qualifying groups. If you are interested in a custom book, including chapters from more than one of our titles, we can provide that service as well.

For details, please contact:
Special Sales Department, Springer Publishing Company, LLC
11 West 42nd Street, 15th Floor, New York, NY 10036-8002
Phone: 877-687-7476 or 212-431-4370; Fax: 212-941-7842
E-mail: sales@springerpub.com

Printed in the United States of America by McNaughton & Gunn.

I would like to dedicate this book to the Heavenly Father who has given me guidance and strength in life's adventures. Also I would like to give credit to my students both old and new, my colleagues, and Gloria Hynes, my mentor and friend.

—Mary A. Miller

First and foremost, to the Lord, our Father, who was ever present and continues to offer guidance. To my loving husband, Waynne, and to my family who sacrificed time spent together to allow for my personal growth. To the nursing profession, which provides the opportunity to help others in new and wonderful ways.

—Deborah C. Wirwicz

CONTENTS

FOREWORD

Becoming a successful medical–surgical clinical instructor is not typically a skill that we are born with. Being a great bedside nurse, occupational health nurse, home health nurse, or any role in nursing does not equate to being an exceptional instructor without, first, learning, being mentored, and practicing the role. As it was during your first year out of nursing school—nervous, excited, unsure—these same feelings may surface once again as you begin your new role as a clinical instructor. How do you begin to prepare for clinical rotations as an instructor? How do you handle students who are having difficulty with the practicum, attendance, or may not be a "good fit" for the profession? How do you negotiate a contract? How do you matriculate a group of 5 to 10 student nurses through hospital orientation? Well, if you ask any of these questions, this book is for you.

Mary A. Miller and Deborah C. Wirwicz have a combined 60 years of nursing experience and more than 20 years as clinical instructors. These exceptional, passionate nurses met over lunch and decided to write this book to help other nurses who are considering or have chosen to become clinical instructors. The authors offer pragmatic information so that you can hone your own craft and have a blueprint to follow. Words of experience, clinical case studies, and pearls and perils of the role are discussed in this book. This valuable resource provides practical advice, direction, and resources about the role of medical–surgical clinical instructor. This concise reference provides a framework to prepare for clinical teaching, organizing, clinical assessment, clinical rotations, and how to deal with students who are in jeopardy of failing or are "troubled." Helpful and relevant tables, pre- and postconference preparation and questions, and activities are also provided in this book.

Simply having students learn the materials is hard enough. But for nursing students to really learn, think, act, problem solve, and critically think is challenging. We all can recall that one clinical instructor and cite the many reasons that that individual was such an exceptional instructor, clinician, and mentor. This book helps organize your thinking and teaching methods to become that one exceptional clinical instructor.

In 2010, the Institute of Medicine (IOM) published a landmark report, titled *The Future of Nursing: Leading Change, Advancing Health*, regarding the transformation of nursing. This important document provided an action-oriented blueprint for improving health care. In addition, the Affordable Care Act, enacted in 2010, emphasized that nurses can and should play a fundamental role in the transformation in today's complex, evolving health care system. Nurses, the largest segment of the health care workforce who are on the front lines of patient care, must be fully engaged with other professions and become professional partners in this transformation.

As patient acuity in hospital settings increases and patients are discharged from hospitals sooner, as the population increases and grows older with more chronic illnesses, the need for nurses will continue to skyrocket. Exceptional clinical instructors are imperative to transition student nurses to competent nurses.

Every day, a nurse makes a difference to a patient, a client, a family member, or a community. Now, you are embarking on affecting patient care on a much greater scale by empowering, educating, and inspiring new nurses. What a wonderful opportunity you have chosen!

Nancy M. Steffan, MS, RN, CCRN, CRNP
Professor, Catholic University of America
Washington, DC
ICU, Suburban Hospital/Johns Hopkins
Bethesda, Maryland

PREFACE

There are increasingly more adjunct teaching positions for which instructors are needed—but the BSN- or MSN-degree nurse, although knowledgeable in his or her own area, may be uncertain as to how or what to teach in a clinical setting. This book offers ideas and resources to help the advanced medical–surgical (Med–Surg II) clinical instructor succeed in this challenging area of teaching.

You may be asking yourself, "Can I be a clinical instructor?" The answer is YES!!! This book contains all the direction and resource materials you need to perform the role of a Med–Surg II clinical instructor.

You CAN Teach ADVANCED Med–Surg Nursing! offers the new clinical instructor a continuation of the medical–surgical learning process. Students will build on previously learned knowledge and skills and incorporate critical thinking into their practice. Week-to-week instruction and resource materials, along with medication quizzes and student learning activities, will help the instructor be sure that the students are learning new knowledge and skills.

Reading each week's activities ahead of time will guarantee that you, the instructor, are prepared for that particular week's activities and learning experiences. Students will be required to submit assignments as directed each week. As a clinical instructor, you will be required to review and grade these assignments. Based on your predetermined objectives, those based on weekly handouts, this should be relatively simple. Having the students keep weekly journals can be a helpful tool for the students; however, weekly journals can also help the clinical instructor discover the weaknesses and strengths of the student. A weekly journal also allows daily feedback on the student's learning experience. Weekly journals can be submitted as notebooks or can be done online; both options should be explained to the students.

Care plan and medication forms are included along with medication administration guidelines. Resources for each body system, which are the learning materials handed out each week based on that week's specific topic, and ancillary PowerPoints and forms from the book are provided. Delegation and patient teaching are also included topics.

Each clinical week is prepared and sequestered to provide the clinical instructor with enough material to teach without covering the same topic twice.

Instructors will discover this book takes the work out of working in the clinical area. Each preconference and postconference topic is planned out. Makeup assignments for those students who miss a clinical class are also included. Projects for days when the clinical unit may be too busy or inclement weather may cause a cancelation of the didactic class are also provided. **Ancillary materials to support these classes and new instructors can be obtained by emailing textbook@springerpub.com.**

Chapter 1: Description and explanation of the role of the medical–surgical clinical nursing instructor: Included are discussions of a typical adjunct professor contract, self-assessments, faculty observations, student preceptor evaluations, site evaluations, relevant forms, and a detailed discussion of strategies for dealing with challenges faced by the first-year instructor.

Chapter 2: Performing effective student evaluations: Instructions on evaluating a student's strengths and weaknesses, directions on documenting student progress, including sample forms and templates, and discussions of coaching strategies and interventions are included.

Chapter 3: Overview of the medical–surgical course: Describes learning required of the student and lists the required skills to master during the medical–surgical course. These skills are presented in the comprehensive skills checklist, which outlines and explains the necessary didactic skills. A sample course syllabus, including a weekly teaching plan, is also provided.

Chapter 4: Pre- and postconference expectations and activities are addressed. Forms to be used by the instructor and the students are presented and explained. Care plans and modified physical assessment guidelines are discussed. Math and vocabulary skills assessments are also included.

Chapter 5: Nursing assessments and patient data collection activities are discussed as the first tier of the nursing process. Concept mapping and development of critical thinking skills that serve as the foundation for establishing treatment goals, interventions, and evaluations are introduced.

Chapter 6: Nursing assessment challenges when caring for patients with sensory deficits, including detailed step-by-step assessment procedures for the visual, auditory, and nasal systems as well as discussion of related conditions and treatment.

Chapter 7: Understanding how patients experience pain, including pain mechanisms, classifications, and assessments and scales. Included are a discussion of the impact of culture, genetics, and disease on pain, and a summary of medications and treatments for pain, including alternative therapies.

Chapter 8: The growth characteristics, causes, risk factors, diagnosis, and treatment of cancer are examined in the first half of this chapter. Treatment methods, including surgery, radiotherapy, and chemotherapy and its side effects are presented and analyzed in the text and in case studies. In a separate discussion, the topic of death and dying is explored, in detail, with a focus on nursing understanding and support for the patient and family, the stages of coming to grips with dying, criteria for establishing brain death, and postmortem care.

Chapter 9: An introduction to fluids and electrolytes, including the organs and the acid–base balance mechanisms that maintain homeostasis, is presented in this chapter. Nursing interventions for the many conditions related to these systems are presented in a detailed fashion, with an emphasis on assessing signs and symptoms, understanding causes, treatments, and interpreting lab test results.

Chapter 10: An introduction to geriatric patient care, including nursing assessment of physiological and mental changes associated with aging; patient education in relation to age-related communication and learning challenges; theories of aging; adjustments to changed physical, emotional, and social circumstances; and care and support issues for the elderly patient and caregiver.

Chapter 11: Assessment procedures and diagnostic tests related to musculoskeletal system diseases and disorders are discussed. Introduction to the structure and function of muscles, bones, and joints; an overview of the causes, symptoms, and treatment of osteoarthritis, osteoporosis, and other bone disorders; and diagnosis and treatment for bone fractures and related complications, as well as other musculoskeletal system injuries, including sprains and strains.

Chapter 12: Introduction to pharmacology and patient safety, the importance of lab work in understanding specific patient responses to medications, and the potential for drug interactions and toxicities. Also discussed are the principles of safe medication administration (including the "five rights"), patient education, and recognizing and treating drug toxicities.

Chapter 13: Foundations of critical care nursing: Discussion of the anatomy, physiology, and electrophysiology of the heart; assessment of heart function (including EKG analysis); and diagnosis and treatment of irregular heart conditions. Discussion of the respiratory system, the brain, and renal system conditions and treatments as well as an overview of complex health issues and critical care situations.

Chapter 14: Introduction to emergency nursing, including assessment, treatment, and decision-making skills used by emergency room and rapid response nurses. This chapter discusses emergency levels and triage decisions; assessment and treatment of illicit and illegal drug emergencies; and emergent nursing situations stemming from a broad array of cardiovascular diseases and conditions, trauma, and shock.

Chapter 15: Introduction to hematology and the endocrine system, including a broad survey of related disorders and diseases and their diagnoses and treatment (especially in regard to liver, bowel, and neurological diseases). Also included are extensive discussions of autoimmune disorders and diseases as well as diabetes. A discussion of nursing issues related to blood transfusions and infectious diseases is also included.

Chapter 16: Introduction to the male and female reproductive systems, how they function, and their respective disorders and diseases, with emphasis on assessment, diagnosis, and treatment. Related topics discussed in this chapter include conception, contraception, the role of hormones, age-related disorders, cancer, sexually transmitted diseases, and HIV/AIDS.

Chapter 17: A framework is presented for transitioning from school into the role of professional nurse with emphasis on defining career goals and establishing a professional identity. Included are a number of specific suggestions to guide students through the job application process including reference letters, résumés and cover letters, interviews, and licensing exams. The midterm and final evaluation tool and criteria are also presented.

Chapter 18: Meeting required didactic hours and makeup exercises for missed and cancelled clinical classes are covered.

Mary A. Miller
Deborah C. Wirwicz

PART I

INTRODUCTION TO THE ROLE OF THE ADVANCED MEDICAL–SURGICAL CLINICAL INSTRUCTOR

Chapter 1

INSTRUCTOR CONTRACTS AND EVALUATIONS

This chapter examines:

- Role of the adjunct medical–surgical clinical nursing instructor
- Typical adjunct professor contract
- Self-assessments and evaluation forms
- Strategies for dealing with challenges faced by the first-year instructor

An adjunct instructor is a part-time instructor without the benefits of full-time employment. The adjunct instructor is held to the same standards of teaching as a full-time instructor. However, an adjunct is not required to perform committee work, which is usually a requirement of a full-time instructor.

The adjunct instructor is required to sign a contract with the institution of higher learning for which they are teaching. The contract guarantees payment to the instructor provided that the terms of the contract are met. The contract will specifically state a length of time for which the contract is in effect as well as what class or classes are being taught. Teaching semesters are typically 14 weeks in length, during which time the class meets one day each week. Summer sessions, however, typically run 8 weeks, and classes are held twice a week during this time.

Clinical instructors must establish clear class objectives and effective methods to impart knowledge to their students. Upon completion of the semester, it is common practice for instructors to complete self-assessments. The clinical instructor's teaching philosophy and methods will be evaluated by the instructor's peers, who will complete evaluation forms and submit them to the institution. In addition, students are strongly encouraged to evaluate the clinical instructor or assigned preceptor, if applicable. A preceptor is defined as a professor or experienced nurse who will train the students and provide specialized experience. For example, there are some clinical classes in which the professor assigns students to an experienced nurse who works in a particular field such as intravenous (IV) therapy, endoscopy, and so on.

Both instructors and students are required to evaluate the clinical site at the conclusion of the class. These evaluations allow the institution of higher learning to determine whether it should continue to use that particular site as a clinical learning environment.

THE CONTRACT

A contract is entered into between the educational institution and the instructor. The contract will describe the terms and responsibilities of employment of the adjunct professor. A sample of a typical contract follows.

SAMPLE ADJUNCT PROFESSOR CONTRACT

A. Employment

This contract shall have a fixed duration of one semester, which will automatically expire at the end of this term. This contract establishes a temporary employment and does not carry with it any future obligations.

B. Duties and responsibilities

The employee's responsibility to the school under the terms of this contract is to serve as an adjunct professor who will be employed for the course(s) listed in this contract and will be required to perform normal teaching, documentation, and advisory duties in accordance with the faculty handbook and other academic and college policies. The employee is required to submit a course syllabus for each course covered by this contract to faculty services and the students at least 1 week prior to the start of the course. The employee is to submit course attendance rosters, midterm grades, and final grades by the academic calendar deadlines noted on the syllabus. The employee is required to set up and check an e-mail account on a regular basis.

C. Position and termination of employee

Employment is an at-will relationship and can be terminated at any time. Reasons can include failure to submit enrollment verification and midterm and final grades; failure to teach material in an acceptable manner; or improper conduct. The employee will give the nursing school sufficient notice of not less than 2 weeks, and monetary compensation will end at termination.

SELF-ASSESSMENT AND EVALUATIONS/OBSERVATIONS

Full- and part-time faculty regularly participate in self-assessments and invite colleagues to observe their teaching to strengthen their instructional skills and to advance actual and constant excellence in instruction. Administrators also observe classes, fostering a friendly atmosphere that promotes dynamic teaching that keeps students at the center.

As part of this assessment process, faculty members should develop a brief self-assessment that they can share with those of their colleagues who focus on promoting excellent teaching. Faculty members should share specific information about the observation with the students. Observation by colleagues using a standard rubric to provide feedback establishes goals and objectives particular to their academic discipline and to the unit itself.

SAMPLE PRE-EVALUATION QUESTIONS

A self-assessment form and observation form follow.

Self-assessment: In reflecting on your role as an instructor, please discuss the following questions. Each response should be one page or less.

1. What are your strengths as a professor?
2. In what areas would you like to advance as a professor?
3. What suggestions do you have for improving your course?

Observation: In reflecting on the class you have chosen to observe, please address the following items. Each response should be one page or less.

1. Briefly describe the students in the course—their demographics, experiences, and attitudes.
2. What are the goals and objectives for the class being observed?
3. How will you know if students are learning what you intended them to learn?
4. What other background information does the observer need to know to be able to follow the class and provide meaningful feedback to you as an instructor?

Sample Self-Assessment Form

The adjunct professor should complete and share this form prior to the peer/administrative observation of a specific class.

Name of faculty member:

Date:

Course title/number:

Number of students:

	Never	Occasionally	Usually	Always
1. Provides an up-to-date syllabus, correct assignments, and additional readings; maintains submission dates; and provides clearly-stated course objectives and goals				
2. Uses the syllabus as a tool for guiding and communicating with students				
3. Posts and maintains a communication pathway with the students by in-person meetings or university e-mail				
4. Follows school policies and procedures related to missed classes, plagiarism, and mid-semester advising				
5. Remains current with developments in nursing, and shares developments in class discussions and projects				
6. Provides timely feedback to students				

Comments:

_____

_____

_____

_____

_____

_____

Sample Observation Form

The evaluator should complete this form after observing the class and then discuss the results with the faculty member.

Name of faculty member:

Name of evaluator:

Date:

Course title/number:

Number of students present:

Category	Approaches standard (1)	Meets standard (2)	Exceeds standard (3)	Rating
Knowledge of content	Professor displays basic content and professional knowledge, but familiarity with nursing's most recent developments is not apparent.	Professor displays solid content and professional knowledge, makes appropriate connections to prior learning, and shows some familiarity with nursing's most recent developments.	Professor displays broad content knowledge and makes appropriate connections to prior learning. Professor demonstrates awareness of nursing developments and encourages students to understand and learn more about evidence-based practices.	
Objectives	Objectives are vague, conflicting, or not related to the topics addressed in class or in real-life situations.	Objectives are significant and clearly communicated to students, relate to the syllabus as well as to the topics addressed in class, have real-life implications, and show connections to current trends in nursing.	Objectives are clear, concise, and appropriately aligned to evidence-based practices. The instructor generates interest and enthusiasm in students.	
Organization of classroom	Classroom is not organized in a way that engages student learning. Professor appears unprepared for class, does not begin and end on time, vaguely explains assignments and activities, and attempts to but does not make good use of class time.	Classroom organization reflects the different modes of learning to engage student learning. Professor appears to have planned the lesson and is prepared for class, begins and ends on time, clearly communicates assignments and activities, and makes effective use of class time.	Professor is well prepared and highly organized and uses instructional knowledge and tools to maximize and encourage student learning within and beyond the classroom. Activities and discussion engage students so that there is optimal time management.	

Category	Approaches standard (1)	Meets standard (2)	Exceeds standard (3)	Rating
Appropriate teaching methods, including the use of technology	Professor does not make the best selection of instructional strategies and does not show awareness of how to teach to multiple learning styles. Instructor attempts to integrate technology and collaboration but the implementation is not effective.	Professor selects appropriate instructional strategies and implements them effectively, integrates technology and collaboration well; demonstrates an awareness of how to teach to multiple learning styles.	Professor selects instructional strategies that best match the objectives and implements them with ease, employs the use of technology and collaboration in ways that enhance learning; effectively teaches to multiple learning styles.	
Uses formal or informal assessment	Professor attempts to but does clearly determine what students have learned.	Professor uses informal and/or formal assessments to ensure that students are learning.	Professor embeds assessments in the lesson and uses them effectively to further student learning.	
Faculty interaction with students	Professor engages some but not all students in classroom activities and discussions, attempts to communicate concepts and ideas but is not always clear, and does not demonstrate concern for students.	Professor engages all students in classroom activities and discussions, communicates concepts and ideas in clear ways using professional language and logical progressions, and demonstrates respect for individuals.	Professor works with students as they explore new material, raise questions, and make connections to real-life situations; students correspond with other health professionals in a clear and organized manner; and establishes a culture of mutual respect for multiple views.	

Comments:

_____

_____

_____

_____

_____

_____

Nursing Program Evaluation Form

Nursing students should fill out this form to provide feedback on their experience with the preceptor.

Preceptor: _____ Course: _____

Date: _____ Site: _____

Completed by: _____

Please circle the most appropriate answer that best describes your viewpoint regarding your preceptor experience. Space is provided after each statement if you choose to add any written comment.

1. Did the preceptor smooth the progress of the orientation process?

   Never   Occasionally   Always

   Comment: _____

2. Did the preceptor show expertise in his or her nursing role?

   Never   Occasionally   Always

   Comment: _____

3. Did the preceptor work in partnership and assist you in planning learning objectives and experiences?

   Never   Occasionally   Always

   Comment: _____

4. Did the preceptor provide immediate and appropriate feedback?

   Never   Occasionally   Always

   Comment: _____

5. Did the preceptor provide resources to the student and facilitate learning?

   Never   Occasionally   Always

   Comment: _____

6. Did the preceptor direct the student through critical thinking and decision making?

   Never   Occasionally   Always

   Comment: _____

7. Did the preceptor consider the students' limitations according to the students' level of training?

   Never   Occasionally   Always

   Comment: _____

8. Did the preceptor encourage questions and offer constructive comments?

   Never   Occasionally   Always

   Comment: _____

9. Did the preceptor use good communication skills?

   Never   Occasionally   Always

   Comment: _____

10. Did the preceptor exhibit a caring and respectful attitude?

Never   Occasionally   Always

Comment: _____

General Comments: Please comment on how this preceptor assisted you to develop your clinical learning experience.

1. Do you recommend this preceptor for other students?

YES   NO

Why or why not? _____

2. Did this clinical setting provide accommodation of learning activities for student learning:

YES   NO

Why or why not? _____

3. Were the course objectives realistic, and how could they be improved?

_____

4. The following worked well in this clinical: _____

_____

5. The following did not work well in this clinical: _____

_____

Do not sign your name. Thank you for your comments.

Clinical Facility Evaluation Form

Nursing students and faculty members should fill out this form to provide feedback to the learning institution on their experience with the clinical facility.

Name of clinical facility:

Course:

Completed by: ☐ Student   ☐ Faculty

Please circle the most appropriate answer that best describes your opinion regarding the clinical site. Space is provided after each statement if you choose to add any additional comments.

1. Was this clinical agency pertinent to the expected clinical experience?

Never   Occasionally   Always

Comment: _____

2. Were the facilities adequate and available to achieve the clinical objectives?

Never   Occasionally   Always

Comment: _____

3. Were there sufficient and appropriate learning opportunities available to meet the objectives?

Never   Occasionally   Always

Comment: _____

4. Was there an adequate number of patients to meet the learning objectives?

Never   Occasionally   Always

Comment: _____

5. Were the types of patients varied in terms of age, types of problems, and so on?

Never   Occasionally   Always

Comment: _____

6. Was the support staff helpful and accepting of students?

Never   Occasionally   Always

Comment: _____

7. Were instructional materials and community resources available to supplement learning (i.e., pamphlets, outside-class opportunities, etc.)?

Never   Occasionally   Always

Comment: _____

8. Were the philosophy, the mission, and the goals of the clinical site relevant to caring?

Never   Occasionally   Always

9. Were the philosophy, the mission, and the goals of the clinical site relevant to health promotion and disease prevention?

Never   Occasionally   Always

10. Were the philosophy, the mission, and the goals of the clinical site relevant to sociocultural diversity?

Never   Occasionally   Always

11. Were the philosophy, the mission, and the goals of the clinical site relevant to safe practices and competent patient care?

Never   Occasionally   Always

12. How far did you travel from home to the clinical site?

Mileage:_____

13. How accessible was the site to public transportation?

Distance:_____

General Comments:

1. List ways in which this clinical site provided a good clinical experience for the student:

_____

2. List areas in which this clinical site might need improvement in order to provide optimal student learning:

_____

3. Do you suggest this clinical site for other students?

YES   NO

Why or why not? _____

_____

If you are a member of the faculty, please sign and date.
Signature: _____ Date: _____

If additional space is needed, please use the back of this sheet.

THE FIRST YEAR AS A CLINICAL INSTRUCTOR

The following outline is a conceptual road map the first-year clinical instructor can follow to achieve success in preparing the course, navigating the all-important first class meeting, and mastering effective student-focused teaching practices.

I. Have or write a philosophy of what you want to achieve as a teacher. Objectives should be achievable and relevant to your teaching responsibilities, such as to instill in your students critical thinking skills, the acquisition of lifelong learning skills, and the ability to function efficiently in a hospital setting. Define your area of responsibility as compared to your students' responsibilities. Improve the education of students in your field by involving discussions of articles in academic journals or published by professional organizations.

II. Create a climate of mutual respect and trust. Do not threaten the students with their grades. Focus on essential knowledge, skills, and attitudes. This makes students eager to learn.

III. Prepare possible topics for discussion during the initial student conference
   A. Student goals and perception of strengths and areas of improvement
   B. Previous clinical evaluation (if applicable) and what the student did to improve his or her weaknesses
   C. Areas of knowledge building or improvement, including time management, organization, skill performance, priority setting, and clinical written work

IV. Prepare to meet the students for the first time
   A. Be prepared and organized. Arrive early to create an open atmosphere. Students are anxious, so keep the first meeting short and purposeful.
   B. State your expectations clearly and concisely. Set boundaries and offer expected outcomes to pass the course. Provide examples of satisfactory and unsatisfactory performances.

V. Select assignments based on specific course outcomes, abilities and learning needs of each student, prior student experiences, number of patients, and patient availability.

VI. Be aware of common student stressors
   A. Harming a patient or making a mistake
   B. Assimilating new nursing skills
   C. Getting "kicked out" of the nursing program
   D. Being observed and evaluated
   E. Feeling a lack of understanding, being overwhelmed, or being frozen with fear
   F. Being unfamiliar with a specialized hospital or unit
   G. Being uncertain of expectations

VII. Prepare to coach students effectively
    A. Provide a learning atmosphere that encourages students to ask questions and to expect honest feedback, teaches how to solve problems, provides challenging experiences that optimize student learning, and fosters mutual respect
    B. Maintain a calm environment
    C. Be consistent when performing procedures
    D. Do not belittle the students when they do not know the answers
    E. Identify student strengths but also identify weaknesses in a nonthreatening manner.
    F. Foster student participation and questions

VIII. Tips for effective questioning
    A. Phrase questions clearly and distinctly
    B. Ask questions in a logical order; wait before expecting a response
    C. Maintain eye contact and listen attentively
    D. Do not interrupt students

IX. Be aware of different types of questions
    A. Lower level questions focus on recall; for example, What is the action of _____? How has the medication affected the patient's blood pressure?
    B. Higher level questions focus more on critical thinking, for example: What would you do differently? What interventions would be effective for this patient? What would you teach the patient? What factors may have caused their noncompliance?
    C. Incorrect student responses
        1. Determine whether the student lacks knowledge or whether he or she is not prepared for the clinical experience.
        2. Determine consequences: Can the student find the correct information, or does he or she need to be sent home from clinical because of this deficiency?

X. Tips for effective teaching
    A. How do you know that the students are prepared? Is the preparation work complete? Prioritize patient care: Are the students mentally and physically able to safely deliver care? Explain the level of care to be performed: The student should be able to do a full unassisted assessment, ascertain the patency of IVs, and ensure that the right orders are being initiated for the patient. The student should be able to understand the correlation of lab results with resulting medical interventions. The student should be able to accurately interpret and calculate vital signs such as mean arterial pressure (MAP), pulse pressure, pulse deficit, and so on.
    B. Different styles of learning: Visual, auditory, and tactile
        1. Visual: Use visual demonstrations, for example, color code laboratory values
        2. Auditory: Talk through the steps to be performed; think aloud
        3. Tactile: Provide hands-on learning

XI. Observe skills performance
    A. Advanced nursing student
    The advanced nursing student should be able to take an assignment of two to three patients and be able to provide all the required care including procedures, medication administration, charting, and addressing in collaboration with the primary nurse any problems that may occur.
        1. The advanced student must verbalize to the instructor the steps before he or she understands the skill.
        2. The student needs to review the skill before performing the skill. Or have they performed the skill successfully before? If the student has performed the skill before, always observe for the first time as a new instructor.
        3. Gather all the necessary supplies and review the skill before entering the patient room.
        4. Introduce the student and yourself to the patient and explain the procedure that is to be done.
        5. In order for the student to become confident, independent, and reassured, the clinical instructor should stand near the procedure or interaction of care of the patient in case nonverbal cues need to be given to the student.

6. Intervene if you feel the procedure is being jeopardized, but make it feel natural to the student and the patient. Do not berate the student in front of the patient.
7. Analyze how the procedure went and provide tips for improvement.
8. If a student denies the mistake or makes excuses, watch the student closely during future procedures.
9. If a student is unqualified for a procedure, develop an action plan and have the student practice the procedure in a skills laboratory. Recheck the student's performance before the student returns to the clinical site.

Chapter 2

EFFECTIVE STUDENT EVALUATIONS

This chapter examines:

- Performing effective student evaluations
- Evaluating a student's strengths and weaknesses
- Documenting student progress
- Coaching strategies and interventions

ANECDOTAL NOTES AND STUDENT EVALUATIONS

As the instructor, it is your fundamental responsibility to provide daily assessments on your students' progress. The success of your students depends on this.

Verbal feedback must be given immediately and often. Always start with the positive aspects of the students' performance. Have every student evaluate his or her performance and determine with the student whether there is any room for improvement. Never submit any written feedback on a student that has not been previously discussed with that student.

It is your responsibility to write down your immediate thoughts and observations of each student in an objective, anecdotal format after any interaction, whether positive or negative. An Anecdotal Notes form is supplied that you can use to record these evaluations. (A phrase list to more precisely address students' strengths and weaknesses is also provided.) These notes can help you write a more accurate and objective evaluation of the student's performance. Dating each entry enables you to evaluate the student's progression over time. For each day of clinical, you must discuss these entries with the student, and the student must then initial the evaluation form.

Anecdotal Notes Form

Student:	
Date	Students must be able to discuss the patient's medical diagnosis, laboratory values, medications, tests, and treatments. Compare with the textbook content. Students must be able to list nursing diagnoses in order of priority, discuss nursing interventions and rationales, and perform nursing care safely and professionally.
	Patient initials: Student initials:
	Patient initials: Student initials:
	Patient initials: Student initials:
	Patient initials: Student initials:
	Patient initials: Student initials:

SAMPLE ACTION VERBS

Sample action verbs will help to describe the students' actions while in the clinical setting. The following is a brief list that can be incorporated into the instructor's assessment of the students.

Communication: addressed, articulated, clarified, collaborated, consulted, directed, explained, interacted, interpreted, listened, observed, participated, presented, referred, resolved, suggested, translated

Helping: advocated, arranged, addressed, clarified, collaborated, demonstrated, diagnosed, educated, encouraged, facilitated, guided, intervened, motivated, prevented, provided, referred, supported

Strengths: was responsible, performed, managed, coordinated, team player, was efficient, was professional, organized, was accurate, reviewed, analyzed, managed time effectively, was timely in completing

Teaching: advised, clarified, communicated, coordinated, encouraged, evaluated, explained, individualized, instructed, motivated

IDENTIFYING, DOCUMENTING, AND CONDUCTING INTERVENTIONS FOR STUDENTS WITH PERFORMANCE DEFICIENCIES

The following outline will help you identify and address behaviors or patterns of behavior that require documentation and intervention.

I. Characteristics
  A. Minimal or last-minute preparation of paperwork
  B. Unable to explain the plan of care
  C. Lack of reliable cited references
  D. Easily distracted
II. Appearance and behaviors
  A. Excessive nervousness
  B. Shows up late with numerous excuses
  C. Dress-code violations: excessive jewelry, unkempt uniform
  D. Complains of being bored
  E. Unauthorized cell phone use
III. Communication
  A. The student repeats what you say
  B. "I'm not sure what you mean"
  C. "I did not have time to look that up"
  D. "I could not find that information"
IV. Descriptions to use when documenting student performance deficiencies
  A. Unsafe, violates basic safety principles
  B. Lacks confidence, efficiency
  C. Requires continuous verbal and physical cues
  D. Does not follow instructions
  E. Written paperwork absent, incomplete, or inaccurate
V. Examples of professional misconduct by students
  A. Not identifying patient before giving medication
  B. Leaving the floor or patient without notifying instructor
  C. Attendance problems or tardiness patterns
  D. Insubordination or lack of respect to others
  E. Lack of accountability for actions
  F. Physically unable to perform patient care because of lack of sleep or use of substances
VI. Examples of student deficiencies in patient care
  A. Not able to demonstrate proficiency with clinical skills
  B. Unable to prioritize patient care activities

        C. Poor time management
        D. Unable to perform assessments appropriately and safely
        E. Not familiar with standard operating procedures
        F. Not prepared to perform basic nursing skills without continuous monitoring or assistance
    VII. Faculty responsibilities
        A. Identify and address behaviors immediately
        B. Report documentation to superior or ask for advice
        C. Discuss observations with student immediately to allow for remediation
        D. Identify behaviors and interventions
        E. Evaluate student fairly and in a timely manner

HOW TO COUNSEL A STUDENT

Here are some helpful tips to use when counseling students regarding their performance deficiencies.

- Use nonconfrontational approaches: Avoid using "You did…" or "You did not…." To solve a problem effectively, the instructor first needs to listen and understand where the student is coming from, establish what the facts are, and then explore the options and brainstorm how to resolve the situation.
- Students may be unaware of their clinical weaknesses or areas of concern. It is important to discuss these issues with students while giving them insight into how they can achieve their own goals. You might say, "I see that you are having difficulty with your organizational skills. What can I do to help you?" Providing encouragement and assistance to students to attend the clinical laboratory to practice their skills can be used as part of the action plan.
- If the problem persists, document any counseling with the student, even though it seems insignificant. Always counsel the student at the end of the shift in private. Document any phone messages and keep e-mails that the student may have sent you and place them in the student's file. Make certain that the student's advisor and the director of nursing are aware of the problem.
- An action plan should be initiated as soon as possible. Avoid discussing problems with the student in front of administrative faculty, such as a course coordinator, clinical lab coordinator, or nursing director. Student information is confidential and students must provide written permission for you to share with others (including other students and interdisciplinary team members not directly involved in the care of said student's patients, such as the course coordinator, the clinical laboratory coordinator, or the nursing director). Obtain information from the institutional student handbook and refer to the counseling form.
- If this is a sentinel event, which is an unexpected outcome for a patient in which the student or instructor is involved, document the event's who, what, when, where, why, and how.
- If you are uncomfortable counseling a student, you can have another faculty member present. If the student becomes agitated, listen to your gut feeling and protect yourself. Try to diffuse the situation or exit quickly. Do not underestimate threats. If you are threatened in any way, take security measures.
- The student may appeal or file a grievance for any decision taken. This underscores the importance of maintaining full and accurate records of student performance and teacher–student discussions.

CLINICAL REMEDIATION

Clinical instructors may refer any student who needs additional clinical practice to the on-campus clinical laboratory.

Clinical Laboratory Referral Form

When a student exhibits behaviors that require corrective actions, the instructor initiates an evaluation tool to create an action plan and notifies the laboratory coordinator.

The laboratory coordinator will provide activities to correct and improve student performance. The laboratory coordinator, the course coordinator, and the clinical instructor will assess the student's progress and determine whether further remediation and/or probation are required.

LEARNING CONTRACT

The learning contract is a more formalized feedback process to address deficiencies in student performance. The contract should be written before the meeting with the student. Regular follow-up meetings should be scheduled. Make certain that the planned remediation process aligns with existing academic regulations and policies before implementation. An effective learning contract will have the following components:

1. Learning objectives (What are you going to learn?)
2. Learning resources and strategies (How are you going to learn it?)
3. Target dates to meet objectives
4. Sources of evidence for learning
5. Criteria for evaluating evidence (How are you going to know that you have learned?)
6. Consequences if objectives are not met
7. Student and faculty signatures

PROBATION

Placing a student on probation requires forms to be completed and signed by the student, the clinical instructor, the course coordinator, and the program director. All copies will be added to the student's formal academic file.

Chapter 3

LEARNING REQUIREMENTS AND SYLLABUS PREPARATION

This chapter examines:

- Student learning and skills requirements
- Course syllabus

SKILLS CHECKLIST AND COURSE PREPARATION

At the start of their clinical classes, nursing students need an overview of the numerous skills they must acquire before they can graduate into the field of nursing. The skills checklist outlines all the steps required for acquiring each skill. The students will find these lists helpful. A copy of the skills checklist appears at the end of this chapter.

Every individual has a different learning style and some may feel overwhelmed by the many tasks required to master this material. Instruct the students to print out the tasks, review the skills beforehand, and bring them to the hospital. Most health care facilities have a skills book that is useful for reviewing nursing skills. In addition, most schools have a list of mandatory skills that must be completed satisfactorily for successful graduation.

As the student completes the task, the performance level of the activity (pass or fail) is initialed and dated by the instructor. This will provide the student with the opportunity to immediately identify any weaknesses and, if necessary, remediate them in the laboratory. The instructor should review the deficiencies and provide opportunities for the student to improve performance by observing or participating in the particular activity.

The skills checklist required for both Medical–Surgical I and Medical–Surgical II is included at the end of this chapter. Inform the students that the skills checklist will be used for both clinical classes and can be used as a reference in both courses. Each clinical class will have its own unique set of opportunities to practice these skills depending on the type of facility, its degree of specialization, and the range of patient health issues.

RESOURCES

Most nursing students have books from their own nursing educational program that may be used as a resource. Often the institution of higher learning will recommend or provide the references and resources on which the clinical and theoretical classes are based. The following suggestions may be helpful to the new clinical instructor:

1. *Winningham's Critical Thinking Cases in Nursing, Medical–Surgical, Pediatric, Maternity, and Psychiatric,* Fifth Edition, by Mariann Harding, Julie S. Snyder, and Barbara A. Preusser. (2012). Elsevier.
2. *Math Calculations for Pharmacy Technicians: A Worktext,* Second Edition, by Robert M. Fulcher and Eugenia M. Fulcher. (2012). Elsevier.
3. *Taylor's Clinical Nursing Skills: A Nursing Process Approach,* Third Edition, by Pamela Lynn. (2010). Wolters Kluwer Health.

BEFORE THE CLINICAL CLASS BEGINS

First-time instructors may not be aware that clinical sites often have requirements that must be met prior to granting permission for the instructor and the students to enter the clinical areas. Examples of such requirements may be proof of additional vaccinations or completion of the health care modules located on the facility's website. Once the additional requirements are met, the facility will often arrange a time for the clinical group to obtain name badges. Be aware that some facilities do allow the students and the instructors to use their school identification name badges.

Become familiar with the facility's requirements such as what time report begins and whether a computer training course is required to chart or give medications. Clarify whether students may shadow other interdisciplinary staff such as respiratory and intravenous (IV) therapy staff, whether they may observe in the operating room, and the process to arrange the shadowing. Make an appointment to meet with the unit manager and become familiar with the unit's routine. Some schools require a 4-hour unit orientation. It is also prudent to inquire where students should park and whether there is a fee for parking. This information should be passed onto the students prior to the first clinical class.

The clinical instructor is obligated to present a syllabus for each course. Many times the theory instructor will forward the completed theory syllabus to the clinical instructor. The clinical instructor can modify the syllabus and submit the revised version to the students. A discussion of syllabus preparation and a detailed example of a syllabus follow later in this chapter.

WEEK 1 LOGISTICS

Week 1 should be a time for students to become familiar with the assigned clinical site and the assigned clinical unit. The clinical instructor should notify students where the group will initially meet and the designated time to arrive. It is helpful for the students to receive a tour of the facility.

If name badges are required by the clinical facility, it may be necessary to arrange a specific time during regular business hours (Monday through Friday) to obtain the badges. This information should be conveyed to weekend students because they may need to arrange time off from a job or to arrange child care during the week in order to obtain the name badge. Students should be informed that name badges are required at all times when on the clinical site.

Touring the facility, students will learn the location and hours of the cafeteria, where public restrooms are located, and where the facility's entrances and exits are located. Students should learn where the laboratory, respiratory department, IV therapy department, and radiology department are located. It is also important to know where the nursing office and the human resources department are located.

SYLLABUS PREPARATION

On the syllabus it is necessary to include your name; a way to contact you directly, such as a cell phone number; and the rules or regulations that you feel should be followed in class. Each syllabus offers an outline that guides the weekly class through various systems or projects. Discuss with the clinical group the syllabus, your expectations, and the clinical objectives. The syllabus should also list those items that you will use to determine grades (e.g., the midterm paper and the final exam) as well as the percentage of the grade that each item is worth.

Participation is usually counted as part of the grade. However, what participation is and how it will be assessed must be defined in the syllabus. Class rules, guidelines, and policies may be covered in the student handbook. Guidelines to address cell phone/smartphone use, laptops, tardiness, respecting others, talking in class, and paying attention should be addressed during the initial meeting.

SAMPLE COURSE SYLLABUS

Course title:

Course number:

Session: (Spring, Summer, Fall, Winter)

Location: Where the clinical will be held. Always include the address of and directions to the hospital.

Meeting time and day: Be sure to include when clinicals will start and end.

Credits: Usually can be found in the school catalog.

Minimum passing grade: 78%

Prerequisites: The advisor will look at the student's record to ensure that all the necessary courses have been completed before registering for this class.

Instructor: Add your name and college e-mail address (Note: your personal e-mail address is not recommended.)

Weather delays, closings, and emergencies: Information regarding school delays and closings should be inserted. Weather hotlines are usually listed in the student handbook. Remind students to check the hotline for information. Frequently the nursing instructor has to make an independent decision on cancelling clinical because schools may not make a decision the day before expected bad weather. Clinicals usually start at 6:30 a.m., so if bad weather is anticipated, there must be an early cancellation of class. If the nursing instructor needs to cancel a class, there may be a specified telephone number that must be notified. If the nursing instructor cancels a class, a makeup assignment is assigned to supplement the loss of clinical hours. Makeup assignments are discussed in Chapter 18 of this book.

Course Description (Example):

Fall 2014, Day

NUR 303C/Medical–Surgical Clinical

Credit: 2.0

This course provides a hands-on opportunity for the nursing student to integrate theory and application of nursing knowledge and skills and to determine outcomes of the patient. The student will be provided with the opportunity to perform in the role of nurse with the guidance and direction of a clinical nursing instructor or preceptor. Students will be encouraged to integrate learned knowledge and skills into the clinical setting.

Course objectives: On completion of this course, the student will be able to:
- Apply theoretical knowledge and skills learned
- Incorporate critical thinking
- Incorporate evidence-based practice into nursing practice
- Deliver nursing care in a safe and competent manner
- Demonstrate delegation skills
- Verbalize professional career goals

Methods of instruction: Skill demonstration (inclusive of group discussion, observation, etc.)

Important notes:
- The student is responsible to attend all clinical classes and arrive on time.
- The student should arrive at clinical in a properly fitting school uniform and labcoat, with identification badges, bandage scissors, black and red pens, a watch with a second hand, a calculator, and a penlight. Hair must be neat and pulled back. Beards should be trimmed. No artificial nails are allowed. Jewelry should be limited. Perfume should be avoided.
- Instruct the students not to bring valuables. There may not be any secure storage places for the students in clinical.
- Any missed clinical class will require makeup hours.

Required text: As required per academic facility

Additional reading: As assigned per instructor

Methods of instruction:

It is important that students understand the instructions given in a clinical setting will vary from classroom teaching. Clinical instruction will be inclusive of demonstrations and direct observation and evaluation of student knowledge and skills. Students will develop effective communications skills by interacting with patients and interdisciplinary team members. Constructive feedback will be given by the clinical instructor to ensure that the student maintains the highest quality of patient care and safety. Students will be given the opportunity to voice their clinical experiences in a weekly journal and during postconferences. Documentation and medication administration proficiency are key components to safe nursing practice. It may have been several semesters since the student has completed the pharmacology course. Therefore, students are expected to complete medication forms and nursing care plans weekly. Students will be given weekly handouts to promote learning and critical-thinking skills. Students must demonstrate professional behavior, effective communication, and compliance with rules, regulations, and facility policies, including the dress code and attendance policy. Attendance and punctuality are mandatory.

Grades:

Many nursing clinical courses are documented with a pass or fail grade. Other schools will document student performance on a grading system that will assess and accumulate the points outlined in the syllabus. An example of a grading table follows.

Calculation of Letter Grades	
96–100	A
93–95	A–
90–92	B+
87–89	B
84–86	B–
83–85	C+
84–81	C
80–78	C–
77.9 or below	F

Assignments:

Any assignments that need a more in-depth explanation should be discussed in a separate space.

Assignments	Points/Percentage
Description of each assignment	Explain or indicate how point or percentage allocations will be calculated into the final grade.
Attendance/tardiness Professionalism Preparedness Participation Documentation and assigned paperwork	60%
Objectives Individual projects	20%
Clinical performance evaluation Medication knowledge	20%
Total points/percentage	100%

		Class Calendar		
Week #	Date	Topic	Assignment	Due Date
Week 1		Clinical orientation	Scavenger hunt Contact information Review expectations, clinical goals	
Week 2		Nursing assessment Concept mapping	Weekly journals, care plans, concept mapping	
Week 3		Sensory deficits and assessments	Sensory deficit exercise Situation exercise	
Week 4		Pain assessment and management	Pain interview exercise Pain research exercise	
Week 5		Cancer Death and dying	Cancer screening brochure	
Week 6		Fluids and electrolytes	Fluids and electrolytes handout	
Week 7		Midterm evaluation, Geriatric nursing	Elder survey	
Week 8		Musculoskeletal system	Musculoskeletal system exercise	
Week 9		Pharmacology and laboratory	Pharmacology exercise Medication survey	
Week 10		Critical care nursing	Anatomy exercise	
Week 11		Emergency nursing	Emergency nurse exercise Crash cart exercise	
Week 12		Hematology and endocrine system	Hematology exercise Endocrine matching exercise	
Week 13		Reproductive system	Body surface area calculation quiz Reproductive system quiz	
Week 14		Final clinical class, Professional identity	Group gratuity unit party	

The clinical instructor is required to document attendance in the enrollment verification form and then weekly thereafter. Midterm grades must be submitted. Often the instructor's paycheck will not be released until the grades are submitted for both midterm and final evaluations.

Important dates to list in the syllabus are the courses add/drop dates, date for final withdrawal, and holidays.

Additional course information and classroom or clinical site policies should be listed:

- Students unable to attend clinical must notify the instructor via e-mail or phone *prior* to the beginning of clinical class.
- Grades will be based on participation, attendance, preparation, and submitted assignments.
- Unexcused absence from more than two classes over the 14-week semester or more than one class over the course of the 8-week semester may result in failing the course. If an illness occurs, the student is encouraged to withdraw instead of failing the clinical. According to school policies, failure of a class and/or clinical will result

in failure of both. There is a specified number of courses that students can fail before being dismissed from the program.

- Clinical courses have set mandatory hours. Makeup assignments will be required for all missed clinical time. Any student who fails to attend 20% of the total clinical hours required will receive a grade of "F" for the course or will be asked to withdraw from the course and repeat the class in the subsequent semester.

Examinations: Examinations are to be taken as scheduled. If a student must miss an exam due to extraordinary circumstances, the student is expected to do the following:

- Notify the instructor *prior* to the exam. The instructor and student can then arrange an alternative date for the examination to be administered. The student must bring in appropriate documentation for missing the examination.
- Any student given permission to reschedule the exam must make up that exam within 1 week of the missed examination. Failure to do so will result in a forfeit of exam points.
- Makeup exams will not be the same version of the missed examination.

ASSIGNMENTS

Students are responsible for submitting assignments at the beginning of class on the due date specified in the course syllabus.

- Any student seeking to submit an assignment at another time must obtain permission in advance.
- Written assignments must be submitted to the instructor at the designated time, unless otherwise arranged by the instructor.
- Points per day may be deducted for assignments submitted late without permission from the instructor.
- Assignments more than 5 days late will not be accepted. The grade will be 0.

Communication: Most instructors use e-mail as the major method of communication. Information important to students may be sent via e-mail. Students should check their e-mail twice daily at a minimum. Instructors and students should make every attempt to respond to e-mail communication in a punctual manner.

STUDENT HANDBOOK

Plagiarism

The student handbook will define "plagiarism." Plagiarism, whether unintentional or intentional, will be subject to possible dismissal from the program, and the assignment or examination in question will receive no credit.

Responsibilities

Responsibilities of the instructor:

- Provide clinical site and unit orientation. The nursing instructor should verify that the students in class are valid students and actually enrolled. This information is available on the school website.
- Be available in the clinical area or by telephone or pager (for students shadowing)
- Provide weekly critical feedback to the students on their performance
- Confirm clinical objectives with each student weekly
- Provide a written midterm and final evaluation conference with each student
- Provide a written evaluation of the clinical site to the institution of higher learning

Responsibilities of the student:

- Develop weekly objectives specific to the clinical site and obtain instructor's approval.

- Seek out learning opportunities
- Be prepared for each clinical experience
- Present self in a professional manner
- Participate in evaluation process

If a clinical preceptor is assigned, the clinical preceptor should:

- Volunteer to participate in the clinical learning experience
- Be willing to be accountable for the student
- Provide mentorship to the student
- Allow the student to perform skills that the student has demonstrated previously
- Encourage the student to demonstrate new clinical skills so the student can observe technique and skill
- Assume the role of advisor and resource for student
- Evaluate the student and submit an evaluation to instructor

Skills Checklist for Medical–Surgical Clinical

Student: _____

Instructor: _____

Skill	Date	Pass/Fail	Remediation
Verify order Patient record Assess steps and materials needed for procedure			
Identify, gather, and prepare equipment and supplies			
Obtain appropriate equipment: Stethoscope, thermometer, probe cover, age-appropriate blood pressure cuff, pulse oximetry, watch, Dynamap charting, flow sheets			
Vital signs			
■ Pulse rate, quality, rhythm, and appropriate sites ■ Respiratory rate and quality ■ Blood pressure: Manual and palpation ■ Blood pressure: Electronic Dynamap ■ auscultation ■ Temperature: Axilla, oral, rectal, tympanic ■ Pulse oximetry (O_2 saturation) and factors that change O_2 saturation ■ Observe for condition or change in condition			
Instruction			

■ Perioperative care and mobility
■ Preoperative preparation and consents
■ Postoperative teaching
■ Postanesthesia care
■ Positioning:
    ■ Supine, prone, lateral, jack-knife, lithotomy, and Fowler's
    ■ Trendelenburg/reverse Trendelenburg
Time out/boarding pass
Preprocedure shave/skin prep
Checklist for surgery			

Safety			
Restraints/safety devices: Ordering, applying, releasing extremities involved, behavior, and care of patient (nutrition, circulation, elimination) Fall prevention, care of confused patient, patient education and documentation, reporting			

(continued)

Skill	Date	Pass/Fail	Remediation
Health history interview			
■ Biographical and demographic information ■ Current health problem ■ Height and weight **Symptom analysis** ■ Onset, location, duration, characteristic, associated manifestation, radiation, and treatment ■ Past health history, surgical history, family health history ■ Health care maintenance ■ Medication use ■ Domestic violence			
Psychosocial history			

■ Risk factors, assessment, appearance, motor activity, behavior, mental status, levels of consciousness, orientation, mood (subjective description) and affect (observable, outward demeanor)
■ Speech, communication, thought processes and content, social history (personal habits), occupational exposure, life stressors, and lifestyle (socioeconomic factors)
  ■ Sexuality
  ■ Learning preferences: Visual, auditory, or other
  ■ Health beliefs: Assessment (cause of illness)
  ■ Health promotion and health-risk appraisal
  ■ Review of systems
  ■ Cultural assessment: Language and communication process, level of ethnic identity, influence of religion, views about discrimination, network support, habits, customs and beliefs			

Physical assessment			
The student will perform the examination using inspection, auscultation, palpation, and percussion in appropriate order **Skin, hair, nails** ■ Color of skin, scars, rashes, or lesions ■ Clubbing ■ Lice or scabs ■ Texture of hair **Eyes, vision** ■ Symmetry and alignment ■ Abnormalities in eyelids ■ Eyebrow distribution ■ Observation of sclera and conjunctiva ■ Symmetry of pupil and iris ■ Extra-ocular movements and cranial nerves ■ Constriction and accommodation of both pupils **Ears** ■ Drainage/symmetry **Nose and sinuses** ■ Color ■ Drainage ■ Loss of smell ■ Pain over sinuses **Mouth and throat** ■ Symmetry ■ Color of mucosa ■ Tongue dysfunction ■ Teeth ■ Parotid gland			

Skill	Date	Pass/Fail	Remediation
Neck and neck vessels ■ Jugular venous ■ Distention ■ Enlargement of cervical nodes ■ Thyroid assessment ■ Carotid auscultation			
Lungs ■ Breathing patterns ■ Use of accessory muscles ■ Skin and nail-bed color ■ Ability to speak ■ Adventitious sounds ■ Spine abnormalities ■ Palpation ■ Tactile fremitus ■ Percussion			
Heart ■ Observation ■ Jugular venous distension (JVD) ■ Point of maximal impulse (PMI) ■ Auscultation ■ Clicks, murmurs, rubs, aortic, pulmonic, tricuspid, mitral valve closure			
Breast and axilla (male and female) ■ Anatomy and symmetry ■ Any masses, drainage, pain, discoloration ■ Palpation ■ Lymph nodes			
Abdomen ■ Color of skin, scars, rashes or lesions ■ Abdominal contour, symmetry, and position of umbilicus ■ Umbilical herniation and enlarged inguinal lymph nodes or masses ■ Bowel sounds in all quadrants ■ Presence of bruits, ascites ■ Percussion ■ Palpation findings ■ Rectum (hemorrhoids, fissures, prolapse)			
Musculoskeletal ■ Inspect overall appearance ■ Observe gait and balance ■ Perform Romberg test ■ Observe spine from lateral and posterior curvatures ■ Palpate along spine ■ Inspect and palpate skin, joints, and muscle groups of upper and lower extremities ■ Joint abnormalities ■ Test muscle strength and range of motion of all limbs ■ Check pulses ■ Inspect hair distribution and skin discoloration on legs ■ Identify presence of edema			
Neurologic ■ Mental status testing ■ Cranial nerve testing ■ Muscle strength			

(continued)

Skill	Date	Pass/Fail	Remediation
■ Level of consciousness (LOC): Glasgow Coma Scale ■ Affect, mood, and memory ■ Are cranial nerves intact? ■ Gait, balance, and coordination in upper and lower extremities ■ Findings of sensory testing: Light touch and sharp and dull discrimination ■ Deep tendon reflexes and Babinski reflex **Genitourinary** ■ Male: Any drainage, bulges in inguinal area, any penile or scrotal abnormalities, any skin abnormalities, opening of the urethra ■ Female: Any drainage, vaginal abnormalities, prolapse, opening of the urethra **General assessment** Appropriate use of instrumentation Assessment of older adult			
Infection control			
■ Hand washing, antibacterial soap application ■ Standard/universal precautions ■ Clean gloving ■ Sterile gloving ■ Sharps disposal ■ Contaminated material disposal ■ Isolation technique (masking, gowning, and gloving for contact, droplet, enteric, reverse, and airborne isolation) ■ Surgical asepsis ■ Sterile technique/sterile field ■ Cleaning bodily fluid spills, ■ Using material safety data sheet (MSDS) **Toileting** ■ Use of bedpan and fracture pan ■ Use of urinal ■ Use of commode ■ Measuring urinary hat ■ Insertion of Foley catheter in male and female ■ Care and maintenance of Foley, supra pubic, and Texas catheter ■ Condom catheter application ■ Flexi-seal fecal insertion and maintenance **Hygiene** ■ Bed bath, shower ■ Oral care: Conscious and unconscious patient ■ Care of dentures, retainers, bridges ■ Shaving ■ Shampooing and hair care ■ Nail care ■ Care of prosthetics (eyeglasses, contacts, eye prosthesis, hearing aid, artificial limbs) ■ Eye, ear, and nose care			
Mobility, immobility, and positioning			
Body mechanics of the patients and students Body alignment and indications ■ Dorsal recumbent ■ Prone ■ Sims' ■ Fowler's ■ Knee–chest			

Skill	Date	Pass/Fail	Remediation
■ Dorsal lithotomy ■ Turning patient every 2 hours ■ Transferring patient using proper body mechanics to bed, stretcher, or chair ■ Use of devices such as egg-crate mattresses, foam mattress pads, and cushions to relieve pressure sores ■ Active and passive range of motion ■ Ambulation ■ Use of wheelchair, crutches, cane, walker, and Hoyer lift ■ Maintenance of traction equipment			
Bed making ■ Making an occupied bed, an unoccupied bed, and a postoperative bed ■ Use of the call bell ■ Transporting a patient			
Intake & output calculations and recording ■ Net balance calculations			
Cold and heat application ■ Hypothermic blanket ■ Hyperthermia blanket (bear hugger) ■ K-heating pad ■ Ice packs			
Genitourinary ■ Intermittent catheter ■ Insertion/removal of indwelling catheter ■ Catheter irrigation ■ Continuous bladder irrigation ■ Catheter care: Indwelling, condom, suprapubic ■ Perineal care ■ Assist with Pap smear ■ Assist with pelvic examination			
Tubes and drains ■ Insertion of nasogastric tube ■ Nasogastric tube maintenance such as checking placement and gastric residual ■ Gastrostomy tube maintenance ■ Initiating tube feedings via tube-feeding devices such as a kangaroo pump ■ Bolus tube feedings ■ Maintenance of drainage collection devices: Jackson Pratt drains, Hemovac, Penrose drains			
Respiratory care ■ Pulse oximetry ■ Nebulizer ■ Use of incentive spirometer (IS) ■ Use of Ambu bag/mask ■ Use of nasal cannula, 100% nonrebreather (NRB), and Ventimask ■ Turn, cough, and deep breathe (TCDB) ■ Closed chest tube drainage system to suction/water and care ■ Chest tube insertion site care ■ Tracheostomy care ■ Postural drainage			

(continued)

Skill	Date	Pass/Fail	Remediation
Arterial blood gas ■ Metabolic acidosis ■ Metabolic alkalosis ■ Respiratory acidosis ■ Respiratory alkalosis ■ Tracheal, oral, and nasal suctioning and care of patient ■ Chest physiotherapy			
Bowel elimination ■ Enema (retention/soap suds) ■ Selection/application of ostomy appliance ■ Ostomy pouch care: Teaching measurement of stoma, burping, preventing infections, attaching and cleaning pouch ■ Stoma skin prep and cleansing, application of powder ■ Ostomy irrigation ■ Removal of impactions ■ Suppository			
Nutrition			
■ Gravity feedings: Enteral gastrostomy/jejunostomy/nasogastric ■ Insertion/maintenance of enteral feeding tube ■ Removal of feeding tube (not gastrostomy tube) ■ Feeding pump ■ Feeding a patient ■ Aspiration precautions ■ Gastric lavage			
Wound management			
■ Pressure ulcer prevention ■ Clean dressing change ■ Superficial dressing change (dry, gauze, topical wound products) ■ Deep wound packing ■ Wet-to-dry dressing change ■ Sterile dressing change ■ Wound irrigation ■ Suture/staple/Steri-Strips removal ■ Wound vacuum-assisted closure (VAC) maintenance ■ Maintenance of specialty bed			

PART II

BASICS OF CLINICAL TEACHING AND STUDENT EVALUATION

Chapter 4

FIRST DAY OF CLINICAL: EXPECTATIONS, FORMS, AND ASSESSMENTS

This chapter examines:

- Pre- and postconference expectations and activities
- Forms to be used by the professor and the students
- Care plans and modified physical assessment guidelines
- Math and vocabulary skills assessments

THE INITIAL CLASS MEETING

Prior to the first class, make copies of the syllabus, contact information sheet, weekly attendance sheet, scavenger hunt sheets, chart check form, guidelines for care plans, care plan form, math quiz, vocabulary quiz, medication forms, and resource materials.

The first meeting may be awkward. The students will try to discover what type of an instructor you are (i.e., strict or lenient) and how you teach. It will be up to you as the instructor to set the tone for the class.

Guidelines included in the syllabus should be discussed or reinforced. For example, you should clarify whether being tardy for more than two classes will count as one absence and whether being tardy will be included in the grading system. Emphasize that students should notify the instructor prior to any class if unable to attend that class.

Students should be told what equipment and supplies they will require during their clinical class. You should also review with them professional appearance rules. Many health care facilities do not allow artificial nails or nail polish (some do allow clear). Hair must be clean and off the shoulders. No streaks of pink or green. Male nurses with a beard or a mustache must be told that the beard or mustache must be neat, clean, and trimmed. Minimum jewelry is to be worn. Usually a wedding band and stud earrings may be worn. Religious necklaces have to be worn discreetly. Tattoos must not be seen. School uniforms must be clean and ironed. Shoes must be white and clean. A laboratory jacket is optional. Students should be informed that most health care facilities do not offer storage space for student items. Students are encouraged to carry only the supplies that are needed. All valuables should be left at home or locked in the student's car.

The initial form that students should complete is the contact information form. At some point in the future you may need to contact your students to cancel a class or to notify them that the class will be delayed. Obtaining the students' contact information now it will make this process flow more smoothly in the future. It is suggested that each student provide a cell phone number. It is strongly suggested that it be a requirement that the students check their school e-mail twice daily (once in the morning and once in the afternoon) to ensure that any changes in class schedules or assignments are received and acknowledged.

It is also wise to find out what types of health care experiences the students may have had. Not all students will have had the same experiences in their previous clinical classes. Some hospitals provide clinical students a broader set of patient health conditions than do others. It may be of benefit for the students to be paired in the first few weeks of clinical classes.

It is customary to hold a preconference and postconference session with each weekly clinical class. Each chapter in this book that is devoted to a specific clinical class will have its own unique pre- and postconference agendas and outlines of handouts and items that should be collected.

Patient assignments will be made during the weekly preconference. Instructors can determine patient assignments by using several methods. One method is for the instructor to arrive on the unit several hours before the scheduled clinical time and discuss with the night charge nurse potential patient care assignments. A second method is for the clinical group to arrive after the morning report and to discuss patient assignments with the morning charge nurse or the unit manager. The final method employed occurs when the instructor arrives on the unit a day prior to the clinical class and carefully reads each chart to evaluate which patient or patients may provide good learning experiences for the students. However, a word of warning: Given the rapid movement of patients within the hospital, the selected patients may be slated for transfer or discharge at any time.

WEEK 1 PRECONFERENCE

Hand out:
- Syllabus
- Contact information form
- Math quiz
- Care plan form
- Sample medication form
- Chart check
- Both scavenger hunts
- Vocabulary quiz

Collect:
- Contact information sheet (when completed)
- Math quiz (when completed)

Have each student sign, date, and time the weekly attendance sign-in sheet at the start of the class. Ensure that the attendance sheet is signed, dated, and timed each week. Contact information sheets should be completed by each student and returned to the clinical instructor during preconference.

The math quiz should be completed and returned prior to ending preconference. Instruct students that quizzes must be completed independently.

Medical–Surgical II students should be able to perform a physical assessment independently. The clinical instructor should make time to observe each student during an assessment to ensure that the student is able to perform this procedure correctly. This chapter introduces detailed guidelines for conducting modified physical assessments that balance obtaining the information required for health care interventions against the limited time available to the students in clinical classes. This discussion will help prepare students for the physical assessment and concept mapping activities that are the focus of Chapter 5.

After preconference, the first day will be acclimation to the hospital and auxiliary units that the students will be using, which were discussed in Chapter 3. The students will be given a brief tour of the health care facility followed by a self-directed scavenger hunt on their assigned units. The students may have other necessary paperwork to complete as well as the scavenger hunt. Sections of the paper or electronic charts will be reviewed to ascertain where to find information as well as to ensure that the students' passwords will work. A certain part of the unit is usually assigned to the students so that normal activity on the unit is not affected. Badges may also be required the first day after preconference and before entry to the unit.

The nursing instructor will guide the students on how to and what to give in a report to the primary nurses assigned to their particular patients. Report will consist of the patient assessment by the student, vital signs, blood sugar, how the patient tolerated activity, any new skin breakdown, and other pertinent information. If a student was unable to complete a certain task, such as a wound change or treatment, that too must also be relayed. Students should be informed on the clinical day plan: preconference, patient assignments (if applicable), and designated tasks required. Inform the students that they must report off (give updated report of care provided and condition of assigned patient) to the primary nurse by noon. They will either have 1 hour for lunch or the instructor may choose to have two 15-minute breaks and a half-hour lunch break. A designated place to meet should be announced prior to students entering the clinical area.

Contact Information Form

1. Name: _____

2. Best way to contact you: _____

　　Please provide a telephone number: _____

　　Please provide your e-mail address: _____

3. Field of nursing you are interested in: _____

4. What experience do you have? _____

5. What type of knowledge do you feel you have? _____

6. What do you feel are your weak areas? _____

7. What is the best way for you to learn? _____

8. What do you feel is the best way for a clinical instructor to help you learn?

_____

_____

_____

_____

MONITORING ATTENDANCE

Every educational program has a specific attendance time requirement. To ensure accurate documentation of attendance, two attendance sheets are included.

The first attendance sheet is a weekly attendance sheet that must be copied weekly by the instructor for each of the instructor's clinical classes. Students must sign the weekly attendance sheets, which provide the instructor with the students' time of arrival and proof of attendance.

Weekly Attendance Sheet for Course _____

Date	Time	Student name

The second attendance sheet is a record that the clinical instructor uses to keep track of absences, tardiness, and makeup assignments for clinical absences. The clinical instructor may benefit from entering an "A" for "absent" and a "T" for "tardy."

The absent student will be required to "make up" the missed clinical hours with an assignment chosen by the clinical instructor. Sample makeup assignments are included in Chapter 18 of this book. Clinical instructors may choose their own way of acknowledging that the makeup assignment has been completed. For example, the clinical instructor may choose to document an assigned makeup assignment with an "M." Once the makeup assignment has been completed, the "M" may be changed to "C" for "completed."

Attendance Record Sheet

	Week 1	Week 2	Week 3	Week 4	Week 5	Week 6	Week 7	Week 8	Week 9
Date									
Name									

	Week 10	Week 11	Week 12	Week 13	Week 14
Date					
Name					

CLINICAL DAY 1

The instructor will pass out the scavenger hunt sheets, the chart check exercise form, the guidelines for care plans, the care plan form, the medication form, the math quiz, and the vocabulary quiz during preconference. The following sections introduce these items and explain how they will be used by the students.

SCAVENGER HUNT

It is necessary to learn the layout of the clinical site. The scavenger hunt is conducted on the first class day while the students do not have any assigned patients. It must be completed before postconference. The students will gather the information without disturbing staff or the routine of the unit. The instructor will be available to help guide the students. Discussion of issues concerning the unit, the scavenger hunt, and the codes to the different locked rooms on the unit (such as supplies, nutrition, conference room) will take place in postconference. A scavenger hunt is a wonderful tool for both the students and the instructor to use to find not only the useful equipment but also the necessary resources and numbers for emergencies.

UNIT SCAVENGER HUNT

1. Where do you find contact numbers? That is, housekeeping, pharmacy, the nursing supervisor. How do you use paging system?
2. Who is responsible to respond to codes?
3. How do you report a condition to infection control/disease?
4. What are the most frequent medication administration times (based on the pharmacy)?
5. What do you do if you have a missing medication dose?
6. How do you contact case management or the social worker? Under what circumstances would you need to?
7. How do you implement a referral for another health care department or doctor?
8. Where do you find the list of unapproved abbreviations that must not be used?
9. Who contacts the MD, if necessary? How is the MD contacted?
10. Where do you find the policies and procedures manual on your assigned unit?
11. Where is the staff bathroom on your assigned unit?
12. What do you do if you need another name band?
13. Where do you obtain clean linens? Where are dirty linens placed?
14. How do you find out who the patient care technician (PCT) is for your assigned patients?
15. How do you discover who is the charge RN for your assigned unit?
16. How do you reach the respiratory therapist if your patient is having difficulty in breathing (DIB)?
17. What do you do if your patient's IV is infiltrated?
18. What do you do if there is a suspicious character lingering in the hallway?
19. Whom do you notify if you notice a staff member placing narcotics in his or her pocket?
20. What do you do in case of a fire on your assigned unit?
21. Where do you find the visitor information for your assigned unit?
22. How do you contact the organ and tissue consortium if your patient is an impending death or dies?
23. How do you answer the unit telephone on your assigned unit?
24. What do you do if you have questions about the unit you are on?
25. Where do you obtain your ordered unit of PRBC (packed red blood cells) for your assigned patient?
26. Where is the library?
27. Where is the pharmacy?
28. Where is the laboratory?
29. Where is the cafeteria?
30. Where is the telemetry area?
31. Where is the security office?
32. Where is the nursing office?
33. Where is the admissions office?
34. Where is the physical therapy office?
35. Where is the nursing education office?

EQUIPMENT SCAVENGER HUNT

1. Where are the IV pumps located?
2. Where are the feeding pumps located?
3. Where is the blood pressure equipment located?
4. Where are the thermometers located?
5. Where are the portable oxygen tanks located?
6. Where are the wheel chairs located?
7. Where is the ice machine located?
8. Where is the glucose monitoring equipment located?
9. Where is the code cart located?
10. Where is the patient lifting equipment located?
11. Where is the IV-start equipment located?
12. Where is the EKG machine located?

CHART CHECK EXERCISE

The chart check exercise will help students learn how to read the patient's chart. It is a useful tool that promotes critical thinking. Discovering why the patient came to the facility and examining the patient's past medical history, medications, laboratory tests, or other tests will help the student learn to gather pertinent data. It is also a necessary information tool when the student begins concept mapping, which is introduced during Week 2.

Chart Check

Question	Yes	No
Was the diagnosis clear? Explain.		
Did you find charting that was conflicting or confusing? Explain.		
Were there health issues that were not addressed? Explain.		
Did the physician's order seem appropriate for the patient's condition? Explain.		
Were the orders legible?		
Were there progress notes that were illegible?		
Did other disciplines chart appropriately? Explain.		
Were pain issues addressed initially?		
Did you find some charting or information confusing? Give details.		
Were the orders dated and timed by all disciplines?		
Did the patient have a deep vein thrombosis (DVT) prophylaxis ordered?		
Is the patient activity level specified?		
Find the policies and procedures manual. Look up two policies and summarize whether the policies are clearly written or whether they are confusing.		
If you had to call a Code Blue, how easy would it be? What would you do?		
When looking at the patient's chart, how can you determine who is the primary doctor?		

List the various sections in the chart:

1. _____

2. _____

3. _____

4. _____

5. _____

6. _____

7. _____

8. _____

9. _____

10. _____

11. _____

12. _____

13. _____

14. _____

15. _____

CARE PLANS

Assigning a weekly care plan helps the student to understand the rationale for prioritizing health problems and the appropriate nursing interventions as well as the signs and symptoms to observe or monitor to ensure the nursing interventions are effective. The care plan forms can help guide the student through the nursing process.

Care plans may be assigned in several ways. Short-term goal care plans can be assigned to demonstrate effective nursing interventions. For example, the care plan to improve physical mobility may be completed on Day 1 when the patient moves from the bed to the chair or performs active range of motion.

Short-term and long-term care plans can help the student learn to evaluate outcomes and to recognize that not all health problems can be resolved within the facility or on the unit. For example, a long-term care plan goal may be initiated but the nursing student may not see the achieved goal. Often long-term goals include home care, rehabilitation, or when the patient should follow up with the patient's physician status post-discharge.

Care plans can be assigned based on scenarios or a disease process. Concept mapping teaches the student how to prioritize and what interventions may need to be completed for each nursing diagnosis. Clinical instructors may find it frustrating trying to find patient assignments that offer a variety of learning experiences. Clinical groups are often assigned to a specific unit within a health care organization. Those specific units may be, for example, a cardiac unit or an oncology unit. Being assigned exclusively to these types of units limits the range of the students' learning experiences.

It may benefit the student if the clinical instructor chooses to assign the student a scenario or disease process with a specific problem for which the student can then develop and base the care plan. Initially, students need to be taught how to collect data. A data-collection tool, labeled "physical assessment form," is included in Chapter 5. The data collection tool will assist the students in collecting subjective and objective data as well as in prioritizing the findings. Students should be informed that when completing care plans, the interventions they specify should be specific as to who may be performing the task or action. A sample care plan template is also included in this chapter and should be copied and given to the students to assist in learning the proper format.

Care Plan Guidelines

Date: _____ Student name: _____

Patient initials: _____ Room number: _____

Nursing Diagnosis	Outcome	Interventions	Rationale	Evaluation
Related to: (use pathophysiology) As evidenced by: Subjective: (List patient complaint for selected problem) Objective: Use all sources. Assessment, test results, and chart information. May need to obtain data from patient's family and friends.	List outcomes expected. Goals should be measurable, specific, and have a time frame (when to begin date and end date).	Nursing interventions should state who will perform the desired intervention, when the intervention will be performed, and how the intervention will be performed. Each intervention should be listed separately.	List rationale for each intervention. Resource or reference must be included for each intervention.	Evaluate each individual intervention. Document whether the intervention was effective or whether there is a need for re-evaluation. Note how effectiveness was determined.

MEDICATION EXERCISES

One or two medication exercises are included in every clinical week chapter, which are to be passed out during each preconference session. Each medication exercise names a particular medication and instructs the students to research and discuss lab tests associated with that medication, potential food interactions, and required patient education specific to that medication, as well as other related issues. The following sample form shows the full range of topics students will research and discuss. Obtaining information

Sample Medication Form

Listed in the vertical box is a medication. For each of the remaining boxes, list the following:

Box 1: List a laboratory result you would need to monitor. Explain the significance of the laboratory test to the medication.

Box 2: List one food that may interact with the medication. Explain the significance of the food item to the medication.

Box 3: List one patient educational instruction you would give to the patient regarding the medication. Explain the significance of the instruction to the medication.

List other educational information you could provide this patient. Are there websites you can refer to? What about travel overseas and health issues? How should the medication be stored? Does the medication being administered interfere with other medications?

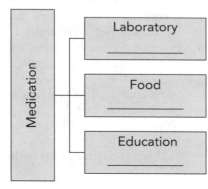

on patients who travel outside of the country is important. It is wise to educate patients on websites that may assist travelers, before they travel to a foreign country, if medications are lost or if they become ill.

CALCULATION AND CONVERSION SKILLS

A math quiz is to be given during the preconference to verify that the students can adequately perform calculations and conversions.

Math Quiz

1. Using the following conversion guide, convert the following temperatures.

$$C = \frac{F - 32}{1.8} \qquad C = (F - 32) \times 5/9$$

   a. 99.5°F = _____C
   b. 100.5°F = _____C
   c. The doctor orders Tylenol 650 mg orally for a temperature greater than 38.6°C. Your patient's temperature is 101.5°F. What dose would you give, if any?
   _____.

2. Using the following conversion guide, convert the following weights.
   Pounds × 2.2 = kg
   a. The patient weighs 110 pounds = _____ kg
   b. The patient weighs 312 pounds = _____ kg

3. In preparation for a colonoscopy, the patient must drink one 8-ounce glass of bowel cleanser every half hour. You receive 1 gallon of the bowel cleanser. The patient must be NPO [nothing by mouth] at midnight. At what time should the patient begin drinking to complete the gallon before midnight?
   _____.

4. Your patient has an elevated sodium level of 152. The doctor orders the patient to increase the oral intake of free water to reduce the sodium level. The doctor orders 96 ounces of water daily. How many cups per day will the patient need to drink?
   _____.

5. Convert the following:
   a. 1,000 mg = _____g
   b. 2.5 g = _____mg
   c. 0.025 mg = _____ mcg
   d. 1.25 mg = _____ mcg
   e. 5,000 mcg = _____ mg
   f. 250 mcg = _____ mg

6. Using the supplied conversion guide, convert the following heights.
   1 inch = 2.54 cm   1 foot = 12 inches
   a. 5 feet 6 inches = _____ cm
   b. 6 feet 2 inches = _____ cm

7. The doctor orders Xanax 0.25 mg orally every night at bedtime. The dose available is 250 mcg tablets. What dose will you give? _____.

8. The doctor orders Dilantin 300 mg orally every afternoon. The dose available is 100 mg caplets. What dose will you give? _____.

9. The doctor orders amiodarone 400 mg orally daily. The dose available is 100 mg tablets. What dose will you give? _____.

10. The doctor orders Vasotec 5 mg orally daily. The dose available is 10 mg tablets. What dose will you give? _____.

11. The doctor orders 1,000 mg of Rocephin IV daily. How many grams of Rocephin would you administer? _____.

12. The doctor orders Synthroid 0.150 mg orally daily. You have 75 mcg tablets. What dose will you give? _____.

13. The doctor orders methylprednisolone 125 mg IVP Q12H. The dose available is 250 mg/5 mL. How many mL will you administer?

_____.

14. The doctor orders digoxin 0.125 mg IV. The dose available is 5 mg/1 mL. How many mL will you administer? _____.

15. The doctor orders 1,500 mL D5.45 normal saline to infuse over 8 hours. Infusion set = 15 gtts/min. How many drops a minute will you run the IVF?

_____.

16. The doctor orders 2 L of NS to run over 12 hours. The gtt factor is 20 gtts/min. How many drops/minute will you run the IVF? _____.

17. Add the following:
    a. 250 + 75 = _____.
    b. 375 + 35 = _____.

18. Subtract the following:
    a. 500 − 250 = _____.
    b. 750 − 375 = _____.

19. Multiply the following:
    a. 125 × 5 = _____.
    b. 250 × 50 = _____.

20. Divide the following:
    a. 250 ÷ 5 = _____.
    b. 20 ÷ 0.9 = _____.

21. A patient is receiving ampicillin 500 mg orally every 6 hours. One hour after administration the patient is complaining of pruritis and hives are present. Diphenhydramine (Benadryl) 75 mg elixir is ordered. The pharmacy has supplied 12.5 mg per teaspoon. How many tablespoons would the nurse administer?

_____.

22. Vancomycin 1.5 grams IV is ordered daily. The pharmacy has evaluated that kidney functions for this client are deteriorating and the creatinine has climbed to 2.6 mg/dL and has determined that the dose needs to be decreased to 500 mg and has to be rescheduled to every 36 hours after the last dose. The last dose was given yesterday, 6/3, at 2100. When is the next dose due?

_____.

23. A Tylenol overdose has been admitted and the antidote Mucomyst (Acetylcysteine) IV has been ordered. The loading dose is 150 mg/kg in 200 ml of D5W to be administered over 20 minutes using an IV infusion pump and micro-drip tubing. The patient weighs 164 pounds. What rate would the nurse set on the IV pump? Round up the kg to the tenth. How many mg would be given?

_____.

24. A patient has received 4 mg of morphine after surgery and the respirations have dropped to a rate of 8 per minute. The nurse is unable to arouse the client and has a standing order for narcan 0.1 mg IV. The dose is supplied in vials that are 0.4 mg/ml. What dose would be given and what size syringe would the nurse utilize?

_____.

25. A patient with anxiety has been admitted with seizures due to a possible benzodiazepine overdose. The antidote Romazicon (flumazenil) is ordered. A dose of 0.2 mg is ordered to be administered intravenously over 15 seconds. Pharmacy has sent 0.1mg / 1 ml vial. What dose would the nurse administer?

_____.

Answers to Math Quiz

1. Using the following conversion guide, convert the following temperatures.

$$C = \frac{F - 32}{1.8} \qquad C = (F - 32) \times 5/9$$

   a. 99.5°F = __37.5__ C
   b. 100.5°F = __38.06__ C
   c. The doctor orders Tylenol 650 mg orally for a temperature greater than 38.6°C. Your patient's temperature is 101.5°F. What dose would you give, if any? __None__

2. Using the following conversion guide, convert the following weights.
   Pounds × 2.2 = kg
   a. The patient weighs 110 pounds = __49.895__ kg
   b. The patient weighs 312 pounds = __141.818__ kg

3. In preparation for a colonoscopy, the patient must drink one 8-ounce glass of bowel cleanser every half hour. You receive 1 gallon of the bowel cleanser. The patient must be NPO [nothing by mouth] at midnight. At what time should the patient begin drinking to complete the gallon before midnight?
   __4 p.m.__ One gallon equals 128 ounces. The patient will be drinking 16 ounces in an hour (8 ounces every 30 minutes × 2). 128 ounces/16 ounces/hr = 8 hours. 12 midnight minus 8 hours would be 4 p.m.

4. Your patient has an elevated sodium level of 152. The doctor orders the patient to increase the oral intake of free water to reduce the sodium level. The doctor orders 96 ounces of water daily. How many cups per day will the patient need to drink?
   __12 cups daily__
   There are 8 ounces in one cup, so 96 ounces/8 ounces/cup = 12 cups.

5. Convert the following:
   a. 1,000 mg = __1 g__
   b. 2.5 g = __2,500 mg__
   c. 0.025 mg = __25 mcg__
   d. 1.25 mg = __1,250 mcg__
   e. 5,000 mcg = __5 mg__
   f. 250 mcg = __0.25 mg__

6. Using the supplied conversion guide, convert the following heights.
   1 inch = 2.54 cm   1 foot = 12 inches
   a. 5 feet 6 inches = 167.64 cm
   b. 6 feet 2 inches = 187.96 cm

7. The doctor orders Xanax 0.25 mg orally every night at bedtime. The dose available is 250 mcg tablets. What dose will you give? __One tablet__

8. The doctor orders Dilantin 300 mg orally every afternoon. The dose available is 100 mg caplets. What dose will you give? __Three caplets__

9. The doctor orders amiodarone 400 mg orally daily. The dose available is 100 mg tablets. What dose will you give? __Four tablets__

10. The doctor orders Vasotec 5 mg otally daily. The dose available is 10 mg tablets. What dose will you give? __1/2 tablet__

11. The doctor orders 1,000 mg of Rocephin IV daily. How many grams of Rocephin would you administer? __1 g__

12. The doctor orders Synthroid 0.150 mg orally daily. You have 75 mcg tablets. What dose will you give? __Two tablets__

13. The doctor orders methylprednisolone 125 mg IVP Q12H. The dose available is 250 mg/5 mL. How many mL will you administer? __2.5 mL__

14. The doctor orders digoxin 0.125 mg IV. The dose available is 500 mcg/1 mL. How many mL will you administer? __0.25 mL = 0.125 mg or 125 mcg__

15. The doctor orders 1,500 mL D5.45 NS to infuse over 8 hours. Infusion set = 15 gtts/min. How many drops a minute will you run the IVF? 47 gtts/min

16. The doctor orders 2 L of NS to run over 12 hours. The gtt factor is 20 gtts/min. How many drops/minute will you run the IVF? 67 gtts/min

17. Add the following:
   a. 250 + 75 = 325
   b. 375 + 35 = 410

18. Subtract the following:
   a. 500 − 250 = 250
   b. 750 − 375 = 375

19. Multiply the following:
   a. 125 × 5 = 625
   b. 250 × 50 = 12,500

20. Divide the following:
   a. 250 ÷ 5 = 50
   b. 20 ÷ 0.9 = 22.2

21. The nurse would administer 2 tablespoons. The prescription calls for 75 mg so $75mg \times tsp (5ml) = 2$ tbsp or 30 ml 12.5 mg

22. There are 24 hours in a day; 6/3 at 2100, to 6/5, at 0900 is 36 hours so the dose should be rescheduled for that time.

23. $\dfrac{164 \text{ pounds}}{2.2 \text{ pounds}} \times 1 \text{ kg} = 74.6 \text{ kg}$ 150mg × 74.6 kg = 11,190 mg/kg

Total volume/ml $\dfrac{200 \text{ ml}}{20 \text{ min}} \times \dfrac{60 \text{ min}}{1 \text{ hr}} = 600$ ml/hr

24. $\dfrac{0.1 \text{ mg}}{0.4 \text{ mg/ml}} = 0.25$ ml. To adequately withdraw and administer the dose, a 1-ml or a 3-ml syringe should be used for accuracy.

25. $\dfrac{0.1 \text{ mg}}{0.2 \text{ mg}} \times 1 \text{ ml} = 0.5$ ml

MEDICAL TERMINOLOGY SKILLS

Make copies of the vocabulary quiz. Hand out one vocabulary quiz to each student during preconference. Students may need to review their vocabulary to ensure that they can accurately define words that will describe the patient's condition. The vocabulary quiz is due by Week 2 preconference.

Students must realize that learning and understanding medical terminology are essential to participating in the nursing program. How health care personnel communicate the physical findings of the patient must be conveyed in a language that all caregivers can understand. For this reason, students should be quizzed on terminology to ensure a complete understanding of the frequently used terms.

Vocabulary Quiz

Define the following words. Return to your instructor by next week's preconference.

Abduction	Atrophy
Accountability	Autonomy
Acupuncture	Beneficence
Adduction	Biot's
Advocate	Blanching
Analysis	Borborygmi
Anorexia	Chancre
Aphasia	Cheyne-Stokes
Atelectasis	Crackles

Culture
Cyanosis
Dehiscence
Dementia
Deontology
Depression
Diffusion
Distention
Dorsiflexion
Edema
Emboli
Empathy
Ethnicity
Evisceration
Excoriation
Exudate
Fidelity
Hemorrhage
Homeopathic
Hypoxemia
Iatrogenesis
Idiopathic
Induration
Inference
Infiltrate
In situ
Justice
Kyphosis
Lethargy
Lordosis

Maximal impulse
Narcolepsy
Neglect
Neuropathy
Nodule
Nonmaleficence
Oliguria
Pallor
Palpation
Paralytic ileus
Perfusion
Peristalsis
Pigmentation
Plantar flexion
Polyuria
Prioritizing
Pulse deficit
Pulse pressure
Referral
Regurgitation
Resiliency
Slough
Stenosis
Syncope
Synergistic
Thrombocytopenia
Thrombus
Turgor
Utilitarianism
Valsalva maneuver

Answers to Vocabulary Quiz

Abduction: To move away from the median plane (mid-section) of the body

Accountability: The responsibility taken on by health care professionals for patient care

Acupuncture: Technique of inserting fine needles at specific points

Adduction: To move toward the median plane (mid-section) of the body

Advocate: A person who supports or speaks in favor of another

Analysis: The examination of body components or parts and the results of that examination

Anorexia: Loss of appetite

Aphasia: Loss or impairment of ability to use or understand language

Atelectasis: A collapsed lung

Atrophy: A wasting away or decrease in size

Autonomy: To function independently

Beneficence: Basic principle emphasizing doing what is best for the patient

Biot's: A pattern of breathing characterized by several short breaths followed by a long, irregular period of apnea

Blanching: To lose color

Borborygmi: rumbling sounds caused by the movement of gas in the intestine

Chancre: The primary sore or ulcer at the site of entry of a pathogen

Cheyne-Stokes: Breathing pattern characterized by up to a minute of apnea followed by a gradual increase in depth and frequency of respirations

Crackles: Abnormal lung sounds, also known as rales, that produce popping sounds

Culture: The shared customs, beliefs, language, and way of life of a particular people

Cyanosis: A bluish discoloration due to deficient oxygenation

Dehiscence: A bursting open of the surgical wound

Dementia: A chronic and progressive disorder of the mental processes

Deontology: The study or theory of moral obligation or duty

Depression: A state of excessive sadness

Diffusion: The process by which molecules move from a region of high concentration to an area of lower concentration

Distention: To enlarge from internal pressure; to swell

Dorsiflexion: Flexing in an upward direction

Edema: Excessive buildup of fluid in the tissue

Emboli: A mass (solid, gas, or liquid) circulating in the blood or lymphatic vessels

Empathy: The ability to understand and be sensitive to the feelings of another

Ethnicity: Affiliation with a particular group based on shared physical or cultural identity

Evisceration: Removal of the organ(s)

Excoriation: Abrasion of the skin

Exudate: The fluid released into superficial lesions or areas of inflammation

Fidelity: Faithfulness or loyalty; conforming to truth or fact

Hemorrhage: Significant loss of blood

Homeopathic: Administering a minute dose of medication

Hypoxemia: Abnormally low concentration of oxygen in the arterial blood

Idiopathic: Illness of unknown etiology

Iatrogenesis: A harm caused by the medical profession that was preventable

Induration: An area of hardened tissue

Inference: A conclusion arrived at from given premises or observations

Infiltrate: To pass into or through a substance or space

In situ: In the normal place without invading the surrounding tissue

Justice: The quality of being just, impartial, or fair

Kyphosis: Exaggerated outward curvature of the spine

Lethargy: Abnormal drowsiness or mental sluggishness

Lordosis: Abnormal forward curvature of the spine

Maximal impulse: Location to auscultate the best heart sounds

Narcolepsy: Condition of brief recurrent attacks of daytime sleepiness

Neglect: To fail to care for, pay little or no attention to, or leave undone

Neuropathy: Any disease of the nerves

Nodule: A small abnormal swelling or aggregation of cells

Nonmaleficence: The principal of not doing something that causes harm

Oliguria: Urine output less than 400 mL/daily

Pallor: Lack of color; paleness

Palpation: To examine by application of the hands or fingers to the body surface

Paralytic ileus: Paralysis of the intestine; causes swelling and pain

Perfusion: The circulation of blood through tissue

Peristalsis: Wave-like involuntary contractions of the digestive tract

Pigmentation: Coloration resulting from deposit of pigments

Plantar flexion: Movement of the foot; to flex the foot or toes downward

Polyuria: Excessive amount of urination

Prioritizing: To organize tasks or goals; placing most important task first

Pulse deficit: Condition in which the pulse at the radial artery is less than that of the heart

Pulse pressure: The difference between the systolic and diastolic blood pressure

Referral: Sending to another for consultation or service

Regurgitation: Backward flow

Resiliency: The ease with which a patient recovers from shock, stress, depression, and so on

Slough: Dead tissue separating from the living tissue

Stenosis: Abnormal narrowing of a blood vessel or tube in an organ

Syncope: A short and usually sudden loss of consciousness

Synergistic: The action of two or more drugs working together is greater than the sum of their actions working alone

Thrombocytopenia: Abnormal decrease in the number of platelets

Thrombus: A blood clot that adheres to the wall of a blood vessel or organ

Turgor: The rigidity of a cell due to swelling with fluid; the elasticity of the skin

Utilitarianism: A theory; to achieve the greatest benefit for the greatest number

Valsalva maneuver: Attempting to exhale with the nose, mouth, and glottis closed; the maneuver of bearing down; may cause a drop in blood pressure and heart rate

WEEKLY JOURNAL

It is helpful to have each student complete a weekly journal to document the student's weekly learning experience(s). The journal may be completed online or via notebook sheets. The clinical instructor may choose which works best. The journal entry should include the date, the clinical course number, and an entry for each clinical day's activity.

Students should be encouraged to include their learning experiences and their feelings regarding said experiences. This documentation can help the clinical instructor gauge what type of learning experiences are effective learning tools for the students and which are not.

Journals can also reflect over time how far the students have come in their professional growth and knowledge development.

PERFORMING A PHYSICAL ASSESSMENT

A nursing student must learn the process of completing a thorough physical assessment. The guidelines on performing a complete and thorough physical assessment should be provided in the medical–surgical textbook chosen for the particular nursing program. This knowledge and this skill set are tested in the college's skills laboratory under observation by the clinical or theoretical instructor. During clinical courses, however, the student must learn to perform a physical assessment that not only provides information supportive of the patient's need for health care intervention but also is not so time-consuming that it monopolizes all the student's time. The instructor should review in preconference how to perform a modified assessment. The modified assessment guideline should be passed out when the instructor gives out the daily assignment and should be collected in postconference with discussion of findings. The instructor should observe each student when performing a physical assessment to evaluate the student's skills. Before the student performs the assessment, the student should be able to voice any findings that they may have observed with the patient. For example, if the patient has been admitted with a left-hemorrhagic stroke, the student may notice right-sided deficits or neglect, lethargy, and so on. Disease processes will usually present with a set of symptoms and treatments. Therefore, the clinical instructor should stress the importance of knowing how to perform a modified physical assessment.

The following guidelines are included to offer an example of a modified physical assessment.

MODIFIED PHYSICAL ASSESSMENT GUIDELINES

The student should knock on the patient's door or stand outside the curtain to ask permission to enter the patient's personal space. Knocking is a sign of respect and will also allow the patient to deny entry in the event the patient requires privacy (e.g., the patient may be using a commode or a urinal). Once inside the room, the student should introduce himself or herself.

> **Student:** "Good morning, my name is Deborah, and I will be your student nurse from 7:00 a.m. until 3:00 p.m. For the next half hour, I will be performing a physical assessment. Can you tell me your name?"
> **Patient:** "Jane Doe"
> **Student:** "How are you feeling today?"
> **Patient:** [Whatever the patient states next may dictate how the student proceeds].
> **Student:** "What is your birth date?"
> **Patient:** [Month, day, and year]
> **Student:** "What day is it today?"
> **Patient:** [Current date]

If the patient is able to make eye contact and answer appropriately, it can be determined that the patient is alert and oriented.

Students should wash their hands prior to beginning the physical portion of the assessment. Washing hands serves two purposes: to prevent the spread of pathogens and also to warm the hands prior to touching the patient's skin.

Student: "I will be shining a light in your eyes to assess pupil response." The room should be darkened as much as possible prior to performing the pupillary response assessment. [Perform the test.] The student should explain that a pupillary change can indicate a change in the neurological system. It should be noted that the patient may have had eye surgery, which can alter the shape of the iris. If the iris is irregular and does not react, the student should investigate whether this event is normal or a new onset. After the pupillary assessment, the student should turn on the lights to allow better observation for the remainder of the assessment. The visual acuity of the patient is not tested in the modified assessment. Assess whether the patient's eyelids are equal or unequal. A drooping eyelid is called *ptosis*. The conjunctiva and sclera should be assessed for color, moisture, and edema. Accommodation is tested by holding a pencil approximately 12 inches away from the patient's nose. Instruct the patient to keep his or her eyes on the pencil. Slowly move the pencil toward the patient's nose. The patient should be able to follow the pencil to the nose and back to its original starting position.

Student: "I will now test your strength [the student must place two fingers of each hand into the patient's hands]. I need you to squeeze my fingers and then release my fingers." The strength of each hand should be documented. Are the strengths equal? Did the patient follow simple commands (i.e., squeeze and release)? The student should place his or her hands on the bottom of the patient's feet. "Push on my hands as if you are pushing on a gas pedal." The student should then place his or her hands on top of the toes and dorsal portion of the patient's feet. "Pull your toes toward you." The strength of the feet should again be assessed, including whether equal or unequal, and documented accordingly.

The student can then assess the capillary refill time by pressing firmly on the patient's nail bed. The nail bed should initially blanch when pressed, and then return to normal color when released. A normal response would be a capillary refill time of less than 3 seconds. The skin temperature can be assessed simultaneously. The patient's skin may feel warm, cool, hot, or cold.

Ask the patient to smile. This will allow the student to assess whether the face is symmetrical. A patient with a history of a cerebrovascular accident (CVA) may have an asymmetrical face. Obtain a set of vital signs. Take the blood pressure in each arm and compare the findings. If the blood pressure is higher in one arm, use the arm with the higher pressure to take blood pressure readings from this point on. Use the appropriate-size blood pressure cuff. If time permits, it is always helpful to obtain blood pressure readings with the patient lying, sitting, and standing.

Obtaining an accurate temperature is not easy. Research has not yet determined which route is more accurate. Tympanic temperatures may be inaccurate if the nurse has not been shown the proper way to insert the tympanic probe or to wait a few seconds prior to taking the temperature. Rectal temperatures can be the more accurate but are inconvenient and often refused by the adult patient. Rectal temperatures are also avoided to prevent stimulation of the vagus nerve (parasympathetic nervous system). Older adults may have ill-fitting dentures or missing teeth, making oral temperatures inaccurate. Axillary temperatures in the elderly or thin adults may read lower than normal due to less muscle or skin available to make good contact with the thermometer probe. It is therefore in the nurse's discretion to determine the temperature route that will offer the more accurate reading.

Respirations should be taken while the patient believes the pulse is being assessed. Most adults will alter their respirations if they are aware the respirations are being monitored. The student should observe whether the patient is breathing normally or has labored breathing. Is the patient using accessory muscles? Are the nares flared?

Unless the pulse is irregular, it should be taken for 15 seconds and then multiplied by 4 to obtain a 60-second count. If the pulse is irregular, the pulse should be counted for a full minute. The student can assess the strength of the pulse. Is the pulse slightly irregular when the patient takes a deep breath? If the pulse is irregular, the student should ask the patient whether an irregular heart rate is normal. In this case, the apical heart rate is required and a pulse deficit must be performed. A patient with atrial fibrillation will have an irregular heart rate.

Next, the skin on the face, head, and neck should be examined. The student should feel the scalp for irregularities. Is the patient bald? Is the hair thinning? Does the patient have scars or acne? Palpate the lymph nodes (preauricular, submandibular, anterior cervical, and submental). Assess the ears. The use of an otoscope can be used to perform a complete ear assessment, but often this is omitted by the bedside nurse unless the patient is admitted with an ear-related health issue. The patient should be asked whether he or she has any hearing difficulties. Elderly patients may be hard of hearing, may use hearing aids, or may be deaf in one or both ears.

The student should assess the nose and sinuses. Is the septum midline? Does the patient have congestion? The otoscope can be used to assess the nostrils, but this test is often omitted by the bedside nurse unless the patient is admitted with a respiratory-related health issue. The student should palpate the sinuses. Are the sinuses tender or painful to palpation? Is there nasal drainage? Are the external nares red and swollen?

Assess the mouth. Ask the patient to open his or her mouth. Is the mouth moist or dry? With a gloved hand and a tongue blade, assess the buccal pockets (cheeks) of the mouth. Assess for ulcers or lesions. Using a penlight or an otoscope, shine the light to the pharynx and ask the patient to say, "ah." Assess the posterior portion of the mouth. Is there redness, drainage, swelling, or white patches?

Assess the throat and neck. Is the trachea midline? Are the carotid pulses present bilaterally? Palpate only one carotid pulse at a time to prevent baroreceptor reflex, which will cause hypotension. Using the bell of the stethoscope, the student should auscultate the carotid arteries. Instruct the patient to exhale and hold while you are auscultating the carotid. A bruit should not be heard bilaterally. A bruit may indicate carotid occlusion. Is the thyroid gland palpable? To assess, stand behind the patient, place the index and middle fingers on the thyroid gland, and ask the patient to swallow. This procedure will allow the thyroid to move. Does the patient have a goiter?

Explain to the patient you will need to inspect the chest. To maintain privacy, have a towel available to cover the chest before removing the patient's gown down to the waist in order to auscultate the lungs. The patient should be in a 45-degree angle or sitting upright. Using the diaphragm of the stethoscope, place the stethoscope in the areas marked on the diagram to assess the lung sounds (see answers to breath sound ausculation quiz on p. 52). Also ensure that the students listen posteriorly for adventitious breath sounds.

Instruct the patient to take a deep breath and blow out each time the stethoscope is moved to a new location. The student will be comparing the left lung with the right lung, both anteriorly and posteriorly. Move the stethoscope to the various positions (note diagram) and auscultate for normal air exchange. Take note of any abnormalities, such as wheezes, rhonchi, rales, or crackles. The student should note whether the patient has difficulty taking in a deep breath or has difficulty exhaling. Note whether the chest is symmetrical when the patient inhales and exhales. Note whether the trachea is midline. When auscultating a female patient, the student may be required to move the breast. It is recommended to use the dorsal aspect of the hand to prevent the patient from feeling uncomfortable or violated.

When the student palpates the chest, abnormal sounds should be documented. The patient may have hyperresonant sounds if the patient has a history of emphysema. The patient may have dull sounds in the presence of a pleural effusion or pneumonia. The student should note the shape of the patient's chest. Is the chest barrel shaped or pigeon shaped? It is appropriate to assess peripheral pulses at this time. Assess the radial, dorsalis pedis, and tibial pulses. If the patient has a below-the-knee amputation, assess the popliteal pulse. Femoral pulses can also be assessed at this time, but this step may be reserved for when the student assesses the genital area.

It is appropriate to move to the cardiovascular examination while the patient's gown is lowered. Using the diaphragm, place the stethoscope on the second intercostal space to the right of the sternum (aortic valve). Next place the stethoscope on the second intercostal space to the left of the sternum (pulmonic valve). Next place the stethoscope at the third intercostal space to the left of the sternum (Erb's point). This is usually the point of maximum impulse (PMI) and where apical pulses are taken. Place the stethoscope at the fourth intercostal space to the left of the sternum (tricuspid valve). Next place the stethoscope at the fifth intercostal space to the left of the sternum (mitral valve). Request the patient lie on his or her left side. Place the stethoscope at the PMI. This will make it easier to detect an S3 or S4 heart sound or murmurs.

Observe whether the breasts are symmetrical. It is not uncommon for women with large breasts to have one breast larger than the other. The larger breast is usually on the dominant side. Note the character of the skin. Is the skin smooth, or is it orange peel–like, which is a potential sign of cancer? Is there any dimpling, which is another potential sign of cancer? Has the patient had reconstructive surgery? Does the male patient exhibit signs of gynecomastia (enlarged breasts)? Place the gown back into the upright position. Cover the patient with the sheet up to and including the symphysis pubis. Explain to the patient you will be assessing the abdomen.

> **KEY NOTE:** A physical assessment is performed in the following order: inspection, palpation, percussion, and then auscultation, except when assessing the gastrointestinal system. When assessing the gastrointestinal system, it is necessary to inspect, auscultate, percuss, and then palpate.

Prior to performing this assessment, it is wise to ask the patient whether he or she needs to urinate, because palpation on the abdominal wall may result in discomfort if the patient has a full bladder.

Inspect the skin of the abdomen. Look for scars (surgical or injury), striae, rashes, or hernias. Ask the patient for correlating information concerning scars such as surgeries if they were not documented on the history and the physical. Observe whether there are pulsations (may indicate an abdominal aneurysm). Is the abdomen flat, protuberant, rounded, distended, or obese? Using the diaphragm of the stethoscope, listen to the abdominal sounds in each of the four quadrants (right upper, left upper, right lower, and left lower). Are the bowel sounds normal, hypoactive, or hyperactive? Percuss the abdomen. The bowel may sound drum like (tympanic) if the patient has a lot of gas or is distended. Deep palpation is usually not performed in the modified physical assessment. It is appropriate to measure the abdominal girth on patients who may have an underlying health issue that bears monitoring (such as ascites in patients with cirrhosis). Rebound tenderness should be reported.

Instruct the patient to lift up the right arm. Ask the patient to move the arm outward, and then across the chest. Instruct the patient to straighten the arm and then turn the entire arm (as if turning a door knob). Repeat this process on the left arm. Instruct the patient to lift the right leg, bend the knee, move the leg toward the left leg, and then outward. Repeat this process with the left leg. If the patient is unable to move the extremity independently, the student should perform passive range of motion on each of the extremities to assess the strength, motion, and presence of pain on movement. The patient's spine should be assessed for the presence of kyphosis, lordosis, or scoliosis.

The genitourinary assessment can be very embarrassing for both the student and the patient. The student should explain to the patient that it is necessary to assess the skin and structures of the genitourinary system. In the female, the student should assess the labia for hair distribution, swelling, bruising, ulcers, or lesions. With gloved hands, open the labia to examine the urinary meatus. Inspect the vaginal opening for redness, vesicles, ulcers, or discharge. The rectum should be inspected for the presence of hemorrhoids. In the male patient, the penis should be inspected for proper physiological development. Hypospadias, or a growth defect in the development of the urinary meatus, may be noted. The scrotal sac should be inspected for lesions, ulcers, vesicles, discharge, or swelling. The femoral pulses can be assessed at this time.

Any abnormal findings need to be presented by the physician first. The nurse can reveal "normal" findings. When there are abnormal findings that the doctor has already discussed with the patient, the nurse can explain and help the patient review the different types of medical treatment that are being recommended. Any concerns will be relayed to the physician. Question the patient whether this condition is a new onset or a previous health issue identified by the patient or the patient's physician. This discussion will allow the patient to continue to build trust and rapport. This also allows the patient to confide in the nurse whether the patient has had previous health issues that were forgotten when the patient's health information was collected.

Breath Sounds Ausculation Quiz

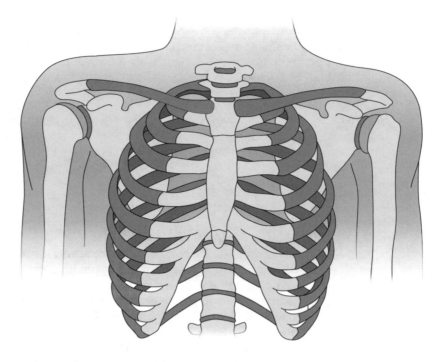

Indicate the areas used for breath sounds ausculation in this image.

Answers to Breath Sounds Ausculation Quiz

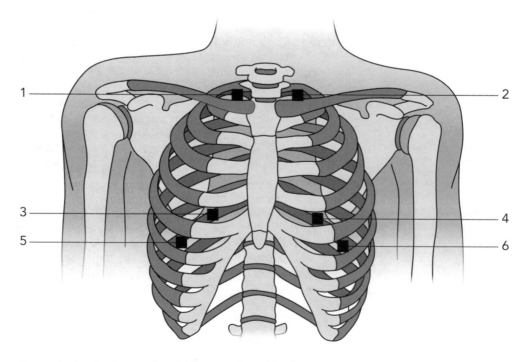

Posteriorly, the lungs should be ausulated in the some areas.

POSTCONFERENCE INSTRUCTIONS

Allow at least 1 hour after each clinical for the discussion of the day's events, patients, diagnoses, nursing care plans, and time management issues (including any issues related to delays in treatment and prioritization), as well as any incidents, reactions with other staff members, and so on. Find a quiet room where patient care can be discussed without disclosure of confidential patient information. This book includes pre-planning exercises and activities based on the students' knowledge levels and skill levels, on the patient population of a specific unit, and on nursing care plan examples. Use the post-conference activities to promote critical thinking and provide learning.

You can invite guest speakers at your clinical site to speak at postconference. You may invite the wound-care specialist, the infectious-disease nurse, the diabetic educator, the IV therapist, the physical therapist, the occupational therapist, and so on. Be mindful that the students may be distracted or tired at the end of the day. Keep postconferences interactive with open-ended questions and engaging behavior.

Encourage the group to identify topics that the students would like more information on.

Create a positive environment and divert negative comments. If there was a negative experience, discuss how to handle the situation. Many students are concerned about a test at school or family problems. It is essential to constantly direct and redirect conversations without becoming a barrier to communication: "I know that you are concerned about the cardiology test tonight, so let's discuss how we would take care of a patient with this disease."

WEEK 1 POSTCONFERENCE

Students in the Medical–Surgical II clinical class should demonstrate their ability to perform appropriately basic nursing skills such as vital signs, activities of daily living, and physical assessments. The nursing instructor should observe each nursing student independently as the student performs these skills on his or her assigned patient. The clinical instructor should not assume the student has gained the appropriate skills until they are proved. Therefore, the instructor should inform the students that they will be monitored throughout the clinical to ensure that they are practicing competent and safe nursing care.

The clinical instructor should also notify the students that each of them will be tested on medications, side effects, desired effects, interactions, and dose calculations (if applicable) prior to being allowed to pass medications or regulate IV fluids on his or her assigned patient. A student who is unable to perform basic medication calculations should be referred to the college or university clinical laboratory for further tutoring and study.

The clinical instructor may be required to attend a computer class at the chosen clinical site to obtain authorization to pass out medications. Be aware, the students may also need to attend these classes. The clinical instructor should plan to allow only one or two students each week to pass out medications to their assigned patients. Attempting to allow the entire group to administrer medications at the same time may make it difficult for the clinical instructor to monitor all students during patient care activities.

The student chosen to administer medications must demonstrate appropriate knowledge of the medications, their side effects, the need for laboratory levels (if applicable), and patient data (blood pressure, heart rate, etc., if applicable) prior to administering the medication to the assigned patient. The prudent clinical instructor will ask the student to provide the preceding information prior to entering the patient care area.

Discuss the vocabulary list with the students. Explain that the complexity of terms and words in the medical profession require the student to basically learn a new language. The medical profession often not only has strange, new words that explain conditions or a disease process but also has many abbreviations. An abbreviation list can be found in the Appendix at the end of this book. It is up to the clinical instructor to determine whether the students should research their own abbreviations or whether the clinical instructor will provide the more common abbreviations to the students.

Notify the students that concept mapping will be discussed next week. It will become evident how the nursing assessment process discussed in this chapter and the concept map can help guide the nurse on gathering patient data and on planning interventions.

Chapter 5

NURSING ASSESSMENTS, CONCEPT MAPPING, AND CRITICAL THINKING

This chapter examines:

- Nursing assessments and patient data collection activities
- Concept mapping and development of critical thinking skills

WEEK 2 PRECONFERENCE

Hand out:
- Medication forms (insulin and digoxin)
- Nursing assessment form (2 copies)
- Concept map template (2 copies)

Collect:
- Vocabulary quiz
- Patient care plan

Students should begin the critical thinking process. Inform them that each week they will be given a minimum of two medication handouts that they will be required to research and complete. Each disease and each medication involve additional data that the nurse must know and understand to ensure adequate patient care and safety. In completing the medication handouts, students will begin to understand the correlation between medications, foods, and laboratory results. This will help the student to become more knowledgeable and will assist the student in performing patient education.

Inform the students that this week each student will be required to choose one of their assigned patient's disease processes. It may be a current disease or one in the patient's medical history. The student will then be required to complete a concept map on the chosen disease process.

Instruct the students to make copies of the physical assessment form and concept map template. Copies of each form will be used during this week's patient care as well as during each subsequent week throughout the clinical course. Inform students that any deficit (i.e., any physical or mental deviation from what should be the normal mental or physiological assessment findings) should be investigated and recorded. Assign each student one patient. During preconference, students will be given instructions on the skills and tasks that will be expected or required of them during patient interactions.

Students will be assigned a patient based on the collaboration between the unit charge nurse and the clinical instructor. Patient assignments are chosen to assist the students to meld theoretical knowledge with didactic knowledge. For example, caring for a patient with a diagnosis of diabetes mellitus can help the student more thoroughly understand the theoretical knowledge concerning diabetes mellitus.

NURSING ASSESSMENT

The nursing assessment, which involves a multitude of skills and steps, is the first tier in the nursing process. The nursing student must recognize that the nursing assessment is the foundation on which the remaining steps in the nursing process are based.

For this reason, the clinical instructor should observe each student performing a physical assessment to ensure proper technique and sequence.

The student must gather information or data. Information may be collected from the patient, the patient's family, the medical record, tests, procedures, and the physical assessment. Information gathered from the medical record should be verified or confirmed to ensure accuracy.

Questions such as why the patient is seeking health care services or what is the patient's chief complaint can assist the student in focusing in on the patient's initial problem. Asking open-ended questions will help the student to gain more information than asking closed-ended questions. An example of an open-ended question is "Tell me about what brought you to the hospital." An example of a closed-ended question is "Were you having abdominal pain?" There are many questions that can aid in obtaining the desired information, such as biographical data, present and past health problems, family health history, environmental history, psychosocial history, and spiritual history.

Interviewing the patient alone often will help the patient feel more comfortable with the nurse and will allow the nurse to screen for abuse without interference. Additional information can be requested from the family when the nurse can sequester the family from the patient. Often the patient may be stoic and not admit that pain has been occurring for weeks or even months. Often, the patient will be alert and oriented × 1 (self), × 2 (self and place), × 3 (self, place, and time), or × 4 (self, place, time, and situation). Cultural behaviors may not present in a familiar pattern. The student must keep in mind that not every culture handles illness or pain with the same physiological characteristics. The family may help give a more complete picture of the patient's health problem.

Example of Physical Assessment Form

Patient name: _____ Age: _____ Diagnosis: _____

Height: _____cm Weight: _____kg Pain: _____

Scale _____

Vital signs: B/P _____HR _____RR _____Temp _____O_2 saturation _____

Neurological: Level of consciousness (LOC): alert/oriented _____ drowsy, lethargic, obtunded, somnolent, or unresponsive

Responds to: Verbal, tactile, noxious, pain, or no response
Postures: _____

Withdraws: Left arm _____, right arm _____, left leg _____, or right leg _____

Able to follow commands _____ Grasp = or ≠
Bilateral lower extremities: push/pull = or ≠

Speech: Clear, garbled, slurred, or aphasic. Facial tone _____ symmetrical/asymmetrical

Pupils: = or ≠   Size: Left ____mm   Right _____mm

History of neurological problems: _____

History of falls: _____ Gait steady: Yes/No   History of dizziness: Yes/No
History of numbness/tingling: _____

Cardiac: Heart sounds: regular/irregular   Murmurs: New/Old

Pulses: Palpable: left radial _____, right radial _____, left dorsalis pedis _____, right dorsalis pedis ____ left posterior tibial _____ right posterior tibial _____. (Enter P for palpable or D for doppled pulse.)

Edema: Location _____

Rate edema: 1+, 2+, 3+, 4+, or anasarca _____

History of cardiac problems: _____

Respiratory: Lung sounds: clear throughout, crackles: location _____, rales: location _____, wheezes (inspiratory or expiratory): location

_____

Respiratory treatments: _____ Type: _____ Frequency: _____
Home O₂: _____ Type: _____ Amount: _____ SOB: _____
DOE: _____ Orthopnea: _____

Sleeps on _____ pillows. Cough: Yes/No; Productive, non-productive

Sputum amount: _____ Color: _____

History of respiratory problems: _____

Gastrointestinal: Positive bowel sounds to all quads: Yes/No
Explain: _____
Hypoactive bowel sounds: _____
Hyperactive bowel sounds: _____

Abdomen: Soft, firm, rigid, tender to palpation: Yes/No. Flat, protuberant, rounded, or obese

Diet: Regular, AHA, ADA, clear liquid, soft, other: _____

Able to feed self: Yes/No. Intake appropriate: Yes/No. Need for dietary consult: Yes/No. Reason for consult: _____

NGT/OGT/PEG/J-tube. Tube feeding type: _____

Defecation: Regular/constipation/ diarrhea/colostomy. Usual bowel regime: Daily; every other day: _____

Does patient require finger sticks AC and HS: Yes/No
Antidiabetic medication: _____

History of GI problems: _____

Genitourinary: Independent voids, Foley, suprapubic catheter, ileostomy, or incontinent: _____

History of hesitancy, frequency, urgency, burning, pain, anuric, polyuric, or oliguric: _____

Dialysis: Hemodialysis, peritoneal dialysis. AV fistula: thrill + or -, bruit + or -, dialysis catheter: _____

Urine character: clear, cloudy, sediment, bloody, or odorous. _____

Urinary output amount: adequate: Yes/No   How many cc/kg: _____

Bladder flat or distended: Yes/No

History of genitourinary problems: _____

Genital: Male: Penis: normal, swollen, normal physical findings: Yes/No
Explain if no: _____

Testes normal: Yes/No. Implants: Yes/No. History of testicular cancer, or prostate cancer: Yes/No

Female: Labia normal: Yes/No. Swollen, red, normal hair distribution

Postmenopausal: Yes/No Menses: regular/irregular Vaginal discharge: Yes/No
Describe: _____

Vaginal odor: Yes/No. Gravida: Number of pregnancies _____
Para (Number of live births): _____

Participates in routine health checks: prostate exam, Pap smear/ mammograms: Yes/No

Results of above tests: normal/ abnormal. Explain: _____

History of genital problems: _____

Musculoskeletal: ROM/PROM. Limitations: Yes/No

Explain _____

Contractures: Yes/No. Location: _____

Joints: Normal/abnormal/swollen/red/painful
Explain _____

Able to ambulate without difficulty: Yes/No
Explain _____

Requires: Wheelchair, walker, cane, or crutches
Explain _____

History of musculoskeletal problems: _____

Integumentary: Skin intact: Yes/No   Pressure ulcer(s): Yes/No

Describe the stage and depth of the wound in centimeters, any tunneling or undermining, any drainage if yes response: _____

Skin: Warm/cool/hot/diaphoretic

Skin color: Appropriate for race: Yes/No
Pale, ashen, cyanotic, jaundice, or mottled

Alterations: Yes/No   Ecchymotic, rash, vesicles, or lesions

Turgor: Good elasticity, poor elasticity, tight, or fragile

Risk level for pressure ulcer: high, medium, or low
Need for wound care consult: Yes/No

Mobility: Immobility, limited, no limitations

IV access: Peripheral, central, or PICC. Site date: _____.
Site assessed: _____
Dry, intact, leaking, or red. Dressing type: gauze, or transparent

History of integumentary problems: _____

Psychological: Behavior: appropriate, inappropriate. Explain: _____
Mood: Appropriate, inappropriate
History of psychological problems: _____

Activities of daily living (ADL): Able to perform ADL: independently, with assist, total care

Current Immunization: Pneumovax: Date administered _____

Flu vaccine: Date administered_____

Tetanus: Date administered _____

Additional notes: _____

CONCEPT MAPPING

Once the patient information has been gathered, the student can begin to organize a concept map. What is a concept map? A concept map is a tool that allows the nurse or nursing student to gather data, analyze the collected data into categories, and then use these finding to determine priority of care.

To begin a concept map, the chief complaint or medical diagnosis is placed in the center of the concept map. Problems or potential problems all stem from the initial complaint or medical diagnosis.

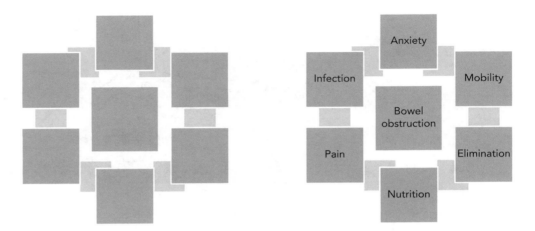

Sample concept map.

As the student begins to look at each section of the concept map, the student must determine what information or data can support an analysis of each problem. For example, one stem box may begin *Pain*: B/P elevated, guarding body part, restless, diaphoretic, moans, tender abdomen, absent bowel sounds, vomiting. Patient admits hasn't eaten in days. Last bowel movement 4 days ago. Takes oxycodone for chronic back pain, which usually causes constipation.

Analysis of each problem must be supported by data. Some data may be used in more than one category, if applicable. The next step in building the concept map is to determine how each stem box interacts or relates to outcomes and interventions.

Concept mapping may seem confusing at first. The concept map is actually a schematic for the nursing process. The concept map will assist the nursing student in learning how to collect, organize, and analyze data. The concept map will teach how to determine what actions or interventions are appropriate for each problem. The concept map will help to determine goals and outcomes. The concept map will also help the student to learn how to communicate important information to the health care or interdisciplinary team.

Let's start from the beginning. The patient comes to the hospital with abdominal pain, which is a symptom. He has been diagnosed with a bowel obstruction, so this is entered in the center of the schematic. The nurse's physical assessment will determine the patient's current status. Information learned from the assessment includes vital signs, pain level (document which pain scale is used), abdominal assessment (tender, hypoactive, absent, or hyperactive bowel sounds), guarding abdomen, vomiting, rigid abdomen, diaphoretic, restless, no bowel movement in 4 days, feels weak, and anorexia.

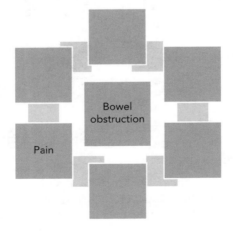

Pain: Tender abdomen, guarding body, diaphoretic, rigid, restless, moans, and blood pressure is elevated.

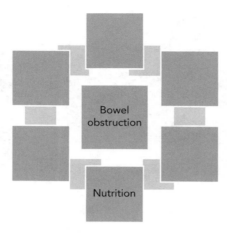

Nutrition: Has not eaten in 5 days. Vomiting, chronic constipation, last bowel movement was 4 days ago, and is diaphoretic.

Is nutrition an issue? Yes. The patient is anorexic and nauseated. He is having insensible losses (fluid losses that cannot be measured) due to his diaphoresis, emesis, and having not eaten for 5 days. As the nursing student continues to gather data for each category, critical thinking begins to develop. The nursing student should review the patient's vital signs to evaluate for hypotension, the lab work to evaluate for renal insufficiency and depleted electrolytes, and the albumin level to evaluate for malnourishment. The student should evaluate for proper skin turgor. Each problem may affect the patient in various ways. What interventions should be initiated for each problem?

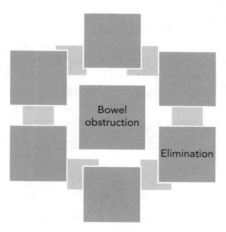

Elimination: Guarding abdomen, vomiting, rigid abdomen, no bowel movement in 4 days, and anorexia.

The patient may have had the bowel obstruction since 4 days ago when the patient first started experiencing symptoms. Diagnostic tests will help determine the cause of the obstruction, such as a tumor, volvulus, or perforation. The potential for septic shock and necrosis of the bowel is increased. Was a lactate level done? When was the last time the patient voided? Is he receiving adequate hydration with current administration of IV fluids? Monitoring intake and output, lab work, and vital signs will help the student to evaluate whether the interventions are effective.

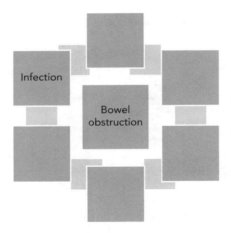

Infection: Does the patient have an elevated temperature? Are the white blood cells elevated? Were blood cultures drawn? The patient also will have a risk for infection because of interventions such as an IV access, any Foley insertion, or any other invasive procedure that could introduce bacteria.

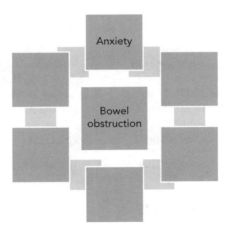

Anxiety: Elevated blood pressure and restless.

Is the patient anxious? Anxiety can interfere with care to the extent that the patient does not listen or understand when the physician attempts to explain the need for surgery. The patient may become anxious because he fears death or the hospital. Some elderly patients may say, "You come to the hospital to die."

Ask the patient whether he has been in the hospital before. How does he usually deal with anxiety? Does his religion prevent him from using any interventions? Has he had surgery before? Has he or his family had any reaction to anesthesia? Did he understand what the physician was saying to him regarding the need for surgery? It is important for the student nurse to be in the room when the physician is discussing medical treatment with the patient. The instructor frequently has to encourage this because students are insecure when the physician questions them. Frequently the client is hesitant to question the physician. The student nurse is frequently required to translate the information that was relayed from the physician.

Once the data are collected, it makes for a clearer picture. The patient has never been hospitalized before. His grandfather died in a hospital 2 years ago. He usually takes oxycodone for his chronic back pain. He was raised Baptist but hasn't attended church in years. He has never had anesthesia and has no idea if his family has ever had a reaction to anesthesia. He is voicing concern: "Do a lot of people have reactions to anesthesia?"

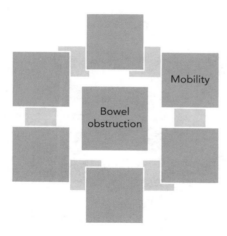

Mobility: The patient feels very weak and restless.

The patient is anxious about anesthesia, so the nurse needs to offer the patient information and reassurance. It is important to address both pre- and postoperative concerns, especially regarding the recovery period, during which the patient may have new incisions, tubes inserted, and so on. The nurse will explain that anesthesia can cause nausea, and the physician can order a patch to help with nausea. Giving the patient information regarding his care and the process of what may happen during the course of his treatment may help to alleviate his anxiety.

Has the patient been able to ambulate to the bathroom by himself? Is the patient steady on his feet when he is standing up? Has the patient been on bed rest?

The patient states that he has become increasingly weak over the past few days. The nurse can determine from this information that the patient has probably experienced decreased mobility for the past 2 to 3 days. Therefore, the patient is at risk for deep vein thrombosis (DVT), pneumonia, and skin integrity issues such as pressure ulcers.

GOALS, INTERVENTIONS, AND EVALUATIONS

Once the data have been collected and entered in the appropriate box, the nurse can determine what the plan and outcomes should be for each problem. Other potential problems include knowledge deficits, fear of surgery, financial fears, alteration in body image, and potential alteration in bowel elimination (colostomy) as well as potential alteration in urinary elimination.

The nurse must now determine the patient goals and outcomes. Listed below are examples of patient goals (decrease or relief of pain) and outcomes (based on an evalvation of the outcome).

(Pain) Goal: **Decrease pain or relieve pain** as evidenced by (AEB) patient stating that the pain has been relieved or is tolerable with a pain level of 3. The goal must be specific to the patient, realistic, and achievable.
Interventions: **Assess** for pain (use pain scale), and **administer** pain medication as ordered. The care plan/concept map should include at least three interventions—one of these should be teaching the patient about medications, treatment plan, and so on. The evaluation may reveal that the outcome is partially met. When an outcome is partially met, the goal and intervention may need revision.
Evaluation (outcome): **Reassess** pain level within 1 hour of administration of pain medication. Determine whether pain goal has been met. There could also be a negative outcome if the patient is unable to comply with interventions.

These key concepts can be summarized as follows:

- Nursing diagnosis (problems) supported with data (AEB).
- The plan is listed as goals. What can the patient measurably achieve within in a certain time limit? Is the patient capable of these goals? The student has to question the patient because the perceived goals may be different than the patient's goals. The patient's planned goal may differ from that of the health care provider. Therefore, the student should inform the patient of the plan for short- and long-term goals. The patient must be an active part in this process.
- The interventions are the planned actions that will help the patient to achieve the intended outcome. This will include preventive measures such as education regarding the abuse of drugs or recognizing noncompliant behavior, implementing measures that will help prevent the extension of the disease, or enrollment in support groups or rehabilitation programs.
- The evaluation (outcome) is based on the patient's response to the intervention. Was the outcome achieved or should it be modified because of current conditions?
- The student should remember that interventions should include medication administration.
- Patient education should also be included in the intervention stage.

For example, the patient with the bowel obstruction had surgery (an anastomosis). What patient education should be included in this patient's plan of care? The nurse should provide patient teaching regarding pain medication, mobility, and incentive spirometry.

To anticipate and address potential problems, the nurse needs to assess the patient for the various risks that may occur as a result of treatment, procedures, hospitalization, medication, and so on.

The nurse can explain that the abdominal muscles and bowel has been cut, the obstruction removed, and the bowel put back together, and this information must be presented in simple terms so that the layperson will understand. Pain medication can help ease the pain and allow for rest. Pain medication can also ease the pain to allow for movement, turning, coughing, and deep breathing.

To recap: The nurse should gather data from the medical record, surgical procedure, advance directive form, laboratory test, procedure notes, and family members. The nurse should note what home medications, including any over-the-counter drugs and herbal supplements, that the patient may have been taking. Understanding the purpose, side effects, and typical dosage of a medication can help the nurse gather more data. The nurse should keep in mind that medications may be listed under brand names, generic names, or as a pharmacy substitution.

Activity levels are often ordered. The nurse may not recognize that an activity level is actually a treatment. If the surgeon orders the patient to ambulate twice daily, it is actually a treatment. The nurse should implement the treatments and document how the patient tolerated the treatment.

Diets and dietary intake are also part of the data collection process. If the patient has severe arthritis, would dietary intake be hindered? Yes. The patient may not be able to feed himself and may be too modest to ask the nurse to help. It is important both to recognize the patient's ability level and to monitor dietary intake. For example, the nutrition department might not deliver a tray, or it might remove the tray without the patient consuming any food. Or, if the patient has a percutaneous endoscopic gastrostomy (PEG), has the dietician ordered an appropriate dietary formula for the patient?

IV fluids are also an intervention. The patient may need electrolytes or medication that will be included in the IV fluids. For example, D5W with 2 amps of bicarbonate, D5/.45 NS with 20 mEq of potassium, Heparin 25,000 units in 500 mL NS, or Levophed 8 mg in 250 mL of D5W.

Nursing students must recognize the correlation between the gathered data, the nursing diagnosis, and the interventions. For example, a woman who had a mastectomy of her left breast not only may have pain issues but also may have an alteration in body image, or anxiety regarding how her husband will view her.

Medication Forms

Listed in the vertical box is a medication. For each of the remaining boxes, list the following:

Box 1: List a laboratory result you would need to monitor. Explain the significance of the laboratory test to the medication.
Box 2: List one food that may interact with the medication. Explain the significance of the food item to the medication.
Box 3: List one patient educational instruction you would give to the patient regarding the medication. Explain the significance of the instruction to the medication.

List other educational information you could provide this patient. Are there websites you can refer to? What about travel overseas and health issues? How should the medication be stored? Does the medication being administered interfere with other medications?

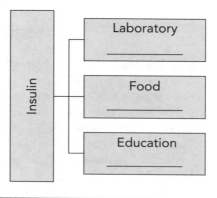

Listed in the vertical box is a medication. For each of the remaining boxes, list the following:

Box 1: List a laboratory result you would need to monitor. Explain the significance of the laboratory test to the medication.
Box 2: List one food that may interact with the medication. Explain the significance of the food item to the medication.
Box 3: List one patient educational instruction you would give to the patient regarding the medication. Explain the significance of the instruction to the medication.

List other educational information you could provide this patient. Are there websites you can refer to? What about travel overseas and health issues? How should the medication be stored? Does the medication being administered interfere with other medications?

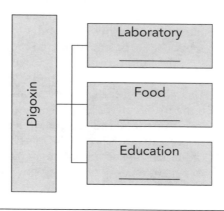

WEEK 2 POSTCONFERENCE

Instruct students to choose one disease process for the assigned concept map. Students should also be instructed to include one potential health issue. Once the concept map is completed, the student should choose one problem related to the disease process on the concept map to use to complete a nursing care plan.

The concept map is used to assist the student to recognize the holistic involvement of a disease. The nursing care plan allows the student to address issues requiring nursing intervention. Concept maps in conjunction with nursing care plans will help the student to develop critical thinking skills.

Ask students to share their patient care experiences. Ask students if anyone encountered any problems that may have caused them some difficulty. What did they do to resolve the problem, and what was the outcome of the intervention? Learning to problem solve is also a learned nursing skill.

Inform the students that the physical assessment form used for the patient assessment should accompany the care plan and concept map when they are turned in next week. This will help to ensure that the student is skilled at assessing the appropriate information related to the patient's disease or health issue.

Inform the students that, beginning Week 3 and for each subsequent week thereafter, all students are required to provide a journal summary of their clinical experience. (The journal may be filled out online or via notebook sheets. The clinical instructor may choose which works best.) The summary should include the problems encountered, what was learned, how the student felt, and any other additional information that would enable the instructor to assist in the learning process of the student.

PART III

TEACHING THE ADVANCED MEDICAL–SURGICAL DISEASE PROCESSES IN A CLINICAL SETTING

SENSORY DEFICITS IN THE ELDERLY AND ASSESSMENTS OF THE VISUAL, AUDITORY, AND NASAL SYSTEMS

This chapter examines:

- Nursing assessment challenges when caring for patients with sensory deficits
- Step-by-step assessment procedures for the visual, auditory, and nasal systems

UNDERSTANDING SENSORY DEFICITS

Week 3 provides education on the senses. Because health and wellness initiatives, health education, and health care interventions assist more people in living longer, nursing education now includes the field of geriatric nursing. With longevity, however, the elderly often experience an alteration of their senses. Deteriorating eyesight, hearing loss, and muscle atrophy can provide challenges for the elderly patient. The nurse must be able to understand the elderly patient's limitations and must provide alternative communication avenues for these patients in order to obtain accurate data and provide appropriate care.

Week 3 allows the clinical instructor to introduce a valuable participation exercise to educate nursing students on sensory loss. For the sensory exercise, the clinical instructor should purchase disposable ear plugs (enough for each student), an inexpensive pair of reading glasses from a local pharmacy, and a stockinet or a blindfold. The students will be addressing surgery with a hearing-impaired patient, so obtain copies of a generalized surgical consent form (one for each student) to use in this exercise.

Students should continue to provide patient care, complete nursing care plans, and complete medication forms, as well as document in their journals.

WEEK 3 PRECONFERENCE

Hand out:
- Sensory deficit exercise
- Medication forms (warfarin and Synthroid)
- Situation exercise

Collect:
- Medication forms (insulin and digoxin)
- Care plan
- Concept map
- Physical assessment form

Inform the students that the sensory exercise will help them to understand the sensory deficits an elderly patient may experience. Ensure that, for the sensory exercise, there is an area that will allow for ambulation and privacy. Try to arrange for this room to have obstacles normally found in a hospital room or at home.

SENSORY DEFICIT EXERCISE

Note: Students must be paired for this exercise.

1. Student #1 must insert the ear plugs into his or her own ears. Student #2 must now attempt to explain the surgical consent to this patient. (Ask the "patient" to repeat what the nurse said.)
2. Student #3 should apply the reading glasses. Student #4 must attempt to have Student #3 read and sign the surgical consent. If you are unable to obtain a surgical consent, any reading material can be used. Have the student (in the role of the patient with poor eyesight) sign his or her name.
3. Student #5 must be blindfolded. Student #6 must assist this patient in ambulating around the room. Avoid stairs, equipment, or furniture that may cause injury.
4. Student #7 must be blindfolded. Student #8 must attempt to orient this patient to the area.

Have students exchange roles and equipment to ensure each student experiences each patient role (hard of hearing, poor eyesight, and blindness). When the students have completed each patient role, discuss what each student discovered about each sensory deficit. What was the most difficult aspect of obtaining information? What was the most difficult aspect of offering education to the patient with sensory challenges? What alternative would be available to assist these patients? Ask all the students to verbalize what they believe they learned from this exercise.

SITUATION EXERCISE

Each student must choose a health issue (reflex sympathetic dystrophy [RSD], insulin-dependent diabetes mellitus [IDDM], Parkinson's disease, etc.) and an associated sensory deficit. Explain that each student must complete the situation exercise form based on the chosen health issue and the associated sensory deficit, and return the completed form by the next preconference.

SITUATION EXERCISE FORM

Disease: _____

Risk for or Cause of: _____

Patient Education: _____

Compliance	Noncompliance
_____	_____
_____	_____
_____	_____
_____	_____
_____	_____

Complications

_____

_____

_____

_____

ANSWERS TO SITUATION EXERCISE FORM

Disease: Diabetes

Risk for or Cause of: Sensory and visual effect; poor eyesight

Patient Education: Dietary changes needed

Compliance	Noncompliance
Active lifestyle	Sedentary lifestyle
Normal blood sugar control	Abnormal blood sugar levels
Normal vital signs	Abnormal vital signs (hypertension)
Normal skin integrity	Abnormal skin integrity (ulcers)

Complications

Overweight or obesity	Drowsiness
Neuropathy	Dialysis
Renal failure	Amputation
Ulcers	Death
Loss of eye sight	

Medication Forms

Listed in the vertical box is a medication. For each of the remaining boxes, list the following:

Box 1: List a laboratory result you would need to monitor. Explain the significance of the laboratory test to the medication.
Box 2: List one food that may interact with the medication. Explain the significance of the food item to the medication.
Box 3: List one patient educational instruction you would give to the patient regarding the medication. Explain the significance of the instruction to the medication.

List other educational information you could provide this patient. Are there websites you can refer to? What about travel overseas and health issues? How should the medication be stored? Does the medication being administered interfere with other medications?

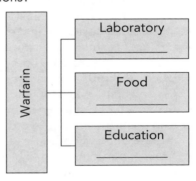

Listed in the vertical box is a medication. For each of the remaining boxes, list the following:

Box 1: List a laboratory result you would need to monitor. Explain the significance of the laboratory test to the medication.

Box 2: List one food that may interact with the medication. Explain the significance of the food item to the medication.

Box 3: List one patient educational instruction you would give to the patient regarding the medication. Explain the significance of the instruction to the medication.

List other educational information you could provide this patient. Are there websites you can refer to? What about travel overseas and health issues? How should the medication be stored? Does the medication being administered interfere with other medications?

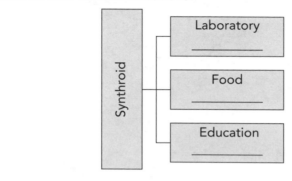

SENSORY ASSESSMENTS

Instruct students to review the anatomy and physiology of the eye, ear, and nose. The following sections explore the steps involved in nursing assessments of the visual, auditory, and nasal systems. These include the conditions affecting these systems and how they are treated and include terminology, nursing interventions, and patient education.

VISUAL SYSTEM

Eye Examination Steps and Terminology
- Assess for symmetry
- Assess for visual acuity
- Eye chart test (patient must stand 20 feet from chart)
- **OD (oculus dexter)** = right eye
- **OS (oculus sinister)** = left eye
- **OU (oculus uterque)** = both eyes
- **Unequal pupils** = anisocoria
- **Consensual** = when light is shone into one pupil, the opposite pupil reacts
- **Extraocular muscle function** = Is the patient able to follow a finger movement from near the nose outward, to the upper left, lower right, upper right, lower left, middle right, and middle left?
- Are the pupils equal in size, round, irregular, and reactive to light?
- Using an ophthalmoscope, the eye can be examined externally as well as several internal structures
- **External structures:** Conjunctiva, sclera, cornea
- **Internal structures:** Iris, lens, retina

Normal Findings
- **Conjunctiva**: Clear with blood vessels
- **Sclera**: White
- **Cornea**: Clear
- **Iris**: Both the same color
- **Optic nerve**: Disc shaped and yellow in color

Visual Problems
- **Color blindness**: Unable to see colors or distinguish color differences
- **Diplopia**: Double vision, weakness, or damage to cranial nerves III, IV, and VI
- **Exophthalmos**: Abnormal bulging of the eyeballs, usually indicative of hyperthyroidism (Graves' disease)
- **Kayser–Fleisher rings**: Rusty-brown ring around edge of the iris and in the rim of the cornea, indicative of Wilson's disease (too much copper accumulation in body)
- **Myopia**: Nearsighted (inability to see far without corrective lenses)
- **Hyperopia**: Farsighted (inability to see near without corrective lenses)
- **Presbyopia**: Decreased or lack of ability to accommodate near objects (requires reading glasses)
- **Astigmatism**: Irregular curvature of cornea
- **Aphakia**: Absence of lens
- **If the patient wears contact lenses, the eyes may be**: red, sensitive, and painful; the patient may have vision problems
- **Ptosis** is a weakness of the eyelids drooping and may indicate eye trauma, neurovascular problems such as stroke, and myasthenia gravis
- **High cholesterol** may exhibit as a white ring around the outer edge of the cornea or the iris may look discolored
- **Yellowing of sclera** indicates jaundice and is an indicator of liver disease

Eye Trauma
- **Blunt eye trauma**: Occurs when the eye is struck with a blunt object
- **Penetrating eye trauma or foreign body eye trauma**: Occurs when fragments enter the eye. Fragments may be made of glass, wood, or metal
- **Chemical eye trauma**: Occurs when the eye is splashed with a solution of acid or alkaline base
- **Thermal eye trauma or burns**: Occur when the eye comes into contact with a hot item or object. This may occur in welding or the cooking of hot oils
- **Hordeolum**: An infection of the sebaceous gland of the eye; a sty
- **Conjunctivitis**: An infection or inflammation of the conjunctiva of one or both eyes; may be contagious

Potential Eye Problems
- **Bacterial infection** of the eye or eyes may be caused by *Staphylococcus aureus* or strep (pink eye)
- **Allergies** may cause the eyes to redden and become watery. Allergens are dependent on the allergies of the patient. Many patients have seasonal allergies (pollen, molds, etc.)
- **Keratitis** is the inflammation or infection of the cornea
- A **corneal ulcer** may be caused by injury (a scratch when rubbing the eye or inserting/removing a contact lens)
- **Cataract** is the development of opacity of the lens
- **Retinopathy** is the vascular deterioration of the retina
- **Retinal detachment** occurs when the retina separates from its correct anatomical area, resulting in a disruption in blood flow; surgical correction may not be possible

- **Macular degeneration** occurs from a deterioration or breakdown of the macula and is uncorrectable
- **Glaucoma** occurs when intraocular pressure occurs (may cause optic nerve damage) resulting in peripheral vision loss

KEY NOTE:
- Intraocular pressure is regulated within the eye by the aqueous humor
- The patient may need medications or eye surgery to correct eye problems
- The patient may need to have the entire eye removed (enucleation) due to cancer
- The patient has to be assessed for the use of contact lenses when admitted to the hospital

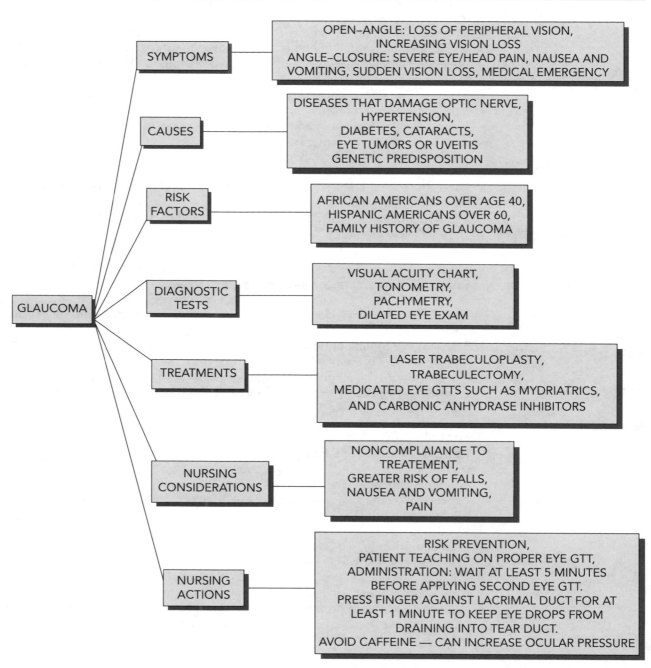

FIGURE 6-1   Example of a concept map.

AUDITORY SYSTEM

The inner ear affects hearing and balance, while the external ear amplifies sound

Ear Examination Steps

First: The patient's ear canal should be inspected to ensure patency.

Second: Gently palpate the external ear to assess for pain.

Third: Using an otoscope, gently lift the auricle upward and back to open the ear canal. Gently insert the otoscope. The otoscope should allow the nurse to visualize the presence of cerumen (earwax). Note the amount and the color of the cerumen. The tympanic membrane should be visualized unless the canal is obstructed by cerumen. The tympanic membrane should be translucent.

Fourth: Hearing acuity should be tested. The nurse should whisper words from a distance of approximately 1 to 2 feet away. Ask the patient to repeat what was whispered.

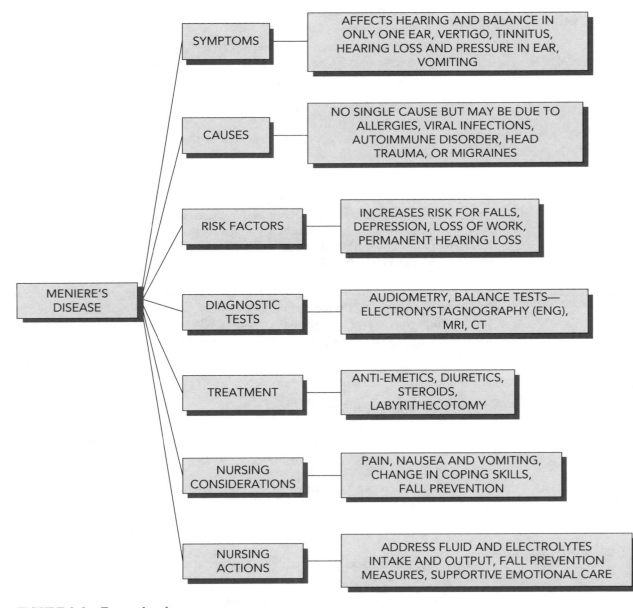

FIGURE 6-2   Example of a concept map.

Auditory System Conditions and Treatments

- **Presbycusis** is the term used to describe the loss of hearing due to the aging process.
- **Tinnitus** is the definition for ringing in the ears. This condition is often caused by excessive aspirin intake.
- **Vertigo** is the term used to describe a spinning sensation.
- **Nystagmus** is a rhythmic motion of the eyes. The etiology of nystagmus may be congenital or late onset. A physician will diagnose the cause. Nystagmus may be associated with labyrinthitis. Labyrinthitis (*itis* = inflammation) causes vertigo.
- **Loud sounds** may cause hearing loss. Using earphones that directly emit loud music into the ears may cause future hearing loss.
- **Medications** (antibiotics, diuretics, chemotherapy drugs, and nonsteroidal anti-inflammatory drugs [NSAIDs]) can be ototoxic and cause hearing loss.
- The temporomandibular joint (TMJ) is affected by **teeth clenching** or **grinding** and may be mistaken for ear pain.
- **Trauma** to the external ear can cause damage to the middle ear resulting in loss of conduction hearing.
- **External otitis** (infection or inflammation) may be caused by the patient inserting objects into the ear canal.
- **Cerumen (earwax)** may block the ear canal, resulting in pain or altered hearing. The physician may suggest an ear irrigation. Cotton-tipped applicators should never be used in the ear canal.
- **Acute otitis media** (blockage of the Eustachian tube) caused by infection (*S. aureus*) is treated with antibiotics. Tympanostomy tube(s) may be placed to decrease pressure and assist with drainage.
- For patients who have had **ear surgery:** The head of the bed should be flat with the surgical ear facing upward. Patient education should include avoiding sudden movements. They should contact their physician if they have worsening pain or become hyperthermic (have the doctor set parameters). Patient must avoid nose blowing (it increases ear pressure). If the patient needs to sneeze or cough, instruct the patient to keep the mouth open to reduce ear pressure. No traveling by airplane.
- **Meniere's disease**, whose etiology is unknown, presents with episodic vertigo. The patient may have hearing loss or tinnitus. It is suggested that endolymphatic hypertension (overproduction of fluid in the inner ear) occurs, resulting in vestibular and cochlear hair cell damage.
- **Acoustic neuroma** is a benign tumor that develops at the junction of the eighth cranial nerve. The tumor usually requires surgical intervention.
- **Benign paroxysmal positional vertigo** (BPPV) is an inner-ear disorder stemming from dislodgement of inner-ear crystals, causing vertigo when the head is repositioned. It is caused by trauma, aging, ear infections, and migraines.

NASAL SYSTEM

Nose Examination Steps

First: Assess the physical appearance of the nose.

Second: Assess the patency of the nares. This can be accomplished by holding one naris closed while asking the patient to breathe in or out. Switch nares and repeat the process.

Next: Using a pen light and a nasal speculum, the nurse inserts the speculum gently. The patient's head should be tilted backward to allow a better visual inspection. The mucus membranes should be moist. The nurse should assess for drainage and note color, amount, and consistency, if present.

Nasal System Conditions and Treatments

Trauma: Trauma to the nose may result in a deviated septum. Trauma may present with edema, epistaxis (nose bleed), or obstruction to one or both nares. If clear liquid is noted in the nares, it should be tested for the presence of glucose. If the clear drainage results in a positive test for glucose, it may indicate a cerebral fluid (CSF) leak.

It should be noted, however, that if the drainage has any blood in it, the glucose test may prove to be a false positive. A nasal fracture may result in raccoon eyes. Raccoon eyes are bilaterally ecchymotic eyes and they are also a sign of skill injury. Rhinoplasty is the surgical repair of the nose. It is not uncommon to have nasal packing (Rhino Rocket packing) inserted into the nasal sinuses to control bleeding. If surgical intervention is necessary, airway management is the primary focus. The nurse should also monitor for pain and signs of infection.

Epistaxis: Epistaxis may occur for many reasons, including trauma, a foreign body, allergies, a tumor, hypertension, or the use of street drugs. Attempt to halt the nose bleed by having the patient sit in the high Fowler's position and lean forward. Compress the soft tissue of both nares for approximately 15 to 20 minutes. If bleeding continues after compression intervention, chemical cauterization or nasal packing may be needed. Nasal packing remains for 48 hours or more. Analgesics should be administered because nasal packing may cause discomfort. Patient teaching should focus on refraining from nose blowing, heavy lifting, or any activity that may increase pressure. If chemical cauterization or nasal packing are unsuccessful, or the patient's condition is not a candidate for these procedures, then the physician may need to insert inflatable catheters (Rhino Rockets) to halt the bleeding. The inflated catheters are positioned against the bleeding source and then inflated to apply pressure. A guide string is taped to the face to prevent dislodgement. Gauze is taped to cover the upper lip and a portion of the nose as a drip pad. The nurse should monitor the skin of the naris that houses the nasal packing. The pressure from the Rhino Rocket may cause decreased perfusion, resulting in necrosis. If this condition presents, the nurse should notify the doctor immediately.

Allergies: Allergies usually present with rhinitis. Rhinitis results in sneezing, watery nasal discharge, watery eyes, and nasal congestion. Causes may be pollen, animal dander, dust, and mold. The patient may complain of a sore throat, hoarseness, cough, headache, or nasal congestion. Patient care is based on interventions to reduce inflammation and symptoms.

Pharyngitis: Pharyngitis is inflammation of the pharynx. The usual complaint is pain or a scratchy throat. The patient may complain of difficulty in swallowing. Pharyngitis caused by a strep infection can cause rheumatic heart disease if not treated with antibiotics. An abscess can develop as a complication of pharyngitis. If an abscess develops, the patient may require a tonsillectomy or an incision and drainage (I&D) of the abscess.

Sleep apnea: Obstructive sleep apnea (OSA) presents when respirations cease for a duration of approximately 20 seconds. When a patient sleeps in the supine position, the tongue or the soft palate relaxes and falls back, resulting in a complete or partial obstruction of the pharynx. This occurrence can result in periods of hypoxemia. It is often reported that the patient has excessively loud snoring. The patient frequently wakes throughout the night, resulting in daytime fatigue. The patient may complain of impaired concentration and loss of memory. A sleep study can reveal the presence of sleep apnea. Treatment includes weight loss for the obese patient, refraining from sedatives or alcohol prior to sleep, or, if necessary, the use of a continuous positive airway pressure (CPAP) device. CPAP is a device that forces oxygen through a mask to maintain an open airway. If the patient's sleep apnea does not improve, a surgical procedure (uvulopalatopharyngoplasty) to remove excessive tissue (that blocks the pharynx) may be necessary.

Tracheostomy

Tracheostomy is a surgical procedure to establish an airway. A stoma is placed in the trachea. This surgical procedure may be performed for several reasons, including long-term ventilation therapy or because of a disease process or injury resulting in an upper airway obstruction. The tracheostomy tube, commonly called a Shiley or

Bivona, has different sizes. The Bivona tracheostomy tube is used for patients with obese necks (Pickwickian syndrome), cervical stenosis, and kyphosis. The nurse is required to have the same size or a smaller size tube (of the same brand) available at the bedside in case of dislodgement or accidental removal.

The tracheostomy is held in place by a balloon that is called a "cuff," which is attached to the end of the tracheostomy tube. When this balloon is inflated, it seals against the trachea, stops the airflow from the mouth, and prevents the patient from talking. The respiratory department will measure the pressure in this cuff because too much pressure will cause tracheal necrosis and possible rupture of the balloon. Underinflation will cause decreased tidal volumes and will allow the patient to talk. Humidification oxygenation needs to be given since the upper airway is bypassed.

There are flaps or a flange attached to the tracheostomy tube that are usually sutured to the skin until the stoma (opening) is established. An obturator is a teardrop-shaped plastic guide that is provided with the tracheostomy set and should be saved to use in case of accidental displacement. "Trach" care requires cleaning around the stoma with sterile normal saline using aseptic technique. The trach ties are adjusted until they are snug but the nurse is still able to fit one to two fingers between the tie and neck. If a Passy-Muir valve is used, the cuff must be deflated before using.

WEEK 3 POSTCONFERENCE

Discuss with the students how they incorporated their learning of sensory deficits into their patient care during this session. Inform students that their weekly journal will be collected next week during preconference and then every week thereafter. Students should be informed that if their journals are submitted electronically their instructor will acknowledge completion of the assignment during preconference. Explain that the journals will be returned to the students during postconference. The required medication handouts, concept map, care plan, and assessment form will be collected during preconference.

Ask for input from the students. Is anyone having difficulty understanding the connection of the disease diagnosis to the additional problems incurred from that chosen problem? Do the students understand how their assessment findings assist them in planning patient care or nursing interventions?

Do the students understand the significance of the medications and how they relate to food, laboratory tests, and patient education?

Inquire whether the students are having difficulty in the theoretical course. Often students are overwhelmed by the amount of assigned homework. Open up the discussion to allow students to voice whether they are having trouble with their assignments. These concerns can be addressed in postconference. The clinical course can be redesigned to allow the students time during postconference to research and discuss the medication assignments during clinical hours.

Chapter 7

UNDERSTANDING, ASSESSING, AND TREATING PAIN

This chapter examines:

- How patients experience pain
- Impact of culture, genetics, and disease on pain
- Summary of medications and treatments for pain

UNDERSTANDING PAIN

Week 4 introduces the study of pain. Pain is a very difficult concept to teach because each person has his or her own way of experiencing and displaying pain. Some patients may be stoic and not exhibit the signs of pain. Patients who are experiencing pain but are intubated or aphasic are unable to express their feelings freely. Various pain scales have been developed to assist nurses in their efforts to accurately assess the patient's pain level. Pain cannot be solely assessed with pain scales; they are used in conjunction with the assessment.

WEEK 4 PRECONFERENCE

Hand out:
- Pain assessment guide
- Pain interview exercise
- Pain research exercise
- Critical thinking cases
- Medication forms (Tylenol and Reglan)

Collect:
- Medication forms (warfarin and Synthroid)
- Concept map
- Care plan
- Physical assessment form
- Weekly journal

Discuss with the students how they assess pain in their assigned patients. Do they use a standardized pain scale? Did the students ask their patients how they handle pain outside of the health care facility? Does the patient have a chronic condition that causes pain? What alternative measures (if any) has the patient used?

Explain to the students that the nursing assessment should always include a pain assessment that explores both pain scales and interventions to manage their pain. Students should ask their patients how they deal with pain (both currently and in the past). Were alternative measures used? What was effective? What is the patient's acceptable pain level?

HOW PAIN IS EXPERIENCED

Many definitions have been given to define pain. Nursing students may often respond, "Pain is what the patient says it is." However, pain can be physiological or psychological in origin.

Pain is the reason that most people seek medical care. Acute pain usually has a sudden onset. Examples of sudden pain include a myocardial infarction (MI) or a cerebrovascular accident (CVA). It is important to understand that chronic pain can be as devastating as acute pain. It is not only a physical complaint but also an emotional one. Some patients must deal with lifelong pain. It can interfere with activities of daily living (ADL), work, and sexual relationships.

Studies indicate that better pain recognition and management are needed. New pain scales (behavioral scales) are available for patients who cannot verbally acknowledge that they may be experiencing pain. An intubated patient and a stroke patient with aphasia are examples of this type of patient. Behavioral pain scales have also been developed for infants and children. Note that in behavioral pain scales the number does not correlate with the verbal rating and should be used in conjuction with an assessment.

Unrelieved pain causes significant changes in the body. Cortisol levels increase due to the increased stress of pain. The heart rate and blood pressure also elevate for the same reason. The patient's immunity decreases, placing the patient at a higher risk for infections. The patient may not eat or take in enough calories, resulting in a decrease in the electrolyte balance. Reduced oral intake due to pain may result in decreased fluid consumption that in turn produces a reduction in urinary output. Lack of sleep due to continuous pain results in a decrease in cognition. Pain has the additional effect of limiting the patient's mobility.

PAIN MECHANISMS

Nociception: The process in which the message of injury is conveyed to the central nervous system (CNS). This process involves transduction, transmission, perception, and modulation.

Transduction: The stimuli (cause of injury) convert to signals. Peripheral nerve endings signal the cause of injury, which results in a release of chemicals that transport the pain signal to the spinal cord.

Transmission: The pain signal travels from the site of injury via peripheral nerve fibers through the dorsal horns of the spinal cord to the thalamus and cerebral cortex.

Dermatomes: Areas of skin innervated by a single spinal cord fiber segment.

Perception: The recognition or realization of pain or injury that results in a response, for example, touching a hot pan handle.

Modulation: A response to painful stimuli, for example, removing one's hand from a hot pan handle.

PAIN CLASSIFICATIONS

Nociceptive: From site of injury to dorsal horns in spinal cord to thalamus and cerebral cortex.

- **Somatic pain:** Achy pain from muscles, bone, and skin
- **Visceral pain:** Pain from organs (e.g., gallbladder or pancreas)
- **Neuropathic pain:** Abnormal pain input. (e.g., phantom pain, reflex sympathetic dystrophy (RSD), or diabetic neuropathy)
- **Acute pain** has sudden onset with known cause. Pain is usually controlled, and the duration of pain is short and usually subsides when the healing is completed
- **Chronic pain** may be characterized as sudden or gradual onset. Chronic pain is pain that persists beyond normal healing. The etiology of the chronic pain may or may not be known. Pain control is attempted but the pain may not cease. Alternative methods to assist in pain control or changing the perception of pain are now being implemented (e.g., massage therapy, aromatherapy, meditation, and herbal therapy as well as traditional methods). Anxiety, fatigue, and depression can increase the perception of pain, but positive attitudes and support from caregivers may reduce the perception of pain.

PAIN ASSESSMENT GUIDE

Pain is currently labeled as a vital sign, along with blood pressure, heart rate, respiratory rate, temperature, and pulse oximetry.

Assessment begins by gathering the following data:

- **Onset:** When did the pain first occur?
- **Location:** Where is the pain? Is it localized, or does it travel (referred pain)? Is it accompanied by other symptoms, such as headache, nausea, and immobility?
- **Characteristic(s):** Toothache-like, stabbing, burning, achy, and so on

PAIN SCALES

- **Number scale:** Usually addresses pain with "0" meaning no pain and "10" meaning severe pain. Each factor is assigned a specific number. The numbers are tallied and compared to a number scale reflective of mild, moderate, or severe pain. Although the total of the pain scale is often associated with a number, it is not the same as a self-report.
- **Facial scale:** Scale begins with a smiling face meaning no pain and ends with a crying face meaning severe pain.
- **Behavioral scale:** This scale contains multiple factors to consider in determining whether the patient has pain. As mentioned earlier, this scale is used for patients who may be intubated or aphasic. The multiple factors include the following: Is the heart rate elevated? Is the blood pressure elevated? Is the respiratory rate elevated? (This may not be true in the patient with chronic pain because the patient has adapted to the pain.) Does the patient moan? Is the patient guarding a body part? Is the patient restless?

INFLUENCES OF CULTURE, GENETICS, AND DISEASE ON PAIN

Pain is not a normal process of aging and it usually indicates a pathological process. Pain assessment/management for the elderly may be complicated because the elderly may be reluctant or cognitively unable to report pain.

Treatment is complicated by the associated pathophysiology of other diseases. For example, individuals with diabetes mellitus will have decreased pain perception due to neuropathy.

In Asian and Native American cultures, patients may prefer to use alternative pain therapies such as herbs, thermal therapies, acupuncture, massage, and meditation. The African American and Hispanic cultures may use prayer as an important factor in pain management.

PAIN TREATMENTS

Medications are often prescribed for pain management. Pain medication may be narcotic or nonnarcotic (e.g., analgesics such as nonsteroidal anti-inflammatory drugs [NSAIDs]). NSAIDs have been linked to gastric bleeding as well as increased risk for MIs and CVAs.

Opioid narcotics may cause respiratory depression. Opioids also cause the slowing of gastric motility, resulting in constipation. Some opioids will lower the seizure threshold, thereby increasing the risks of seizures.

Pain medications may be given via different routes. These include the oral, sublingual, buccal, nasal, rectal, transdermal, intramuscular, intravenous, and spinal routes. If the pain medication is delivered in a patch, the medication patch must be changed as per the institution's policy. Medication patches must be dated and timed when applied. Pain medication patches may take up to 38 hours to absorb, so intermittent (breakthrough) pain medication should be available. Narcotic patches should be disposed of according to hospital policy—usually in the needle disposal box—and witnessed by another nurse. Do not dispose of these medications in the regular trash.

Caution must be applied because of the similarity of drug names, their potency, and the risk for respiratory depression.

Patient-controlled analgesia (PCA) and patient-controlled epidural analgesia (PCEA) are commonly used post-operatively in a hospital setting as well as in trauma patients. The patient controls administration of a premeasured drug. In addition, a basal or continuous rate of opioids can also be administered if ordered by the physician.

Pain medication can have an adverse effect:

- **Tolerance:** The body appears to become less sensitive to the pain medication, resulting in the need for a higher dose to achieve the same comfort level.
- **Dependence:** The body will exhibit signs or symptoms of withdrawal when the drug is halted abruptly. Symptoms may include anxiety, tremors, or diaphoresis.
- **Addiction:** The patient desires to seek narcotics for a purpose other than pain management.

Other conjunctive treatment for pain can include trigger-point injections of anesthetics and steroids into muscles, an intrathecal pain medication pump into the spinal column, and spinal cord stimulators that block pain impulses from traveling to the brain.

> **KEY NOTE:** Pain control is still a necessity for patients who currently abuse drugs or have a history of drug abuse. The underlying key is management of medications to control pain. It is helpful to consult a pain specialist nurse who will evaluate and implement a combination of medications to help manage the patient's pain. Often the combination of a nonnarcotic with a narcotic can achieve greater pain control than one pain medication used alone. A mild sedative administered at the same time as the ordered narcotic can assist in creating a more effective pain-management regime.

ALTERNATIVE THERAPIES

Patients who experience pain may benefit from an alternative therapy such as acupuncture, massage, hypnosis, relaxation, and use of a transcutaneous electrical nerve stimulation (TENS) unit.

- **Acupuncture** is the treatment modality in which a licensed acupuncturist inserts thin needles into the body at designated locations. Patients often seek acupuncturists to alleviate pain. Known as *chi*, this traditional Chinese therapy is used to balance the positive flow of energy. However, acupuncture is thought to stimulate the body to improve pain management and circulation. With a licensed acupuncturist, acupuncture therapy offers minimal risk unless the patient is on a blood thinner or becomes infected due to reusable needles.
- **Massage therapy** is another alternative treatment for pain management. Massage therapy has been shown to benefit the patient by decreasing muscle tension and stress, thereby reducing pain. Massage therapy can also aid the patient with muscular strains. In addition, patients with anxiety may benefit from massage therapy because the warm oils and soothing kneading of the muscles aid in relaxation. Patients should be aware that massage therapy should be used together with, and not in place of, traditional medication interventions.
- **Hypnosis therapy** allows the patient to enter a restful state with increased focus on a designated health problem. A therapist may use images or verbal cues to assist the patient to become relaxed and enter into the hypnotic state. It should be noted, however, not every patient is able to achieve a hypnotic state, often making therapy ineffective. Hypnosis has been used to assist patients to cope with fears, anxiety, and stress, as well as to assist patients making behavioral changes (e.g., smoking cessation). Hypnosis has also been used for treatment of phobias and weight loss.
- **Relaxation therapy** is a technique used to assist the patient in reducing anxiety and tension. Visual imagery encourages the patient to envision a peaceful place. While envisioning the peaceful place, the patient should attempt to relax and eliminate any stress, anxiety, or pain. Meditation is similar to visual imagery because it encourages the patient to focus on breathing or softly verbalizing a particular word or sound (a mantra).

- **A TENS device** is a small device that produces an electrical current to suppress pain signals. Although there is controversy over whether or not the TENS unit will help in pain control, studies have shown that results are individualized. The TENS unit may aid in pain control by directing the focus of the patient to the stimulation of the electrical impulse.

PAIN INTERVIEW EXERCISE

Interview two people (age 62 or older) and enter their answers to the following questions:

Have you ever experienced pain?_____

What was the underlying cause of the pain?_____

What did you do for the pain?_____

Can you describe the pain?_____

_____

_____

_____

_____

Have you attempted alternative therapies? If so, what type?

_____

_____

_____

Did the alternative therapies work? _____

Did you take any medications for the pain? If so, what did you take?

_____

_____

_____

Did you seek medical care for the pain?_____

PAIN RESEARCH EXERCISE

Research evidence-based articles online for the three various types of pain scales. Articles can be reviewed at the National Institutes of Health website or the Online Journal of Issues in Nursing website. Write a short summary for each. List two types of patients or conditions that would be appropriate for each of the various pain scales.

The antidote for an opiate overdose is naloxone (Narcan). An antidote competes for the receptor site, thus preventing the narcotic from binding to the receptor site, resulting in a complete blockage of the narcotic effect. Because Narcan is an opioid antagonist, this drug should be given in smaller doses to prevent severe opioid withdrawal symptoms, such as seizures, pulmonary edema, and severe agitation.

> **KEY NOTE:** Narcotics affect the CNS. Nonnarcotic analgesics affect the peripheral nervous system by reducing the production of a hormone-like substance (prostaglandin). Prostaglandin influences peripheral pain signals

Medication Form

Listed in the vertical box is a medication. For each of the remaining boxes, list the following:

Box 1: List a laboratory result you would need to monitor. Explain the significance of the laboratory test to the medication.

Box 2: List one food that may interact with the medication. Explain the significance of the food item to the medication.

Box 3: List one patient educational instruction you would give to the patient regarding the medication. Explain the significance of the instruction to the medication.

List other educational information you could provide this patient. Are there websites you can refer to? What about travel overseas and health issues? How should the medication be stored?

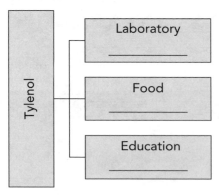

Listed in the vertical box is a medication. For each of the remaining boxes, list the following:

Box 1: List a laboratory result you would need to monitor. Explain the significance of the laboratory test to the medication.

Box 2: List one food that may interact with the medication. Explain the significance of the food item to the medication.

Box 3: List one patient educational instruction you would give to the patient regarding the medication. Explain the significance of the instruction to the medication.

List other educational information you could provide this patient. Are there websites you can refer? What about travel overseas and health issues? How should the medication be stored?

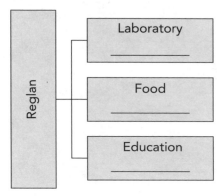

LIST OF PAIN MEDICATIONS

(Not All-Inclusive)	
acetaminophen	ketorolac
aspirin	methadone
buprenorphine	morphine
capsaicin	naproxen
carbamazepine	oxycodone
Celebrex	oxymorphone
codeine	pentazocine
diclofenac	Percocet
etodolac	Percodan
fentanyl	Stadol
hydromorphone	tramadol
ibuprofen	

CRITICAL THINKING CASES

CASE #1

A 52-year-old male of Middle Eastern descent is admitted with diffuse abdominal pain, nausea, vomiting, and abdominal distention over the past 3 to 4 days. Pain has been increasing in intensity over the past days. A computed axial tomography (CAT) scan shows a ruptured sigmoid volvulus with distended bowel loops. Emergency surgery, as well as diagnostic lab tests, were scheduled. Abdominal surgery consisted of a sigmoid resection with primary anastomosis and Hartmann's procedure. Post-operatively, the patient received a PCEA (administration pump for use when returning back to the floor). The medication in the PCEA machine is fentanyl 7,500 mcg/300 mL bag (25 mcg/mL) with bupivacaine 1.25 mg/L double checked by both nurses. The PCEA settings are fentanyl 12.5 mcg demand, lockout 10 minutes, basal 25 mcg/hr, clinician bolus of 25 mcg every 30 minutes not to exceed 0.2 mg/hr. The nurse notices that the epidural tubing has a yellow strip in the tubing. The nurse inspects the patient's back and the PCEA tubing and dressing are intact. The nurse will fill out the PCEA sheet that follows, which is checked by two nurses.

Thirty minutes after the initial assessment, the nurse is evaluating the patient, and the patient complains of feeling less pain relief than earlier. When the nurse checks the

Date/Time PCEA Initiated
1. Delivery rate: _____ml/hr
2. Bolus dose: _____ml
3. Lockout interval: _____minutes
4. Maximum 1-hour limit: _____ml
5. Loading dose: _____ml

PCEA PUMP SETTINGS							PATIENT ASSESSMENT						
Date/ Time	Delivery rate	Bolus dose	Delay	1-hour limit	Number of injections demanded/ delivered	Volume infused	Pain	Sedation	BP	P	RR	Side effect	Initial

pump, she finds that the patient has pushed the button 36 times within a half-hour period.

Answer the following questions and return by preconference next week.

1. Where is the epidural catheter placed?
2. Why is bupivacaine added to the epidural?
3. What are the advantages of PCEA?
4. What are the disadvantages of PCEA?
5. What conditions does the nurse need to evaluate on a continuous basis?
6. The patient received two clinician boluses in the past 4 hours in addition to the original settings. How much fentanyl has the patient received during the first hour?
7. Fill in the PCEA sheet.
8. What causes may prevent the patient from receiving relief from the PCEA administration?
9. What is a volvulus?

ANSWERS TO CASE #1

1. The epidural catheter is inserted into the epidural space between the spinal column and the dura. The epidural catheter is placed and the medication will innervate a particular part of the skin called a dermatome (a part of the skin that derives from a nerve root), which will provide post-op pain relief to that site.

2. Bupivacaine acts as a local anesthetic.

3. PCEA provides improved pain relief over other methods and can improve the patient's outcome. It is frequently used post-operatively for post-op pain, for procedural pain, and for cancer, trauma, and labor pain.

4. PCEA may cause nausea, vomiting, pruritus (itching), hypotension, numbness, hematoma, bleeding, infection, headache, and/or motor weakness as well as paralysis.

5. The nurse needs to monitor the back dressing for hematomas and the line for patency as well as test muscle strength, monitor dermatomes for sensation, and monitor for paresthesia.

6. The PCEA settings are fentanyl 12.5 mcg demand, lockout 10 minutes, basal 25 mcg/hr, clinician bolus of 25 mcg every 30 minutes not to exceed 0.2 mg/hr.
    Two clinician boluses were 25 mcg × 2 = 50 mcg.
    Basal rate of 25 mcg/hr × 1 hour = 25 mcg.
    There are six times (10 minutes lockout) × 1 hour that the patient has pushed within the first hour, which is 6 × 12.5 mcg = 75 mcg.
    Total amount of fentanyl received in first hour is 50 mcg + 25 mcg + 75 mcg = 150 mcg.

7. Filled-in PCEA sheet.

Date/Time PCEA Initiated
1. Delivery rate: ____1____ml/hr
2. Bolus dose: ____1____ml
3. Lockout interval: _____10___minutes
4. Maximum 1-hour limit: ____9____ml
5. Loading dose: ___0____ml

PCEA PUMP SETTINGS							PATIENT ASSESSMENT						
Date/ Time	Delivery rate	Bolus dose	Delay	1-hour limit	Number of injections demanded/ delivered	Volume infused	Pain	Sedation	BP	P	RR	Side effect	Initial
1/12 1300	1	2	10	9	12/9	9	10	1	130/72	110	12	0	mm
1/12 1700	1	0	10	9	36/9	18	18	1	124/76	100	16	0	mm

8. The patient has pushed the button on the PCEA machine more than the allotted dose of six programmed doses in the machine. The patient has pushed the button 36 times and this is recorded in the machine. The nurse needs to investigate why this has occurred. The reasons could be:
   - The PCEA pump is malfunctioning.
   - The nurse is confused over the concentration of the drug (mcg versus mL) and has programmed the pump incorrectly.
   - The demand dose is confused with the basal rate.
   - Wrong lockout on pump.
   - Wrong medication.
   - The patient needs reeducation on the pump.

9. A volvulus is twisting of the large or small intestines that can cause decreased blood flow and ischemia.

CASE #2

The nurse assumes care of a 38-year-old Caucasian female with a history of fibromyalgia who is normally on MS Contin 20 mg orally three times a day at home. The nurse is told in report that the patient, who is admitted for the management of her pain, complains of 10/10 pain in her joints, but is frequently laughing and talking while she is requesting this pain medicine. The nurse giving report feels that the patient is a "drug seeker" and that she really does not have the pain she is reporting. Her lab work and vital signs are all within normal limits, and the patient is currently receiving Vicodin one tablet every 4 hours as needed for pain. She is married and has two children, ages 8 and 10, and is currently on disability because of her diagnosis.
   Answer the following questions and return by preconference next week.

1. What is fibromyalgia?
2. Why would the patient be talking and laughing if she is in so much pain?
3. What kind of changes will occur with chronic pain?
4. What is pain?
5. What are the immediate and long-term goals for this patient?
6. What are the patient's priorities?
7. What other factors might be influencing this patient's pain?

ANSWERS TO CASE #2

1. Fibromyalgia is a chronic, widespread, painful disease that affects the muscles and joints. The symptoms will range from mild to severe weakness, fatigue, insomnia, and muscle trigger points. The cause is unknown. Associated cognitive disorders and psychological issues such as posttraumatic stress disorder are usually present.

2. Chronic pain causes changes to the autonomic nervous system and loss of brain mass. Patients with chronic pain may have adjusted to their condition, so their sympathetic nervous system may have adjusted its response when dealing with pain. This will make the patient appear less stoic to the pain response—the "fight or flight" response usually associated with the sympathetic nervous system.

3. Chronic pain will worsen other physical conditions. There are changes to the fascia, decreasing blood flow to the muscles. Damage may occur to the neurological pathways. There may be increased sensitivity to pain, emotional changes (such as anxiety disorders and depression), and cognitive deficits.

4. Pain is what the patient's perception of pain is. Pain is experienced differently by each person. Pain is usually undertreated.

5. The immediate goals are first to deal with the patient's pain and then to encourage her to seek other modalities for pain relief such as acupuncture, exercise, healthful eating, NSAIDs, use of a TENS unit, family therapy, and caregiver support. Long-term goals include addressing the issues of sleep deprivation, appetite loss, and depression.

6. There may be loss of appetite, lack of sleep, and depression. The patient may be experiencing strained relationships. Psychosomatic issues may cause a patient's pain. There was a change in the type of medication and administration, and it may not be effective in relieving the patient's pain.

7. Emotional responses may intensify the pain. There may be feelings of hopelessness. There may be a cognitive impairment present because of changes caused by chronic pain. Some patients may underrate their pain because of a fear of being labeled as a "drug addict." The nurse's or doctor's perception of the patient's pain may not lead to effectiveness of care. There may be persistent biases concerning tolerance, addiction, and dependency.

WEEK 4 POSTCONFERENCE

Return weekly journals to the students if submitted as hard copy. Students should be informed that if their journals are submitted electronically their instructor will acknowledge completion of the assignment during preconference. Inquire whether the students were able to assess for pain on their assigned patients. Did the students have difficulty determining what pain scale to use?

Instruct the students that when completing the medication exercises, they should include whether the medication may interfere with other medications. It is important to teach the students that they are responsible to ensure that there are no drug incompatibilities when administering medications.

Inform students that Week 7 will also include a mid-term evaluation. Attendance, clinical participation, and assignments will be calculated to determine the student's midterm grade.

Chapter 8

UNDERSTANDING CANCER, CANCER TREATMENTS, AND DEATH AND DYING

This chapter examines:

- Etiology of cancer
- Growth and reproduction phases of normal and malignant cells
- Cancer technology
- Chemotherapy
- Complications, death, and dying

The growth characteristics, causes, risk factors, diagnosis, and treatment of cancer are examined in the first half of this chapter (Week 5). Treatment methods, including surgery, radiotherapy, and chemotherapy and its side effects, are presented and analyzed in the text and case studies. In a separate discussion, the topic of death and dying is explored in detail with a focus on nursing understanding and support for the patient and family, the stages of coming to grips with dying, criteria for establishing brain death, and postmortem care.

Cancer is often thought of as a single disease process. In actuality, cancer is a group of diseases. This week's topics include cancer, cancer treatments, and how cancer develops. Cancer affects different populations and its incidence increases with age. Chemotherapy is coordinated by cell cycles. Chemotherapy medications are designed to attack cancer cells in their various stages of development.

Students should be encouraged to review normal cell growth and the reproduction of both healthy and malignant cells. The student will begin to learn that disease processes often result in the death of a patient. Students should recognize that recovery from a disease is not always possible and that death does not reflect failure on the part of the nurse or the health care team.

WEEK 5 PRECONFERENCE

Hand out:
- Cancer screening brochure exercise
- Cancer cell exercise
- Medication forms (Neupogen and iron)
- Religion exercise
- Cancer care cases
- Death and dying cases

Collect:

- Weekly journals
- Medication forms (Tylenol and Reglan)
- Concept maps
- Care plans
- Physical assessment form
- Pain interview exercise
- Pain research exercise
- Critical thinking cases

Inform students that the main project for this week is creation of a cancer screening brochure. Many computers have programs that allow for brochure development. The students may need to learn how to format (bifold or trifold) and print the brochures (two-sided printing). In addition, there is a research exercise that examines how different religions approach providing care for dying patients and their families.

UNDERSTANDING CANCER

CANCER TERMINOLOGY

Alopecia: Loss of hair

Anemia: Hemoglobin level that is lower than gender norms; below the critical level may be life threatening

Angiogenesis: Ability of cancer cells to secrete substances that stimulate blood vessel growth

Aplastic anemia: Bone marrow does not produce red blood cells (RBCs)

Benign: Not malignant

Biopsy: The removal of cells or tissues for examination under a microscope

Carcinogenic: Cancer causing

Carcinoma: Cancerous tumor (epithelial cells)

Cyst: A fluid-filled sac

Cystitis: Inflammation of the bladder

Dissemination: To spread throughout

Dysphagia: Trouble swallowing

Dysplasia: Various sizes and shapes of cells

Effusion: Fluid leaking from vascular tissue into body cavity or intrapleural space.

Endogenous: Originates from within

Epidemiology: Study of both the distribution of disease and what diseases and health problems are in specified populations

Epistaxis: Nose bleed

Extravasation: Leakage of medication from the vein into the tissue

Gleason Score: Scoring of different stages of prostate cancer

Hyperplasia: Increase in the number of normal cells

Isotope: Radioactive element used in diagnostic procedures and cancer treatments

Jaundice: Yellow skin (may be secondary to hepatic failure)

Leukopenia: Reduced number of leukocytes

Malaise: Generalized feeling of being unwell

Metaplasia: Exchange or replacement of normal cells with a different cell type

Metastasis: Spreading of cancer cells and invasion of other tissues

Nadir: The lowest point of the change to the bone marrow (platelets and white blood cells [WBCs]) that occurs after chemotherapy. Lab work must be constantly monitored since this condition can predispose the patient to infection and bleeding.

NED: No evidence of disease

Neoplasm: Mass of new tissue growth

Oncology: The study of cancer

Petechiae: Mini hemorrhages characterized by small red dots on skin or mucous membranes

Radon seed: A small capsule containing radon that is placed near a cancer lesion (used as a cancer treatment)

Stomatitis: Inflammation of the oral cavity

Septicemia: Systemic infection

TNM: Classification of malignant tumors ("T" for size of tumor, "N" for involvement of lymph nodes, and "M" for metastasis)

Tumor specific antigens: Antigens expressed by the cell surfaces (e.g., PSA is an antigen specific to the prostate)

Vascular access devices (VAD): Central venous devices such as the mediport, Groshong, triple lumen catheter, and peripheral intravascular central catheter (PICC) that are used for administration of vesicant drugs

CELL GROWTH PHASES

G1 phase: RNA and protein synthesis occurs

S phase: DNA synthesis occurs

G2 phase: Mitotic spindle forms; mitosis cell division occurs

G0 phase: Resting phase (cells are dormant)

Differentiation: Maturing of normal cells

Proliferation: Increase in number of new cells; to reproduce

CHARACTERISTICS OF CANCER CELLS

- Cancer is characterized by the uncontrolled growth and spread of abnormal cells.
- Cancer cells are undifferentiated and can return to a previous state.
- Metastasis begins with the development of a tumor (angiogenesis). The tumor requires its own blood supply. As the tumor grows, it produces like cells, which continue to grow abnormally.
- Invasive-like qualities occur in the abnormal cells, resulting in changes in the surrounding tissue. The abnormal cells infiltrate, gaining access into the lymphatic system. These metastases occur in the liver, lung, bone, and brain.
- Abnormal cells may be labeled as lesions, neoplasms, tumors, or cancer.

KEY NOTE: Cancer cells cannot survive without oxygen and nutrients.

CANCER CELL PHASES

There are three distinct cancer cell phases: the initiation phase (DNA changes), the promotion phase (repeated exposure to cancer-causing stimuli), and the progression phase (increase in malignant cell growth). These are discussed in more detail as follows:

- **Phase 1 (initiation phase):** Cancer-causing stimuli cause changes in cellular DNA.
- **Phase 2 (promotion phase):** Exposure to stimuli (which may lay dormant for years) with suppressor genes regulating or preventing cell proliferation. As people age, suppressor genes lose their capability to suppress, and cancer cells then reproduce.
- **Phase 3 (progression phase):** Cancer becomes evident. A cancer tumor must be 1 cm in size to be palpable. A tumor the size of 1 cm contains approximately 1 billion cells.

Cancer cell membrane proteins such as carcinoembryonic antigen (CEA) and alpha-fetoprotein (AFP) can be detected in a serum blood test. These laboratory blood tests are marker tests. The CEA is ordered by the physician after cancer is suspected.

Prevention and early detection are the best interventions relating to cancer. Reducing the risk of cancer is the primary intervention. Examples of primary prevention include reducing exposure to carcinogens such as the sun; smoking cessation; reducing consumption of red meats; and increasing fiber intake while reducing fat intake. Secondary prevention reflects the detection of cancer. Tertiary prevention reflects the care and rehabilitation of cancer.

Risk factors for cancer include the following:

- Heredity
- Stress
- Age
- Gender
- Diet
- Occupation
- Tobacco use
- Obesity
- Sun exposure
- Economic status
- Virus infections hepatitis B and C, HPV

Signs of cancer can include:

- A change in bowel habits
- A sore that fails to heal
- Unusual bleeding
- Thickening of skin or lump in breast
- Difficulty in swallowing
- Change in wart or mole
- Hoarseness or nagging cough

IDENTIFYING CANCER

Various cytologic examinations are used to identify cancer:

- **Exfoliation:** scraping sample (e.g., cervix)
- **Aspiration:** fluid or blood (e.g., bronchial washing)
- **Needle biopsy** (e.g., tumor)
- **Incisional biopsy** (e.g., breast)
- **Excisional biopsy** (e.g., lumpectomy)

KEY NOTE: Radiological examinations provide for the earliest detection.

Various imaging technologies and other tests can also be used to detect cancer. These include x-rays, computed tomography (CT) scans, magnetic resonance imaging (MRI), ultrasonography, radioisotope scanning, angiography, bone marrow aspiration, and tagging of antibodies.

KEY NOTE: A biopsy is the most definitive way to diagnose cancer.

X-ray imaging is a screening tool that is the least expensive method for detecting cancer. Examples include mammograms (breast) and chest x-rays (lung).
CT scan test results provide visualization of the anatomy in cross sections and produce greater accuracy.
MRI is similar to a CT scan, but more expensive. MRI is considered the test of choice for screening cranial and neck tumors. Because of the dangers related to MRI's magnetic qualities, an MRI screening tool must be completed first, before the patient is scanned. Because of the MRI's powerful magnetic field, the patient must be screened to ensure he or she has no metals within the body (metallic implants [intentional or unintentional] such as aneurysm coiling or shrapnel fragments, metal slivers in the patient who is employed as a metal worker, clips, pins, screws, or piercings) because the MRI can heat the metal or draw the metal from the inserted area resulting in pain, injury, or death. The patient should be screened for claustrophobia because of the confining design of the MRI device.

Ultrasonography is useful for imaging prostate and breast cancers.

Radioisotope scanning is used in conjunction with radioactive isotopes. Isotopes target specific cells, rendering those cells more visible.

Angiography is a costly and tedious procedure. Dye is injected into the vascular system near the tumor, and the tumor is visualized under fluoroscopy. Blockage of the dye within the vascular system confirms the location of the tumor. The dye may cause allergic reactions and renal failure.

Tagged antibodies is a procedure that uses radioactive isotopes with specific antibodies that target cancer cells. A nuclear scan can then detect a concentration of the radioisotopes and thereby locate the cancer.

Bone marrow examination is the aspiration of bone marrow (usually from the iliac crest) to evaluate the process of hematopoiesis (development of RBCs).

Tumor markers are molecules in the body that are used to diagnose the presence of a malignancy within the body. Tumor markers may be present in the serum and body fluids. Examples are PSA (detects prostate cancer) or CEA (detects whether the tumor was completely resected). The BRAC gene mutation will identify a risk for breast or ovarian cancer. Bence-Jones protein in the urine confirms multiple myeloma.

Tumors can be benign or malignant. Benign tumors are noninvasive. Malignant tumors are atypical cells that may invade neighboring tissue or organs and spread to different areas of the body. The ability to invade or metastasize is the main characteristic of a malignant, tumor and it is often used to distinguish a malignant tumor from a benign tumor. *In situ* is the term used to describe a preinvasive carcinoma. If discovered and left untreated, the carcinoma will continue to grow and become malignant. The correct terms for the degree of severity indicate the degree of differentiation, as follows:

G1: Slight abnormality
G2: Moderate abnormality
G3: High abnormality (poor differentiation)
G4: High abnormality (difficult to determine area of origin); very poor differentiation

Tumor staging reflects the tumor's growth in size and the progression of the disease process:

T: Size of primary tumor
N: Lymph node involvement
M: Positive or negative for metastasis

TYPES OF CANCERS

Sarcomas: Tissue origin: connective (bone, cartilage, muscle, and fat)
Lymphomas: Tissue origin: lymph node
Carcinoma: Originates in the epithelial layer, which forms the linings of the organs and passageways.
Leukemia: Tissue origin: bone marrow
Multiple myeloma: Tissue origin: bone marrow. It causes osteolytic lesions that weaken the bone, causing pain and increasing the risk of fracture; also causes hypercalcemia; and has vague symptoms.

CANCER TREATMENT

Cancer treatment includes surgical intervention, radiation therapy, chemotherapy, and immunotherapy. Adjunctive therapy is a combination of the different treatment modalities.

Surgical intervention: May be used to resect a tumor or may be used as a diagnostic tool (to diagnose and stage the cancer). Surgical intervention may be curative or palliative. Palliative surgical intervention may be performed to reduce the size of the tumor in order to decrease pain or symptoms of distress. Supportive care may be incorporated into the plan of care at any time. For example, a Keofeed can be inserted to provide nutrition for the patient who cannot eat because of painful mouth ulcers from chemotherapy.

Radiation therapy: There are two types (internal and external):

- **External radiation** is used to treat local cancer growths. Normal cells can recover from radiation therapy. However, cancer cells cannot recover once DNA damage has occurred.
- **Internal radiation (brachytherapy)** is the insertion or implantation of radioactive seeds/material directly into the tumor. Implantation may be temporary or permanent.

KEY NOTE: It is important for the caregiver or nurse to recognize that the patient is radioactive. The nurse must recognize that **time**, **distance**, and **shielding** principles must be used when giving care to the patient with radioactive implants:

- Time spent near the patient should be limited when giving care. Plan care appropriately to minimize exposure to staff.
- Distance should be the greatest possible distance from the patient. The patient should be in a private room.
- Shielding should be used (lead gloves and apron). Monitor for radiation exposure using a film badge (such as those worn by radiology technicians).

Chemotherapy is the term used to describe the use of antineoplastic agents. There are various classes of chemotherapeutic agents:

- **Cell-cycle agents:** Affect cells during reproductive synthesis; effects may not be limited to cancer cells; side effects often include bone marrow depression, thrombocytopenia, and anemia
- **Alkaloids:** Prevent mitosis
- **Alkylating agents:** Inhibit reproduction of cells
- **Antimetabolites:** Replace cancer cell proteins, resulting in cancer cell death
- **Hormonal agents:** Block production of normal hormones in tumors

Chemotherapy can be administered via oral, intramuscular, subcutaneous, intrathecal, or intravascular (IV) routes. A mediport is often inserted to administer IV chemotherapy. Extravasation can occur in peripheral IV sites, resulting in necrosis of tissue and muscles. A central vascular device is required to prevent potential irritations.

When administering chemotherapy, the required personal protective equipment (PPE) would consist of chemo safety gowns and chemo safety gloves. Absorbent pads are required when preparing chemotherapy to prevent leakage. Chemotherapy is eliminated from the body through urine, stool, and emesis; therefore, PPE must be worn to protect the health care worker. The toilet must be flushed twice after patient use. The nurse must maintain PPE safety procedures for up to 48 hours after the chemotherapy regime is completed.

SIDE EFFECTS OF CHEMOTHERAPY

There are several side effects of chemotherapy:

- **Alopecia**: Hair loss
- **Oral complications**: Painful ulcers in the mouth (stomatitis)
- **Thrombocytopenia**: Decreased platelets (chemotherapy may be withheld if the count is less than 100,000); decreased platelets increase the risk of bleeding
- **Genetic defects in first trimester**: Fetal malformations, or may not be evident for years
- **Pain**

- **Fatigue, bleeding**, hematopoietic symptoms (leukopenia, thrombocytopenia, and anemia)
- **Infection**: Prevent with proper hand washing
- **Imbalanced nutrition**: Monitor weight, intake and output, and albumin blood level (normal level 3.5–5)

Listed below are oncology emergencies:

1. **Infection (sepsis)**
2. **Spinal cord compression:** Cancer causes reduction of blood supply to spinal cord and nerves
   Treatment: Laminectomy
3. **SIADH** (syndrome of inappropriate antidiuretic hormone): Too much antidiuretic hormone, causing dilution of the plasma; symptoms include hyponatremia, elevated urine sodium, decreased serum osmolarity, increased water retention, irritability, and headache; sodium less than 120 is an emergency because low sodium creates cerebral edema
   Treatment: Restrict fluids, 3% NSS hypertonic
4. **Hypercalcemia** (normal level 9–10.5)
   Symptoms: Polyuria, nausea/vomiting (N/V), and muscle weakness; late signs include diminished deep tendon reflexes, EKG changes, and paralytic ileus
   Treatment: Calcitonin and glucosteroids
5. **Disseminated intravascular coagulation (DIC):** Caused by gram-negative sepsis; causes extensive blood clots that consume all clotting factors and platelets
   Diagnosis: PT, PTT prolonged; fibrinogen decreased, low platelets, increased fibrin split products
   Treatment: Heparin, antibiotics
6. **Superior vena cava (SVC) syndrome:** Obstructs internal or external SVC; reduces blood flow/cardiac output to heart
   Signs/symptoms: facial edema, dyspnea, and JVD
   Diagnosis: CT scan, x-rays
   Treatment: Airway management, diuretics
7. **Cardiac tamponade:** Fluid accumulates in pericardial sac (more than 15–50 mL)
   Signs/symptoms: Tachycardia, narrowing of pulse pressure, pulsus paradoxus, and muffled heart sounds
   Treatment: Pericardial window
8. **Tumor lysis syndrome:** Destruction of large amount of cells releases intracellular potassium, phosphorus, and uric acid into metabolism
   Treatment: Aggressive IV hydration; monitor weight, intake and output, EKG, and hypotension (low BP)

KEY NOTE: If the WBC result is less than 2,000/mL, the patient is at great risk for infection. Notify the physician. The patient's therapy may need to be modified. If the patient's platelets result is less than 20,000/mL, monitor closely for bleeding. Notify the physician. The physician may order an irradiated platelet transfusion.

ADDITIONAL TREATMENTS

- **Bone marrow transplant:** Patient receives donor bone marrow.
- **Total parenteral nutrition (hyperalimentation):** Cancer patients often present with loss of appetite and fatigue. Physicians may order parental caloric intake. Patients with a peripherally inserted central line (PICC), a central venous catheter (CVC),

or a mediport can have total parenteral nutrition (hyperalimentation). Patients with standard peripheral intravenous catheters can have peripheral parenteral nutrition (PPN).

TPN	PPN
Glucose: 0% to 50%	Glucose: 0% to 10%
Amino acids: 0% to 15%	Amino acids: 0% to 5 %
Multivitamin, electrolytes, and trace elements as determined by physician (based on laboratory results)	Multivitamin, electrolytes, and trace elements as determined by physician (based on laboratory results)
Lipids: 0% to 20 %	Lipids: 0% to 20 %

Hyperalimentation adds calories and the lipids add fat grams needed to support nutritional need. The hyperalimentation consists of IV amino acids (protein), 50% dextrose (carbohydrate), electrolytes, and vitamins and trace elements (and may contain lipids). Two medications, insulin and heparin, may also be added to hyperalimentation. The TPN order is based on the patient's lab work, intake and output, BUN, creatinine and liver function test (LFT) levels, weight, and nutritional demands. TPN needs to be administered through a "dedicated" central line (i.e., nothing else should be given through that IV line), and a micron filter must be used. Because of the high glucose in the TPN, the patient's blood sugar should be checked every 6 hours.

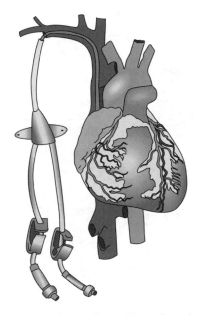

This central venous catheter allows TPN to be infused directly into a large vein. Note the catheter enters into the subclavian vein and ends before entering the right atria.

A PICC line can also be inserted in the brachial area and end before entering the right atria. Both catheters allow for TPN infusion.

FIGURE 8-1   Example of a central venous catheter.

There are two types of TPN infusions: *continuous* (infuses continuously for 24 hours) and *cycling* (shorter times and will gradually be decreased). When a new bag of TPN is to be administered, the solution and additives must be checked by two nurses to ensure that the order and the solution match. If the TPN completes before the next TPN bag is available, a bag of D10W should be initiated to infuse at the same rate to prevent onset of hypoglycemia. If an infusion of TPN runs behind in administration, do not speed up the rate "to catch up."

TPN infusion complications include:

1. Catheter-related sepsis
2. Metabolic complications (prerenal azotemia, gallbladder, and hepatic dysfunction)
3. Mechanical complications (pneumothorax, air embolism, and dysrhythmias)
4. Hyperlipidemia due to lipid infusion
5. Volume overload
6. Malnourished patients, such as anorexia nervosa patients, need hyperalimentation started gradually, due to their starvation state, to prevent a hypermetabolic state

CANCER SCREENING BROCHURE EXERCISE GUIDELINES

Each student should develop a brochure to teach patients about cancer screening. The brochure size should be 8½" by 11", printed on both sides. The brochure can be set up with either a bifold or a trifold format to allow more information to be included. Include the importance of wellness check-ups. Include signs and symptoms to monitor for. Add pictures to aid in the brochure's effect. You may use a nonexistent facility as your health care system's, for example free Skin-Cancer Screening at the Royal Epidermis Clinic. The brochure is due by the next clinical preconference.

CANCER CELL EXERCISE

Label the various phases of cancer cell growth. Return by preconference next week.

Factors that can cause target cells to become abnormal.

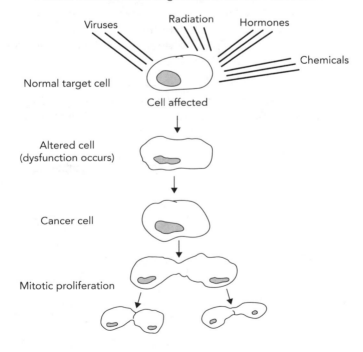

ANSWERS TO CANCER CELL EXERCISE

These factors can cause a target cell to become abnormal.

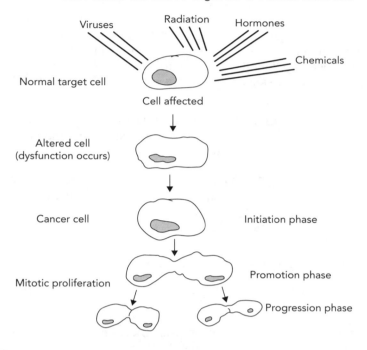

Medication Forms

Listed in the vertical box is a medication. For each of the remaining boxes, list the following:

Box 1: List a laboratory result you would need to monitor. Explain the significance of the laboratory test to the medication.
Box 2: List one food that may interact with the medication. Explain the significance of the food item to the medication.
Box 3: List one patient educational instruction you would give to the patient regarding the medication. Explain the significance of the instruction to the medication.

List other educational information you could provide this patient. Are there websites you can refer to? What about travel overseas and health issues? How should the medication be stored?

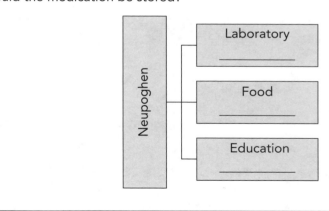

Listed in the vertical box is a medication. For each of the remaining boxes, list the following:

Box 1: List a laboratory result you would need to monitor. Explain the significance of the laboratory test to the medication.
Box 2: List one food that may interact with the medication. Explain the significance of the food item to the medication.
Box 3: List one patient educational instruction you would give to the patient regarding the medication. Explain the significance of the instruction to the medication.

List other educational information you could provide this patient. Are there websites you can refer to? What about travel overseas and health issues? How should the medication be stored?

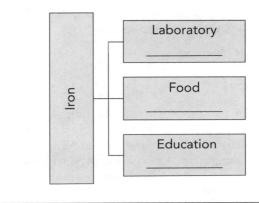

CANCER CARE CASES

Students should read the two case scenarios and answer the questions that follow them. Return by preconference next week.

CASE #1

A 72-year-old Caucasian female is admitted with oat cell carcinoma status postchemotherapy. She is complaining of extreme fatigue and weakness. She has had a decreased appetite and has not eaten for two days. Her lab work consists of WBC 2.3, Hgb 7.8, Hct 21.2, platelets 86,000, sodium 123, potassium 3.6, chloride 101, carbon dioxide 24, calcium 7, and albumin 1.2.

1. What is oat cell carcinoma?
2. What considerations would the nurse evaluate to indicate when a patient needs a blood transfusion?
3. What is the normal platelet count, and what will influence the platelet count?
4. What precautions would you use with a low white count?
5. What antidiuretic abnormalities may occur with oat cell carcinoma?
6. Why does the patient have a low albumin level?

ANSWERS TO CASE #1

1. Oat cell carcinoma is a highly malignant cancer in the lungs that is treated with chemotherapy and radiation.

2. The nurse needs to ask these questions:

   • Is the patient symptomatic? For example, does the patient have a low blood pressure? Does the patient have tachycardia? Does the patient have cool or clammy skin? What is the trend in the hematocrit?

- Is there any evidence of bleeding?
- Is the patient scheduled for any procedure or surgery that is going to cause blood loss?
- Is a blood transfusion going to complicate the prognosis (i.e., might it increase the risk of reoccurrence of cancer)?

3. Normal platelet count is 150,000 to 300,000. Platelet counts are influenced by bleeding, chemotherapy, radiation, and medications such as Plavix, aspirin, or Pepcid.

4. Reverse isolation, which requires protecting the patient from others; no fruits or fresh flowers.

5. The sodium is low and may be indicative of syndrome of inappropriate diuretic hormone (water intoxication). Cancer cells will manufacture and secrete ADH, which will result in extreme dilution of sodium. Low sodium will then cause changes in the neurological system that can lead to seizures and coma. (Remember "too many letters, too much ADH.")

6. Albumin is an indicator of the overall health of the patient and is needed for growth and repair. The patient has not eaten for several days

CASE #2

A 45-year-old female is admitted with extreme fatigue and chest pain. The patient has a past medical history of ovarian cancer in both ovaries with metastasis to the uterus. The patient is being treated with Taxol and Cisplatin, given IV every 3 weeks through a mediport. On assessment the nurse notes numerous ecchymotic and petechiae sites. The patient states that she frequently "bumps" into things. Her skin is cool, she has delayed capillary refill of 4 seconds, RR 24 with O_2 saturation of 91%, BP of 88/60. She is ordered a 250 mL bolus. Her coagulation studies are within normal limits. The patient is ordered 2 units of PRBC and a random unit of platelets. The following lab work is listed:

Sodium 152 mEq/L	WBC 2,000
Potassium 4.8 mEq/L	Hgb 7 g/dL
BUN 30 mg/dL	Hct 21.6
Creatinine 1.5 mg/dL	Platelets 9,000 mm$_3$

1. What is a bolus?
2. What considerations need to be addressed before a blood transfusion?
3. What is ecchymosis and what are petechiae?
4. What does the BUN/Cr ratio mean?
5. Why can a low WBC be dangerous to a patient?
6. What is a random unit of platelets?
7. Why are the sodium and potassium elevated?
8. What is a mediport?

ANSWERS TO CASE #2

1. A bolus is a rapid infusion of isotonic fluids to increase intravascular volume, and is given in this circumstance for hypotension. The patient is anemic and is symptomatic because of low blood pressure and narrowing pulse pressure. It will take time, at least 1 to 2 hours, to crossmatch and the patient is presently symptomatic.

2. The type of IV access needs to be evaluated. There needs to be a large-bore IV to give blood products, preferably an 18 or 20 gauge IV. The patient's cardiac

and respiratory status needs to be addressed, as well as the blood consent, doctor's order, and vital signs. The patient's respiratory status must be assessed for the risk of fluid overload. Because chemotherapy can frequently cause cardiomyopathy, the student should evaluate for any cardiac stress related to a blood transfusion.

3. Ecchymosis is purplish discoloration of the skin caused by ruptured blood vessels. When observing ecchymosis, it is wise to circle the area and to measure the diameter of the extremity to see whether the bleeding increases its size. Petechiae are small, reddish-brown flat spots that appear in the skin or mucous membrane. These skin alterations are due to low platelets and the trauma from the patient bumping into items.

4. BUN is a waste product. Creatinine evaluates the amount of nephron injury. A BUN/Cr ratio will detect conditions that are affecting the kidneys. A normal BUN/Cr ratio is 15 to 1, but when there is decreased blood flow, such as when a patient is in shock, the ratio will increase to 20 to 1. When there is an intrinsic disease such as glomerulonephritis, there will be BUN/Cr ratio of 10:1. This patient's BUN/Cr is 30/1.5, which reflects kidney injury.

5. A lowered WBC can make the patient more susceptible to infection. Neupogen might be ordered to increase the WBC.

6. A random unit of platelets is a collection of up to 6 to 8 units of different donor specimens with the same ABO grouping collected into one bag for transfusion. The survival rate for platelets may last for 3 days, but it may be dependent on the disease process. The physician may order leukocyte-reduced platelets to avoid a transfusion reaction.

7. The sodium and potassium are elevated due to dehydration and hypovolemia.

8. A mediport is a central line catheter implanted under the skin. It is accessed by the nurse using sterile technique and is punctured through the skin with a Huber needle that looks like a fish hook. The mediport is used both for infusion and blood draws.

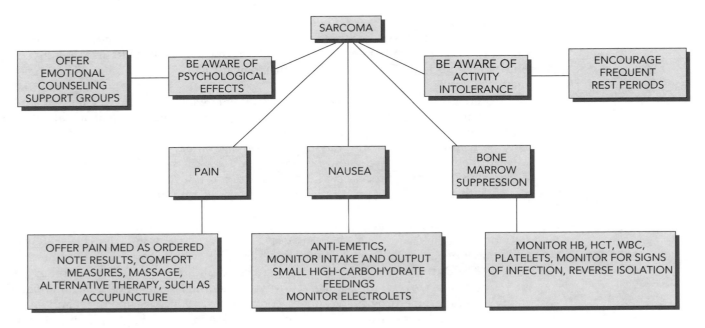

FIGURE 8-2 Example of cancer concept map.

DEATH AND DYING

Death is rarely in the forefront of our minds. Death is usually thought about when a disease process or accident occurs. The thought of death often produces fear in the individual.

Comfort care guidelines direct the nurse on ways to care for the patient who may be dying. Treating symptoms, providing emotional support, and giving bereavement care allow the patient to die in comfort and with dignity. Physiological death occurs when the heart stops or the brain function ceases.

The dying patient has many facets that the nurse must envision holistically. The patient may be experiencing fear related to the impending death. Aspects of the patient's culture may differ from those of the nurse's. The attitude of the patient and patient's family toward death may also differ from that of the nurse.

Often the patient (when coherent) and the patient's family may view death as a passage into the next phase of life. Others, however, may believe that death is the final stage of life. The nurse must discretely gather data from the patient, family, and friends to discern ways to offer the appropriate physiological, emotional, cultural, and spiritual support.

The place or location of death may vary. Some patients prefer to die at home, while others feel comforted by having health care providers nearby. The nurse can maintain activities of daily living (ADL) for the patient, offer emotional support for the patient and the patient's family, and provide pharmaceutical intervention (pain or antinausea medication), as needed.

It is important to allow the patient to verbalize fears and feelings. The weakened patient who is unable to provide self-care may experience many emotions including fear of losing any sense of control, becoming a burden, or humiliation due to incontinence or lack of strength.

Patient and family religious beliefs vary greatly. The health care staff is encouraged to provide support, which generally is appreciated by the patient and the patient's family. Nurses are encouraged to ask the patient and the family what the caregivers can do, provide, or allow in order to support them. This support may include allowing the family to sing hymns at the bedside, bathe the patient, provide clergy, anoint the patient, say prayers, bring in a favorite pet, and so on. Each patient will have his or her own unique needs.

Patients with a known disease process may be well aware of their impending death. In contrast, family members may arrive at the hospital only to find their loved one dying. Sudden onset or sudden death can be difficult for the family to accept, no matter what the underlying cause may be.

There is little doubt that death is accompanied by many emotions. Family members may have regrets or may have difficulty accepting the impending or actual death of their loved one. If the death was caused by a modifiable behavior, family members may be feeling guilty for not having attempted to intervene. There may be anger toward the patient for dying and leaving them. How each family member or friend experiences the dying process is as individualized as it is unique.

Death and the dying process cannot be discussed without mentioning the stages of dying.

When a terminal diagnosis is delivered, the patient may not accept the news. Patients in denial refuse to believe the test results, or they rationalize that a mistake must have been made. Denial can be experienced by the family as well as by the patient. The duration of the denial stage may be an undetermined length of time.

The next stage of dying is anger. However, it should be noted here that, although many experience the progressive stages of dying in sequence, each patient and family may vary in their journey through this process. Anger may reflect an underlying belief of injustice. "I've been a good person; it's not fair!" The patient may lash out. Family and friends may have difficulty supporting the patient during this time because the patient's anger may be inappropriately directed at them.

In the next stage, the patient begins to bargain. The patient is working past the anger stage and attempting to bargain with their deity for a cure or for more time. The bargaining stage may be personalized and it may or may not be seen by family members. The patient may bargain in private or when alone.

The next stage of dying is depression. The patient arrives at the realization of impending death. The patient begins to mourn the ramifications of his or her own passing. They will be unable to provide for their family, will not see the children or grandchildren graduate, and so on. The patient may become silent and withdrawn. The patient may also become frequently fearful of the dying process or of what may happen to him or her after death.

The final stage is acceptance. The patient accepts the inevitable. The patient may voice that he or she is at peace and no longer fears the end. These stages may be experienced by both the patient and the family. However, the process is individualized. The stages may be experienced in either a progressive or random fashion. Certain stages may be revisited or omitted completely. The concept of the stages of dying serves only as a guide to addressing the emotional needs of the patient and the family.

Nurses must offer themselves to the patient and the family by listening to their needs, hearing their fears, and offering emotional support. The nurse may sit in silence nearby or may offer comfort measures such as holding the patient's hand or reading religious material to the patient.

Inquire about clergy. Would the patient and the family like his or her pastor, priest, rabbi, or other spiritual advisor to offer prayers? Listen to the needs of the patient.

As the patient continues the dying process, physiological changes continue. The patient's appetite may become poor, or the patient's cognition may decrease. The nurse should anticipate the patient's needs (mouth care, perineal care, and repositioning) and provide the necessary comforts.

Always remember that the patient should be able to die with dignity. The patient has the right to choose how he or she dies. An advance directive, living will, or MOLST (medical orders for life-sustaining treatment) will direct the health care staff. It is the patient's choice whether full life-support measures should be provided or whether the patient should be allowed to die without extraordinary measures such as resuscitative medications or intubation.

There are procedures that can be used to determine when a patient's condition has deteriorated and brain death has occurred. Many of the brain's functions are controlled by the brainstem. Brain cells do not regenerate; any type of lack of oxygen or metabolic processes can destroy the brain cells. Brain death is determined by clinical criteria that provide physiological proof that the brainstem is no longer able to maintain its function. The patient must not be hypothermic or have a paralyzing disease, and must be screened for medications that might cause a coma (such as barbiturates). The body may continue with regular vital signs, and the patient may just appear to be sleeping. Brain death is a legal finding and must be adequately determined before life-sustaining equipment can be discontinued.

To determine brain death, there are certain criteria that must be met, including coma with cerebral unresponsiveness, apnea, absence of brainstem reflexes (no cough, gag, or corneal reflex).

Apnea is a clinical bedside test determined by the absence of spontaneous respiration in the presence of an adequate CO_2 determined by the patient's arterial blood gases (ABGs).

Absent brainstem reflexes will be determined by pupils that will not react to light and will remain "fixed" or dilated. There should not be any spontaneous eye movements. The patient will be tested by rapid rotation of head from side to side (oculocephalic response). Normally, with an intact brainstem the eyes will look away from the rotation ("doll's eyes"). The corneal reflex will be tested by touching the cornea lightly with cotton. This procedure will normally stimulate a blinking reflex.

A gag reflex is assessed by attempting to elicit a gag by touching the back of the tongue or throat. A caloric test (vestibular stimulation) involves injection of cold or warm fluid into the ears; if there is brain damage, the eyes will not respond to this simulation. A cerebral angiography will also be absent at the circle of Willis.

When death is imminent, medical organizations mandate that the state's organ donation organization should be notified by the nurse. If the patient is considered to be an appropriate organ donor, then the organization will talk to the family about possible organ donation before or after death.

After the patient dies, offer the family time with the patient. The ending of life and the finality of death may bring forth an array of emotions. Provide tissues and privacy to the family and friends. Do assure the family that the health care staff is readily available if needed. Keep in mind, each health care facility has specific paperwork that the next of kin must sign. Be diplomatic and present the paperwork when the time is appropriate (prior to the family leaving).

The nurse provides postmortem care. Maintaining the body is important because rigor mortis (stiffness) occurs several hours after death. Newly graduated nurses may fear providing postmortem care. Support should be given by seasoned nurses or the clinical instructor to ensure the development of professional growth.

> **KEY NOTE:** Some religions do not allow the body to be placed in the morgue. Usually the family will notify the nursing staff of this fact, but it is wise to inquire whether there are any special requests to ensure that the patient's wishes are carried out.

DEATH AND DYING CASES

CASE #1

A 27-year-old male has suffered a gunshot wound to the right temporal region of the head due to a drug deal incident 48 hours ago. The patient is listed as "nondisclosure" because the perpetrator has not been arrested. A CT scan of the head shows fragmentation of the bullet and shows an intracranial epidural hemorrhage with midline shift of ventricles and diffuse edema of right cerebral hemisphere. The patient presents with a BP of 88/60, HR 130, O_2 saturation 98% on PRVC AC 16, TV 500, PEEP 5, and FIO 2% of 50%. Pupils are 6 mm, and coma scale is 3. There are absent brainstem reflexes. A brain flow study is negative, and the patient has been declared brain dead and is being followed by the organ donation service.

Answer the following questions and return by preconference next week.

1. What does it mean when a patient is listed as "nondisclosure"?
2. How would nurses defend themselves and this patient from harm?
3. What are the normal brainstem reflexes?
4. What determinants need to be established before a patient is declared brain dead?
5. What is a brain flow study?
6. What factors are considered when assessing this patient?

ANSWERS TO CASE #1

1. Nondisclosure of a patient means that no information on the condition or location of the patient is disclosed. If this information has been compromised, then the patient may need to be moved to a different location and security notified.
2. Nurses must be aware at all times of their surroundings and who is around the patient. All individuals must have proper identification, even if a person may be wearing a medical uniform. There is usually an emergency button that can be pushed that will result in an immediate security presence.

3. Normal brainstem reflexes are the ability of the pupils to react and accommodate. There will be a corneal, or blink, reflex. There is a cough and gag reflex when stimulated. The patient would be able to breathe on his own efforts.

4. There must be absent brainstem reflexes, apnea, and a persistent unresponsive coma that is irreversible.

5. A brain flow study is used to demonstrate cerebral brain flow. A negative study indicates that there is no cerebral blood flow.

6. Level of consciousness (LOC); the type of cerebral involvement and damage that has occurred; vital signs, especially blood pressure; what the trajectory of the bullet was; and whether there is other organ involvement. If the patient is a donor, then optimal perfusion of the organs will need to be maintained.

CASE #2

An 87-year-old male has suffered a middle cerebral infarct. The patient is maxed out on vasopressors and is deteriorating regarding his blood pressure and heart rate. He has been exhibiting decerebrate movements. He has already been intubated for 7 days. He is a "DNR," but everything else can be initiated. Hospice is being consulted for a terminal wean. BP now is 80/60, and an idioventricular rhythm of 40 is now present.

Answer the following questions and return by preconference next week.

1. What is the significance of a middle cerebral infarct?
2. What does it mean to be "maxed" out on vasopressors?
3. What factors are addressed in a DNR LT order?
4. What is a terminal wean?
5. What is an idioventricular rhythm?
6. What are decerebrate movements?

ANSWERS TO CASE #2

1. The middle cerebral artery is one of the major arteries that supply the brain, so injury to this area can significantly reduce perfusion to the brain, causing increased intracranial pressure and ischemia.

2. Vasopressors are medications that help raise the blood pressure and cardiac contractility. There is a maximum limit for each drug that can be given. Frequently this occurs when interventions are no longer effective in reversing the condition.

3. DNR LT means "do not resuscitate limited therapy." The factors addressed in a DNR LT order, when there is an acute condition that may cause the patient's death, are the interventions the patient or the patient's family that they want or do not want, such as intubation, vasopressors, cardiac compressions, blood transfusions, tube feedings, and so on. Because this is a legally binding agreement that must be complied with, the nurse must be aware of what is allowed and what is not allowed.

4. A terminal wean means that the patient's status is terminal and has specified the patient has no chance to survive. The terminal wean may consist of weaning the patient from the ventilator, that initiating a morphine drip, administering benzodiazepines for anxiety and pain, and keeping the patient comfortable.

5. An idioventricular rhythm, commonly referred to as a dying heart rhythm, will cause severely decreased perfusion. An idioventricular rhythm requires immediate intervention if the patient's condition is viable. It is characterized by a widened QRS and an absent P wave.

6. Decerebrate movements are abnormal posturing of the body characterized by extension of the extremities. This indicates brainstem damage.

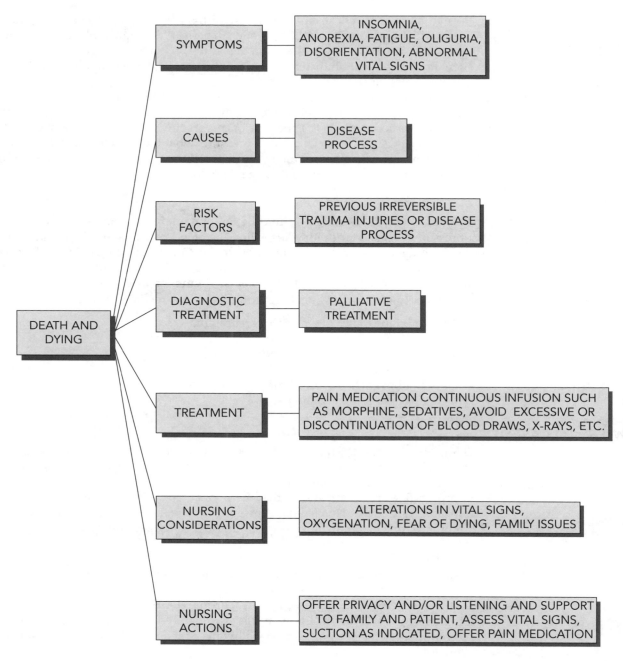

FIGURE 8-3 Example of a concept map.

RELIGION EXERCISE

Research two different religions or life philosophies, such as Judaism, Christianity, Islam, Buddhism, Bahaism, Santeria, Mormonism, Shintoism, atheism, and so on. Answer the following questions for both of your choices based on your findings.

1. List cultural and religious practices offered prior to death.

_____

_____

_____

2. Do these practices assist in supporting the patient and family through the stages of dying? Explain.

_____

_____

_____

3. List the types of postmortem care that the religion supports.

_____

_____

_____

4. List how the religion's beliefs determine the finality of how the body is managed. For example, the role of the funeral home, and burial or cremation.

_____

_____

_____

WEEK 5 POSTCONFERENCE

Return weekly journals to the students.

Discuss with students whether they have had any personal experience with cancer or with death and dying. Ask the students whether they understand why knowing about the stages of death and dying is important for nurses. Explain how recognizing the stage that the patient may be in will assist the nurse to provide appropriate support.

Instruct the students to choose the format for their cancer screening brochure. It can be a bifold or trifold. Each side should be filled with information. The brochure may be in black and white or in color. The choice is up to the student. Students will offer input on the brochures of their fellow students during the Week 6 postconference.

Inquire whether the students have any special religious interventions for a dying patient within their own religion. Inquire whether the students fear caring for a dying patient. Students must learn that dealing with death is integral to caring for patients and their families. Students should attempt to overcome any fears.

Be sure to ask students whether they have any questions that they wish to address.

Conclude the postconference by informing students that they must learn to be objective when it comes to death and dying. Many religions have various practices that may not seem appropriate; however, the practices are based on specific religious beliefs and need to be respected.

Chapter 9

FLUIDS AND ELECTROLYTES AND THE ACID–BASE BALANCE

This chapter examines:

- Fluids and electrolytes
- Nursing interventions for the many conditions related to these systems

Week 6 discusses fluids and electrolytes. Fluids and electrolytes create processes that maintain homeostasis. Understanding fluids and electrolytes will help the student to recognize nursing interventions or potential responses to certain diseases and processes.

The Week 6 discussion also attempts to explain briefly how fluids and electrolytes, acid–base balances, and the organs involved help maintain homeostasis. Students should be encouraged to learn how to determine abnormal arterial blood gas (ABG) and serum electrolyte results.

WEEK 6 PRECONFERENCE

Hand out:
- Medication forms (Aldactone and Lasix)
- Fluid and electrolyte cases
- Laboratory quiz

Collect:
- Medication forms (Neupogen and iron)
- Cancer screening exercise
- Cancer cell exercise
- Death and dying cases
- Physical assessment form
- Journals

Inform students that they will be required to assess and provide a summary of their patient that includes the fluid and electrolyte balance, as well as any changes, or abnormalities. Their summary should also include what interventions would be appropriate in order to ensure stabilization if in fact there is an abnormality. The summary should include a brief medical history and diagnosis, the student's name and date, and it will be collected during the Week 7 preconference.

Medication Forms

Listed in the vertical box is a medication. For each of the remaining boxes, list the following:

Box 1: List a laboratory result you would need to monitor. Explain the significance of the laboratory test to the medication.
Box 2: List one food that may interact with the medication. Explain the significance of the food item to the medication.
Box 3: List one patient educational instruction you would give to the patient regarding the medication. Explain the significance of the instruction to the medication.

List other educational information you could provide this patient. Are there websites you can refer to? What about travel overseas and health issues? How should the medication be stored?

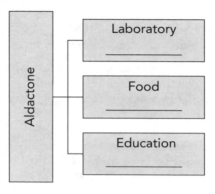

Listed in the vertical box is a medication. For each of the remaining boxes, list the following:

Box 1: List a laboratory result you would need to monitor. Explain the significance of the laboratory test to the medication.
Box 2: List one food that may interact with the medication. Explain the significance of the food item to the medication.
Box 3: List one patient educational instruction you would give to the patient regarding the medication. Explain the significance of the instruction to the medication.

List other educational information you could provide this patient. Are there websites you can refer to? What about travel overseas and health issues? How should the medication be stored?

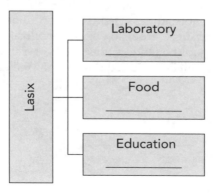

FLUIDS AND ELECTROLYTES

Homeostasis is achieved when the body attempts to maintain an internal balance. Homeostasis requires a stable pH environment of 7.35 to 7.45. When the pH deviates beyond this range, the body responds to maintain stability. The following information will explain how the body attempts to maintain homeostasis.

The body has three major fluid components: the intracellular fluid (ICF), the interstitial fluid (ISF), and the intravascular fluid (IVF).

ICF (within the cell): Contains the necessary nutrients and electrolytes (potassium = K, magnesium = Mg, phosphate = Ph, and chloride = Cl) required to provide cell maintenance and remove wastes

Extracellular fluid (ECF) (ISF [around the cell]) and **IVF** (within the blood vessels): Contain electrolytes (sodium = Na, calcium = Ca, and chloride = Cl)

Normal Electrolyte Values (Serum)

- Sodium: 135 to 145
- Potassium: 3.5 to 4.5
- Chloride: 98 to 108
- Carbon dioxide (CO_2): 22 to 34
- Magnesium: 1.5 to 2.0
- Calcium: 8.5 to 10.5
- Serum osmolarity: 280 to 300 mOsm/kg

MECHANISMS AFFECTING FLUID AND ELECTROLYTE BALANCE

Osmosis: Movement of water or body fluid across a semipermeable membrane; water goes where sodium goes

Diffusion: Movement (passive) of ions from an area of greater concentration to an area of lesser concentration

Osmotic pressure: The amount of pressure required to halt the flow of water across a membrane

Colloid (albumin) pressure, also known as **oncotic pressure:** Pressure exerted in the blood vessels to pull water into the vasculature to maintain a blood pressure

Osmolarity: The number of particles in a solution

Specific gravity: The weight of particles in a solution

Hydrostatic pressure: Provided by the force exerted by the heart

ORGANS OF HOMEOSTASIS

Listed below are the organs that are involved in homeostasis in which the body regulates its internal processes in order to function properly.

Kidneys: Primary organs in maintaining homeostasis; control fluid volume and electrolyte reabsorption and excretion.

Lungs: Regulate CO_2 to maintain acid–base balance.

Adrenal glands: Secrete aldosterone that influences absorption or excretion of fluids and electrolytes (sodium and potassium).

Pituitary gland: Secretes antidiuretic hormone (ADH) to direct reabsorption of fluids.

Parathyroid gland: Maintains balance of serum calcium.

To maintain homeostasis, the body must balance fluids and nutrients while removing waste. The endocrine system secretes hormones to regulate the metabolic function of the body.

The plasma fluid portion of blood includes water, protein, clotting factors, and electrolytes. Serum is the fluid remaining after a blood specimen clots: plasma minus fibrinogen or clotting factors.

There are components surrounding the body's cells that carry nutrients, eliminate waste, and maintain homeostasis. These factors are listed below.

ISF: fluid that surrounds cells (lymph included)

Transcellular fluid (TCF): cerebrospinal fluid, pericardial fluid, pleural fluid, synovial fluid, intraocular fluid, sweat, and digestive fluid. (Note: Body water, or fluid, decreases with age.)

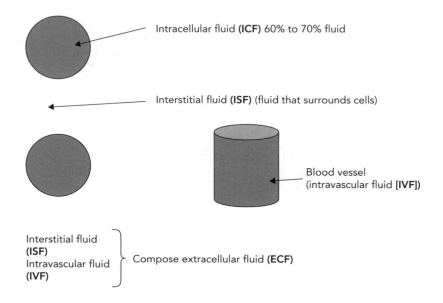

Cations: Ions with positive charge (they give up an electron)

Anions: Ions with a negative charge (they gain an electron)

Univalent ions = balance. For example, the sodium ion (Na+) will join with the chloride ion (Cl⁻).

Diffusion: Factors that influence diffusion are elevated temperature, increased number of particles, and decreased size or weight of particles. An example of diffusion is:

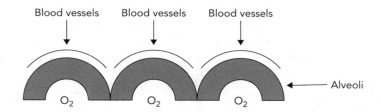

Oxygen moves from an area of higher concentration (within the alveoli) to an area of lower concentration (within the blood vessels). CO_2 moves from an area of higher concentration (within the blood vessels) to an area of lower concentration (within the alveoli).

Facilitated diffusion needs a carrier. Glucose and amino acids require a carrier (protein) to carry them into the cell.

Active transport is the process of moving molecules against a concentration difference with the use of energy. Most electrolytes move by this method. The active transport carrier substance is adenosine triphosphate (ATP).

Renal tubules save sodium and glucose by active transport. When blood sugar is ≥ 200 mg/dL, glucose spills into the urine. The glomeruli reabsorb glucose but have difficulty when glucose levels become too elevated.

Fluids and solutes are filtered within the body and move from an area of high fluid concentration to an area of low fluid concentration by hydrostatic pressure, gravity, and the pressure created by the body's own pumping action: the heart.

Osmotic diuresis: Increased urine output is caused by mannitol, glucose, and contrast dye, which cause a reduction in renal fluid reabsorption.

Osmolarity measures the ratio of water to solutes or the number of particles in each liter of fluid. Sodium (Na+) is the primary determinant of ECF osmolarity. Potassium (K+) is the primary determinant of ICF osmolarity.

Solutions may be isotonic, hypotonic, or hypertonic:

Isotonic is similar to body fluid (0.9NS)
Hypotonic fluid is less than body fluid (0.45NS)
Hypertonic fluid is greater than body fluid (3% NS)

THE KIDNEYS

The kidneys regulate body fluids. Thirst and urinary output help to regulate fluid balance. The kidneys and the lungs promote acid–base balance. The kidneys excrete hydrogen and generate bicarbonate anytime there is an abnormal production of acid that results in acidosis. The kidneys also help to regulate calcium ions to promote the absorption of vitamin D. Vitamin D_3 must be altered by the liver, and then the kidneys, before the gastrointestinal tract can absorb calcium.

Erythropoietin is produced by the kidneys in response to low oxygen delivery levels. The erythropoietin levels control the production of red blood cells that, in turn, carry oxygen to the body.

The average urinary output is 40 to 80 mL/hr. It should be noted that urinary output is often determined by fluid intake. Blood urea nitrogen (BUN) is the waste produced by the kidneys. The Bowman's capsule is the kidney's barrier for filtration. Renal tubules reabsorb sodium, HCO_3, glucose, and amino acids.

Fluid intake results in an increase in blood pressure. The kidneys then excrete sodium and water to reduce the blood pressure to within baseline limits or the circulating volume. The sympathetic nervous system (SNS) provides a response to any rapid changes in the effective circulating volume (ECV).

The body monitors itself with receptors in the carotid sinuses, aortic arch, and renal vessels. If there is a reduction in the circulating volume, the receptors note the decreased pressure in the arterial walls. This reduction causes a change in cardiac output. The body causes vasoconstriction (in the SNS) resulting in increased vascular resistance, promotion of thirst, and signaling the kidneys to reabsorb water and sodium.

The SNS provides vasoconstriction by stimulating an increase in sympathetic tone. This response changes cardiac output and vascular function, resulting in an increase in the blood pressure. Remember, cardiac output (CO) × systemic vascular resistance (SVR) = blood pressure (B/P). The SNS stimulates the release of renin. Renin acts on the angiotensinogen produced in the liver to create angiotensin I. Angiotensin I is converted to angiotensin II.

> **KEY NOTE:** Angiotensin II is a very potent vasoconstrictor.

Kidney diseases may cause problems within the body. Renal stenosis results in decreased perfusion of the kidneys. This decreased perfusion stimulates a release of renin. This process continues until the patient experiences hypertension. The patient may require medication to prevent the conversion of angiotensin I to angiotensin II.

The secretion of aldosterone causes an increase in the reabsorption of sodium and water (depletion of potassium), resulting in raising the blood pressure. Medications such as angiotensin-converting enzyme (ACE) are prescribed to reduce the aldosterone production or secretion, thereby reducing the blood pressure.

When the body is experiencing a hemorrhage, there is a decrease in renal perfusion. The kidneys respond by releasing renin. Renin is converted to angiotensin I, then to angiotensin II. Vasoconstriction occurs and there is a release of aldosterone. Aldosterone signals the kidneys to reabsorb sodium and water. This action results in increased vascular volume, raising the blood pressure. This process is short-acting if the patient is actively hemorrhaging.

When the blood pressure is too high, the hormone atrial natriuretic factor (ANF) is released by the atria. This hormone reduces the blood pressure and vascular volume. When sodium and water levels are elevated, the kidneys respond to the increased filtration rate and reduce the production of renin and aldosterone, thus resulting in vasodilation. ANF is released in response to anything that produces a Starling's law type of stretch.

ADH and thirst aid in the regulation of fluid volume. ECF osmolarity regulates fluid movement in and out of cells.

> **KEY NOTE:** If ECF osmolarity is elevated, the cells shrivel. ↑ Osmolarity = shrivel. If ECF osmolarity is reduced, the cells swell. ↓ Osmolarity = swelling.

Also known as vasopressin, the ADH is an arterial vasoconstrictor. ADH acts on distal tubules in the kidneys to increase reabsorption of water. ADH production is stimulated by serum osmolarity and effective circulating volume (ECV). The hypothalamus is stimulated by increased osmolarity and secretes ADH. ADH is stored in the posterior pituitary gland. Factors that influence the production of ADH are low blood pressure, pain, stress, and certain medications.

Decreased serum osmolarity, decreased fluid volume, and lower blood pressure stimulate thirst. Thirst is the primary response against hyperosmolarity.

> **KEY NOTE:** An alert and oriented patient may be dehydrated but have normal osmolarity levels because he or she is able to drink enough fluid to satisfy the thirst response.

A fluid volume imbalance (hypovolemic shock) occurs when the body can no longer compensate for the loss of fluid.

RELATED INFORMATION

Polyuria (excess urination) can be noted in diabetes insipidus (DI) and can be related to diuretics, or auto-diuresis. Increased urine output = hypokalemia.

Oliguria means that less than 400 mL of urine was excreted in a continuous 24-hour period. Decreased urine output = hyperkalemia.

Anuria means that less than 100 mL of urine was excreted in a continuous 24-hour period.

Urine osmolarity is 50 to 1,400 mOsm/kg. Urine specific gravity is 1.001 to 1.040.

Insensible fluid loss from the lung and skin (sweat) can total up to 10 mL/kg/24 hr.

Above the pylorus (anatomical area where stomach meets intestine) fluid loss is isotonic, but rich in sodium, potassium, chloride, and hydrogen. Below the pylorus fluid loss is isotonic but rich in sodium, potassium, and bicarbonate.

Gastric juices contain hydrochloric acid (HCl). Abnormal loss of gastric fluid (due to gastric suction) results in alkalosis. The lower gastrointestinal fluids contain bile, pancreatic juice, and intestinal secretions. Pancreatic secretions are high in bicarbonate and neutralize acidotic gastric juices. The intestines produce mucous, electrolytes, and digestive enzymes. The intestines are the major site of water and nutrient absorption. Diarrhea is the major cause of loss of lower gastrointestinal fluid and electrolytes. Vomiting results in the loss of upper gastrointestinal fluid and electrolytes.

Third-spacing is a condition that results in fluids not being available to the ICF or ECF. An early clue in recognizing the development of third-spacing is low urine output and edema when adequate fluid intake has occurred.

> **KEY NOTE:** A shift in fluid or cardiac output results in the kidneys holding onto fluids, resulting in low urine output.

FLUID AND ELECTROLYTE IMBALANCES

It is very important to note that electrolyte imbalances can produce physical signs and symptoms that the nurse can recognize. A prudent nurse will acknowledge the importance of identifying those patients who may be at risk of electrolyte imbalances and will closely monitor them to prevent and intercept before significant imbalances occur.

Geriatric patients are less able to concentrate urine and are less able to compensate for fluid losses. Immobile patients (due to CVA, hip fracture, dementia, arthritis, etc.) may have poor fluid intake. Elderly patients may also consciously reduce fluid intake to prevent nocturia, incontinence, or "bothering someone to help me to the bathroom."

Nurses can gather needed data by weighing patients, monitoring intake and output, and asking whether clothing has become tight or loose. If the patient has had an elevated temperature, the body will lose fluid and electrolytes. If the patient is positive for crackles or rhonchi, fluid excess may be present.

If the skin is flushed and dry, the patient may be dehydrated or have a fluid deficit. Poor skin turgor may also reflect ISF loss. Edema may reflect ISF excess. Positive jugular venous distension (JVD) may be reflective of fluid excess. Dry oral mucous membranes are not a true indicator of fluid deficit. The patient may be a mouth breather, which gives a false positive for fluid deficit.

Restlessness and confusion can be the result of a fluid deficit or an electrolyte abnormality. Decreased sodium levels can result in confusion. Decreased magnesium or calcium levels can result in decreased neuromuscular responses (Trousseau's sign and Chvostek's sign).

Trousseau's sign: (Hypocalcemia) induces carpal tunnel symptoms when the blood pressure cuff is inflated above baseline levels for 2 minutes.
Chvostek's sign: (Hypocalcemia) Percussion to the face below the zygomatic bone. Procedure is positive when twitching presents to the ipsilateral face muscles.

Intact skin protects the body from fluid losses. Wounds such as pressure ulcers or burns can rob the body of fluid. Excessive use of diuretics can also deplete the body of needed fluids. Medications (mannitol and dextrose) can inhibit water.

To recap: A patient's low blood pressure causes the body to respond by activating the SNS. The SNS stimulates the production of renin, which causes increased heart rate (tachycardia), increased cardiac contractility (greater pump action), and increased vascular resistance (narrow blood vessels). These measures increase the blood pressure while the renin–angiotensin–aldosterone system causes the retention of sodium and water by the kidneys.

A low blood pressure causes a cardiac response. The heart rate increases to ensure blood (carrying oxygen and nutrients) reaches all tissues. Low blood pressure can cause muscle weakness as well as decreased cerebral perfusion resulting in dizziness, lethargy, confusion, and syncope. Decreased perfusion can result in chest pain or cardiac dysrhythmias reflective of coronary ischemia. Shock occurs when fluid loss is greater than 25% of the intravascular volume.

Hypokalemia = GI loss
Hyperkalemia = Adrenal insufficiency
Hypernatremia = Diabetes insipidus (DI)
Hyponatremia = Fluid excess, syndrome of inappropriate anti-diuretic hormone (SIADH)

NORMAL FLUID BALANCE

Gains		Losses	
Water PO intake	500–1,700 mL	H_2O vapor (lungs and skin)	850–1,200 mL
Water from food	800–1,000 mL	H_2O vapor (GI tract)	50–200 mL
Water/food oxidation	200–300 mL	Urine	600–1,600 mL
	1,500–3,000 mL		1,500–3,000 mL

Insensible fluid losses are lost daily, regardless of the patient's physiological status. The largest amount of fluid loss is the urinary output. Almost all GI fluids are reabsorbed in the small intestine of the healthy person.

> **ECF volume deficit:** Losses of sodium and water (hemorrhage, diarrhea, vomiting, kidney disease, excessive sweating, burns, decreased ADH production, third-spacing, etc.) result in isotonic imbalances and ECF volume deficit.
> *Signs and symptoms:* Weakness, nausea, vomiting, poor skin turgor, furrowed tongue, dry skin, weight loss, and dry mucous membranes.
> *Treatment:* Treat the underlying cause. Restore fluid volume with (0.9NS) isotonic solutions.

ACID–BASE BALANCE

The body consistently attempts to restore or maintain homeostasis. If there is too much acid in the body, the kidneys will secrete bicarbonate into the bloodstream in an attempt to neutralize the excess acid. If there is too much bicarbonate in the blood, the body will increase the level of carbonic acid in an attempt to neutralize the excess bicarbonate.

CO_2 reacts with H_2O under the influence of carbonic anhydrase to produce H_2CO_3 (carbonic acid).

The respiratory to metabolic ratio is as follows:

$$
\begin{array}{lll}
H_2CO_3 & : & NaHCO_3 \\
1\ \text{part} & : & 20\ \text{parts} \\
1.2\ \text{mEq/L} & : & 24\ \text{mEq/L}
\end{array}
$$

Normally the body produces CO_2 at the rate at which the body can eliminate it. If the lungs are unable to eliminate CO_2, the pCO_2 increases. The increased CO_2 is recognized by the respiratory center in the medulla. The medulla stimulates an increase in the respiratory rate to "blow off" the excess CO_2. If the CO_2 is decreased, the medulla may decrease the respiratory rate to assist the body to retain more CO_2.

The kidneys regulate hydrogen concentrations by regulating bicarbonate production, excretion of hydrogen, reabsorption of sodium, and retention of bicarbonate.

ACID–BASE BALANCE IRREGULARITIES
Arterial Blood Gas Interpretation
The ABG is used to evaluate acid–base balance and oxygenation. The key to interpreting ABGs is very simple. First you need the normal values:

NORMAL VALUES

pH	(acid)	< 7.35–7.45 >	(alkaline)
pCO_2	(alkaline)	< 35–45 >	(acid)
HCO_3 22–26	(acid)	< 22–26 >	(alkaline)

STEP 1: Is the pH is normal?

If pH less than 7.35 or greater than 7.45, it is considered **UNCOMPENSATED.**

If pH is 7.35 to 7.45, then it is considered normal or **COMPENSATED.**

STEP 2: Is the pCO_2 and HCO_3 alkaline or acid?

STEP 3: Match the two likes (acid/acid, or alkaline/alkaline).

pCO_2 = respiratory

HCO_3 = metabolic

EXAMPLE 1:

pH	7.31	**acid**
pCO_2	52	**acid** (respiratory)
HCO_3	24	normal (metabolic)

pH: Uncompensated (+) respiratory (+) **acid**osis
(Acid) (Acid)

EXAMPLE 2:

pH	7.59	alkaline
pCO_2	44	normal (respiratory)
HCO_3	35	alkaline (metabolic)

pH: Uncompensated (+) metabolic (+) **alkal**osis

Potential Causes of Abnormal Acid–Base Balances

Respiratory acidosis (increase in CO_2): Caused by disease processes that cause CO_2 retention. Those disease processes may be pulmonary diseases (COPD or pneumonia); respiratory depression from drug ingestion or administration; lung injury; or disorders affecting the respiratory muscles (muscular dystrophy, ALS, Guillain–Barré syndrome, etc.).

Signs and symptoms: Decreased rate and depth of respirations, neurological depression

Treatment: Improve ventilation by using CPAP, BIPAP, intubation, or Lasix in pulmonary edema

Respiratory alkalosis (decrease in CO_2): Caused by hyperventilation; may be any factor or disease process that causes increased respiratory rate; disease processes that cause anxiety, fever, thyrotoxicosis, being intubated (ventilator), or injury to the medulla/respiratory center of the brain

Signs and symptoms: Increased respiratory rate, extremity numbness, muscle spasms, seizures, light-headedness, or loss of consciousness

Treatment: Treat primary cause; correct hypoxia, adjust ventilator settings, or sedate

Metabolic acidosis: An increase in hydrogen caused by metabolic etiology, such as diabetic ketoacidosis, lactic acidosis, or renal insufficiency.

Signs and symptoms: Deep, rapid respirations, increased urinary output, progressive loss of consciousness, decreased serum HCO_3, and hyperkalemia

Treatment: Treat underlying cause; physician may order sodium bicarbonate if pH is too low

Metabolic alkalosis: Above-normal serum bicarbonate levels; causes may be vomiting, gastric suctioning HCl from the stomach, excessive intake of alkaline foods, or excessive ingestion of sodium bicarbonate

Signs and symptoms: Muscle weakness, paralysis, abdominal distention, cardiac arrhythmias, or slow and shallow respirations

Treatment: Treat underlying cause; physician may order Diamox (makes kidneys excrete HCO_3)

ELECTROLYTE ABNORMALITIES

Hyponatremia (hypo-osmolar imbalance) can be caused by poor sodium chloride intake, diuretic usage, increased free water intake, excessive gastrointestinal fluid losses (from vomiting, diarrhea, or gastric suctioning), renal disease, or decreased secretion of aldosterone. Remember this mnemonic saying "**S**alt **S**hould **L**ive **U**p **T**o **I**ts **L**ivelihood" for **S**odium, **S**IADH, **L**oss of GI fluids, **U**rine (renal), **T**hyroid (hypothyroidism), **I**nsufficiency (adrenal), and **L**iver cirrhosis.

Signs and symptoms: Nausea and vomiting, headache, confusion, lethargy, fatigue, restlessness and irritability, muscle weakness, seizures, and decreased consciousness. When sodium levels in the blood become too low, excess water enters cells and causes the cells to swell. The patient will exhibit signs of neurological confusion and deficits when serum sodium levels are low (usually < 115 mEq/L), which will result in intracerebral osmotic fluid shifts and brain edema.

Treatment: Increasing dietary sodium intake or replacement of fluids via IV access (0.9NS), 3% saline hypertonic in small doses, and restricting free water.

Hypernatremia (hyper-osmolar imbalance) can be caused by diuretics, dehydration, DI, or diarrhea

Signs and symptoms: Thirst; elevated temperature; restlessness; coma; concentrated urine; high urine specific gravity; and increased Hgb, Hct, and BUN

Treatment: Increase free water intake or infuse hypotonic solutions such D5W, daily weights, intake and output, and restrict sodium; avoid D5W if the patient has cerebral edema

Potassium deficit: Hypokalemia can be caused by inadequate dietary intake, diabetic acidosis, diuretic usage, steroid therapy, gastrointestinal losses, and increased aldosterone secretions.

Signs and symptoms: Muscle weakness, abdominal distention, paralytic ileus, U wave on the EKG, or cardiac arrhythmias; hypokalemia is a significant cause of digoxin toxicity

Treatment: Increase dietary sources of potassium, or the physician may prescribe potassium chloride

Potassium excess: Hyperkalemia can be caused by renal insufficiency, tissue destruction, excessive intake of potassium-containing foods while taking a potassium-sparing diuretic, or hemolysis.

Signs and symptoms: **R**espiratory depression, (**O**liguria/**A**nuria), **D**ecreased cardiac contractility, dialysis, **M**uscle weakness and reflexes, **P**eaked T waves, **P**rolonged or widened QRS, and **P**rolonged PR

Treatment: Kayexelate, insulin given along with D50 via IV route, dialysis, or calcium chloride IV

Calcium deficit: Hypocalcemia can be caused by inadequate dietary intake, inadequate absorption (vitamin D is necessary), hypoparathyroidism, pancreatitis, excessive blood transfusions (citrate in blood), or elevated phosphorous levels

Signs and symptoms: Muscle cramps, tetany, tingling of fingers, seizures, Trousseau's sign, or Chvostek's sign

> **KEY NOTE:** Think "sats"—**s**pasms and convulsions, **a**rrhythmias, **t**etany, and **s**tridor.

Treatment: Calcium gluconate IV (when condition is critical), or increase dietary intake together with vitamin D

Calcium excess: Hypercalcemia may be caused by excessive calcium intake, hyperparathyroidism, cancer, or prolonged immobilization

Signs and symptoms: Pathological fractures, kidney stones, absent tendon reflexes, cardiac arrest, lack of coordination, abdominal pain, confusion, and sedative effect on CNS

Treatment: Reduce calcium intake or implement progressive mobility.

> **KEY NOTE:** Calcium and phosphorous have an inverse relationship: when phosphorous goes up, calcium goes down, and vice versa.

Hypomagnesemia: Caused by decreased gastrointestinal absorption due to diarrhea, alcoholism, hypokalemia, inadequate dietary intake, laxatives, pancreatitis, and burns

Signs and symptoms: Tremors, tetany, seizures, dysrhythmias, depression, confusion, dysphagia; low magnesium levels will increase digoxin toxicity

Treatment: Give magnesium, take seizure precautions, and check kidney function

Hypermagnesemia: Can be caused by renal failure, magnesium infusion, and antacids

Signs and symptoms: Depresses the CNS, hypotension, facial flushing, muscle weakness, absent deep tendon reflexes, and shallow respirations

Treatment: Dialysis, calcium gluconate, diuretics

Hypoglycemia: Low glucose (blood sugar level less than 70 mg/dL)

Causes: Skipped meals, too much insulin administration or antidiabetic pills, beta blockers, alcohol, too much strenuous activity (list not all inclusive)

Signs and symptoms: Irritability, confusion, diaphoresis, change in level of consciousness, coma, and seizures

Treatment: Depends on symptoms and the alertness of the patient and how low the blood sugar is. Administer 3 or 4 glucose tablets (15 g of carbohydrate, 4 oz. of any fruit juice, or 8 oz. of milk). If unresponsive give D50 IV or glucagon and recheck blood glucose level every 15 minutes for improvement. If glucagon is to be given, first turn patient on side since it might induce nausea and vomiting.

Hyperglycemia: Elevated blood sugar (fasting blood sugar greater than 110 mg/dL [milligrams per deciliter] or blood sugar greater than 180 mg/dL 2 hours post-meal)

Causes: Failure to take insulin or prescribed glucose-lowering medications, ingestion of a high-carbohydrate meal, infection, or increased stress

Signs and symptoms: Headache, increased thirst, frequent urination, and fatigue.

Treatment: Take medication as ordered, increased activity level, and increase oral fluid intake (noncaloric beverages)

Hypophosphatemia: Low phosphate levels in the blood

Causes: Stomach surgery; lack of vitamin D; medications such as Maalox, Amphogel, and Lasix; alcoholism; and low magnesium and high phosphorous levels

Signs and symptoms: Confusion, muscle weakness, diarrhea, nausea, and vomiting

Treatment: Oral or IV phosphorous replacement

Hyperphosphatemia: High phosphate levels in the blood

Causes: Kidney failure, hypoparathyroidism, dietary intake (soda, processed cheese, chocolate, etc.), hemolysis of red blood cells, acidosis, and rhabdomyolysis

Signs and symptoms: Can cause numbness and tingling in the extremities, muscle cramps, memory loss, and convulsions

Treatment: Dietary control, phosphate binders

Hypochloremia: Low chloride levels in the blood

Causes: Fluid loss; diarrhea; medications such as bicarbonate, diuretics, or laxatives; adrenal disease

Signs and symptoms: Low shallow breathing, acidosis, high sodium levels, muscle twitching

Treatment: Avoid caffeine and alcohol, replacement of chloride, stop the offending medication, and evaluate for kidney disease

Hyperchloremia: Elevated chloride in the blood
Causes: Fluid loss; hypernatremia; kidney failure; SIADH; hyperparathyroidism; and drugs such as diuretics, corticosteroids, estrogens
Signs and symptoms: Nausea, vomiting, diarrhea
Treatment: Stop offending medication, start hydration, evaluate for kidney disease

ELECTROLYTE EXERCISE

Complete the following by circling the appropriate answer from the right column. Return by preconference next week.

1. Potassium level of 5.7	hypokalemia, hyperkalemia
2. Sodium level of 119	hyponatremia, hypernatremia
3. Edema reflects interstitial	fluid deficit, fluid excess
4. Excessive urinary output	DI, SIADH
5. ADH is secreted by	hypothalamus, posterior pituitary
6. A pH greater than 7.45 is	acidosis, alkalosis
7. Potassium level of 2.9	hypokalemia, hyperkalemia
8. Sodium level of 150	hyponatremia, hypernatremia
9. Metabolic refers to	lungs, renal
10. Na 156 reflects	dehydration, fluid excess
11. Respiratory rate 42 reflects	hypocapnia, hypercapnia
12. Heart rate 125 reflects	hypovolemia, hypervolemia
13. Urinary output 400 mL/24 hr	polyuria, oliguria
14. Polyuria causes	hypokalemia, hyperkalemia

ANSWERS TO ELECTROLYTE EXERCISE

1. Potassium level of 5.7	hyperkalemia
2. Sodium level of 119	hyponatremia
3. Edema reflects interstitial	fluid excess
4. Excessive urinary output	DI
5. ADH is secreted by	posterior pituitary
6. A pH greater than 7.45 is	alkalosis
7. Potassium level of 2.9	hypokalemia
8. Sodium level of 150	hypernatremia
9. Metabolic refers to	renal
10. Na 156 reflects	dehydration
11. Respiratory rate 42 reflects	hypercapnia
12. Heart rate 125 reflects	hypovolemia
13. Urinary output 400 mL/24 hr	oliguria
14. Polyuria causes	hypokalemia

FLUID AND ELECTROLYTE CASES

CASE #1

Mr. Green, a 78-year-old male, comes to the clinic because he felt his heart racing. You obtain a set of vital signs, which are BP 100/62, HR 140, RR 16, Temp 98.6, and O_2 saturation 94. The cardiac rhythm is sinus tachycardia with frequent PVCs. You ask Mr. Green if he is on any medications. His medications consist of Lasix 40 mg twice a day, Vasotec 10 mg daily, and potassium 20 mEq daily. He swears he takes his medications faithfully. He is on a regular diet. His blood sugar is 163. Mr. Green states he had eaten a large amount of his favorite candy (black licorice) before his heart started racing. His potassium comes back at 3.0 mEq.

Answer the following questions and return by preconference next week.

1. What could be the causes of the high heart rate?
2. What diagnostic tests should be ordered?
3. What pharmaceutical interventions should be given?
4. What patient teaching related to this situation should be done?
5. Should the nurse be concerned about the O_2 saturation?

ANSWERS TO CASE #1

1. This is a trick question. Licorice contains glycyrrhizic acid, which is similar to aldosterone and triggers the body to release potassium. Symptoms will result in severe vomiting, fatigue, and irregular heart rate. Lasix can also cause the body to excrete potassium. It is important to know the contents of the patient's food, medications, and herbal supplements. REMEMBER: NEVER assume the obvious.
2. EKG, electrolyte panel, troponin, CPK MB, and CXR
3. Replace the potassium
4. Dietary teaching
5. No, the respiratory rate is normal, and the patient is not symptomatic. The elderly have reduced lung volumes and may have a lower pulse oxygen.

CASE # 2

A 15-year-old female is admitted with diabetic ketoacidosis. She has been a type 1 diabetic for 12 years. She is admitted with Kussmaul's breathing, lethargy, and nausea. She is an avid runner at school. She has been adjusting her insulin and diet because she was concerned about her weight. She has currently placed herself on a 1,200-calorie-a-day diet. She weighs 58.5 kg and is 165 cm tall.

Lab Work

Na 150	FBS 384	WBC 11	Osmolarity level 350
K 4.0	BUN 34	Hct 42	
Cl 110	Cr 1.2	ABG: pH 7.30, PO_2 80, PCO_2 37, HCO_3 17	
CO2 16	Hb 14	HbA1c 10	

Answer the following questions and return by preconference next week.

1. What do the sodium, osmolarity, Hgb/Hct, and BUN/Cr all have in common?
2. What does the serum CO2 of 16 and the ABG's indicate?
3. What does the HbA1c indicate?

ANSWERS TO CASE #2

1. They are indicators of probable dehydration. The normal osmolarity level is 280 to 300 mOsm/kg, and a level of 350 indicates dehydration. The BUN/Cr ratio is greater than 20:1, which also will be an indicator of dehydration. The sodium level is within parameters, but it is trending to hypernatremia. Hgb and Hct are both elevated, which is another sign of dehydration.

2. Both of these indicate acidosis. Serum CO2 (bicarbonate) is an indicator of acidosis. Normal values:
   pH: Normal: 7.35 to 7.45
   PaCO$_2$ Lungs: Normal: 35 to 45 (alkalosis if below 35, acidosis if above 45)
   HCO$_3$ (bicarbonate) Metabolic: Normal: 22 to 26 mEq/L (acidosis if below 22, alkalosis if above 26)
   Patient ABGs: pH 7.31, PO2 80, PCO2 37, HCO$_3$ 17
   pH_7.31 is acidosis uncompensated.
   PCO2 37 is within normal limits.
   HCO3 17 is acidosis.
   So this uncompensated metabolic acidosis present in diabetic ketoacidosis.
   Metabolic acidosis can be caused by prolonged diarrhea, ingestion of salicylic acid, lactic acid secondary to anaerobic metabolism, or ketone bodies secondary to insulin deficit.

3. HbA1c is elevated and indicates that the glucose has not been controlled over the past 3 months.
   (The important issue regarding the oxygen is to determine (1) whether the patient is hypoxic, and (2) is there another disease process evident? In this case, she is on room air and the oxygen is within normal limits of 80% to 100%; but, if she was on 100% oxygen, that may indicate an acute lung process such as pneumonia.)

BLOOD DRAWS AND TEST TUBE COLORS

Frequently, nurses will be required to draw labs from the patient. As with giving medications, the nurse must use two identifiers to make sure the right lab study, right patient, right time, and right tube are performed properly. Avoid dilution of the blood—if the blood is drawn from a central line, then at least 5 to 10 mL of the blood withdrawn has to be wasted first. In order to prevent false results, tubes need to be drawn in the order presented below. Avoid prolonged use of the tourniquet.

Light blue top: PTT, PT, fibrinogen
Red top: Blood screening, digoxin, lithium
Royal blue top w/o additive: Copper, zinc
Green top: Electrolytes, BMP, Chem 7, comprehensive metabolic panel, LFT, AST, ALT, CPK, C-reactive protein, amylase, LDH
Purple (lavender) top: CBC, sedimentation, BNP
Dark blue top with additive: Heavy metals
Gray top: Ammonia, lactate
Gold top: Digoxin levels

Blood cultures are collected in two different sites at two different times. The site needs to be properly cleaned. Both aerobic and anaerobic bottles should be collected.

LABORATORY QUIZ

You have the following patients. Name the blood tubes needed and return by preconference next week.

1. Mr. ETOH (Alcohol). The doctor wants to check his ammonia level.
2. Ms. Blood Letting. The doctor wants to check her CBC and coagulation.
3. Mr. Endstage. The doctor wants to check his BUN and creatinine.

4. Mrs. Confused. The doctor wants to check her CBC, ELR, PTT, PT, and ammonia level.
5. Mr. Overdose. The doctor wants to check his Tylenol level and his liver enzymes.
6. Mrs. Coumadin. The doctor needs to check her INR level.
7. Mrs. Transfusion. The doctor needs to check a type and crossmatch and a CBC.
8. Ms. Heart Failure. The doctor needs to check her ELR, BNP, and digoxin level.
9. Mr. Septic Blood. The doctor wants cultures × 2 sites and lactate level.

ANSWERS TO LABORATORY QUIZ

1. Gray top
2. Lavender top and light blue top
3. Green top
4. Lavender top, green top, light blue top, gray top
5. Green top
6. Light blue top
7. Lavender top, red top
8. Green top, lavender top, gold top
9. Gray-top tube, four blood culture bottles—two aerobic, two anaerobic

WEEK 6 POSTCONFERENCE

Explain to the students that fluids, electrolytes, and the acid–base balance are the keys to homeostasis and should be thoroughly understood. It would be beneficial for each student to purchase a book or download an application as an additional reference that explains fluids and electrolytes to ensure the student has a clear understanding of how fluids and electrolytes are the key to diagnostic intervention.

Ask students to take note of when they feel the need to drink. Did their body make their mouth dry? Did they recently urinate? Were they stimulated by observation (i.e., a television commercial or someone else drinking)? Ask students to observe how long they go between beverages. Ask the students to take note on the color of their urine. Is it concentrated after they have been sitting for hours or pale and clear? Is there sediment? Is there an odor?

Making students more aware of their own bodies and how they function will help reinforce their understanding of fluids and electrolytes. Reinforce that diuretics do not all work the same way. Some deplete potassium, while others may be potassium spar-ing. Encourage students to research diuretics. Ask students to note signs and symptoms of diuretic overdose and to prepare patient education regarding each diuretic medica-tion. Also, it would be wise to take note of what foods to avoid when taking each of these medications.

Chapter 10

CARING FOR THE GERIATRIC PATIENT

This chapter examines:

- Nursing assessment of physiological and mental changes associated with aging
- Patient education in relation to age-related communication and learning challenges
- Theories of aging; adjustments to changed physical, emotional, and social circumstances
- Care and support issues for the older adult patient and caregiver

Week 7 discusses the geriatric patient. With better health care and positive lifestyle changes, people are living longer. Geriatric nursing is on the rise. As geriatric patients seek health care interventions, the prudent nurse should be aware of those physiological changes occurring in the older adult that may affect safe and appropriate care.

WEEK 7 PRECONFERENCE

Hand out:
- Medication forms (levodopa and Celebrex)
- Survey on elder care
- Elder care case

Collect:
- Cases
- Electrolyte exercise
- Medication forms (Aldactone and Lasix)
- Snapshot summary (students' input and output)
- Concept maps
- Care plans
- Physical assessment form
- Journals

Inform the class that this week will cover geriatrics and the physiological changes that occur with aging. The students should pay close attention to their patients. Instruct the students to observe their patients' skin, reflexes, and any other characteristics they notice that highlight the differences (physiological) between themselves and their patients.

GERIATRICS

Aging is an irreversible process that begins as early as conception. Each person ages at a different rate, with a progression of different signs or symptoms. There are various factors involved with aging that range from genetic factors to modifiable factors such as diet, activity level, stress, and lifestyle habits (smoking and drinking).

As the population ages, chronic health problems may begin to appear, such as hypertension, arthritis, hearing loss, cardiac disease, cataracts, and forgetfulness, as well as depression, dementia, or Alzheimer's disease. Frailty often accompanies the aging process, resulting in falls or injuries that cause the older patient to be dependent on others for support.

Given improvements in safety measures (seatbelts) and health-promotion education (diet, exercise, and antismoking education), people are living longer. It is therefore safe to say that, with the increase in safety measures and health education, there is a corresponding decrease in the mortality rate that contributes to the ever-growing number of older people.

As the population ages, there is a greater likelihood that the growing elder population will need additional supplemental support. Older individuals may need financial support, or they may need food, shelter, or personal assistance with activities of daily living (ADL). A nurse's responsibility is to assess the older patient's ability to function (mentally and physically). The patient's family should offer input to ensure that complete and accurate data are collected. Because each person ages at a different rate, the needs vary from individual to individual.

To gather data, the nurse must first understand how to communicate with an older adult. Due to the physiological and psychological changes associated with aging, the patient may experience a greater degree of farsightedness and have greater difficulty adapting to sharp changes in light. (It would be helpful to review the discussion in Chapter 6 on assessing older patients for sensory deficits.) Older patients lose their ability to hear higher pitched tones. Older people also have greater difficulty coordinating information all at once. Keep the message simple.

With increasing age, adults react more slowly and less accurately to sensory stimulation. Because the central nervous system's capacity to process information is reduced, older people often miss messages if their attention is divided. Don't overload your messages with unnecessary information. Make the message seem familiar. Familiar experiences are easier for older people to process. Older people find comfort and security in seeing and hearing events in the usual way. Repeated exposure to a message reduces the effort needed to interpret it.

Make the message concrete. Older people rely more on concrete than on abstract thinking. Visual aids improve recall for all adults. Take it point by point. When designing a message for an older person, space out each point you wish to make. Older people concentrate on the first part of a message longer than younger people do. If you present information too quickly, the earlier cues will overpower the points you make later. Spacing the message allows older people to process each piece of information individually. While no scientific standard exists, the general rule is the slower, the better.

Give preference to print media. When older adults are allowed to process information at their own rate, their learning abilities improve. Print media lets consumers set their own pace.

Views among the entire adult population about aging are multidimensional, with both positive and negative elements. It is a fact that both younger and older adults show evidence of automatic ageism. Ageism is defined as a negative attitude based on three factors: feelings due to a person's age, stereotypes about what someone is like just because he or she is a certain age, and differential treatment because of a person's advanced age.

The nurse who demonstrates negative attitudes toward an older patient may be misinformed about the aging process and the health care needs of the older adult. The nurse may benefit by gaining knowledge about the normal aging process and by increasing contact with healthy, independent, older adults.

THEORIES OF AGING

Theories of aging (note that this discussion is not all inclusive) can be labeled as biological, psychological, or sociological. Biological theories may include intrinsic (internal) or extrinsic (external) biological theories. One intrinsic theory is based on the premise that a biologic clock triggers specific cell behaviors at a specific time, thus resulting in each species being given a predetermined time to live.

An extrinsic theory is based on the concept that alterations in lymphoid tissues lead to loss of capacity for self-regulation, thus leading to normal or age-related cells being recognized as foreign matter. The body's immune system reacts by forming antibodies to destroy these cells.

Psychological theories discuss the cognitive functional changes related to aging (loss of memory, learning, and problem-solving abilities). Fluid intelligence, also known as fluid reasoning, is the ability to analyze, problem solve, and acquire knowledge. This theory suggests that cognition and fluid intelligence begin to decline during middle age.

Short-term recall memory declines with age; however, long-term recall memory remains constant. Changes in memory may occur when there is a change in the older person's environment.

Sociological theories attempt to explain the aging processes through concepts of age-related socialization changes. The concept of social behavior holds that self-worth is premised on being valued by peers, by society, or on the premise of self-gratification. As the patient ages, life changes may include loss of one's job (retirement or downsizing), loss of family (children are grown), loss of friends (who are dying), and a deteriorating physical state, all resulting in a declining social network.

Theories often begin with basic concepts. One such concept holds that each person has a framework of needs. This concept is based on the premise that as a person ages, his or her needs will change based on various factors. These factors may be based on physical or psychological needs.

ADJUSTING TO AGING

Adjusting to advanced age may be difficult for the aging individual. There are numerous examples of individuals having difficulties: Elderly men climbing ladders to continue home and yard care, or buying a flamboyant automobile. Aging women may be preoccupied with body improvements (plastic surgery, cosmetics, hair dyes, etc.). There are numerous transitions that accompany aging. Roles may change suddenly, upended by the loss of spouse, loss of friends, retirement, a need for supportive care that results in relocation to a long-term care facility, or a reversal of parent–child roles.

Physiological changes may present with postural changes (kyphosis), hyperextension of the neck, loss of skin elasticity, wrinkles, increase in body fat, water loss, sagging skin, fragile skin, decrease in hair growth (scalp hair for men, pubic and axillary hair for women), decrease in muscle strength, reduced heart rate, decreases in kidney filtration function, bone loss, vision changes, and decreased immunity. In addition, slower reproduction of epidermis results in delayed wound healing.

Certain physiological changes associated with aging may also interfere with nutritional requirements. These changes include missing teeth, ill-fitting dentures, xerostomia (lack of sufficient saliva production to aid in swallowing), and atrophic gastritis (lack of HCl production resulting in a lack of iron and vitamin B_{12} absorption that is secondary to consumption of antacids or proton pump inhibitors causing an alkalinizing effect).

Vitamin replacements are needed for the aging because vitamin D is required (600 IU) for maintaining bone mineralization and serum calcium levels at normal levels. Calcium is needed (1,200 mg) for the maintenance of bone density and plasma calcium levels. It is also needed to help prevent depression and poor memory. Vitamin B_{12} is required for the myelin sheath of the central nervous system. A vitamin B_{12} deficiency can cause macrocytic anemia and peripheral neuropathy. Vitamin B_{12} levels should be drawn annually because folic acid supplementation can mask a B_{12} deficiency.

Cholecystokinin plays a key role in facilitating digestion within the small intestine. It is secreted from mucosal epithelial cells in the first segment (duodenum) of the small intestine, and it stimulates delivery into the small intestine of digestive enzymes from the pancreas and bile from the gallbladder. Cholecystokinin is also produced by neurons in the enteric nervous system, and is abundantly distributed in the brain.

Older people may slowly become confused over a long duration or may abruptly demonstrate an acute confused state. Abrupt confused states may present when the older patient has an illness or an acid–base imbalance. The patient may hallucinate, become delusional, or have confusing visual or auditory perceptions. Urinary tract infections, pneumonia, transient ischemic attacks (TIAs), cerebrovascular accidents (CVAs), electrolyte imbalances, narcotics, or nutritional imbalances may be the underlying causes of the acute confusion. The priority interventions for these types of patients are to prevent injuries and to correct the underlying causes of confusion.

It is important to identify those frail and elderly patients who are at risk. When the elderly are hospitalized, the nurse should consider the patient's discharge needs (especially assistance with ADL, placement, and medications) early in the hospital stay. This includes utilizing interdisciplinary teams, special care units, and individuals who focus on the special needs of geriatric patients. Standard protocols exist for screening the hospitalized older adult patient for common at-risk conditions such as urinary tract infection and delirium. Advocate for referral of the patient to appropriate community-based services.

The nurse should ask the following questions when evaluating nursing care interventions for the elderly:

- Is there an identifiable change in ADL, mental status, or disease signs and symptoms?
- Does the patient consider his or her health state to be improved?
- Can the patient and caregiver afford the care that is required?
- Can the nurse document positive changes that support the interventions?

Gender differences may play a key role in evaluating posthospitalization care.

Men are more likely to be living with their spouse, to have health insurance, and to have a higher income after retirement; they are less likely to be involved in caregiving activities, and they generally have fewer chronic health problems than women.

Women are more likely to live alone, simply because—as statistics reflect—women are more likely to experience the loss of their spouses. Women are less likely to have health insurance, but more likely to live in poverty, lack formal work experience, have a lower income, and rely on Social Security as their major source of income. Women are also more likely to be the caregiver of an ill spouse and to have a higher incidence of chronic health problems such as arthritis, hypertension, stroke, and diabetes.

It is important for the nurse to perform a functional assessment of the elderly patient. The functional assessment will identify self-care deficits. Can the patient perform independent ADL? Can the patient cook and clean independently? Is the patient mentally, physically, and financially able to pay the bills? Does hearing loss or vision loss interfere with ADL? Does the patient have impaired mobility? Is the patient at risk for injuries or falls due to underlying disease processes (diabetes, arthritis, or cataracts)? What support system or reserves does the patient have in place? This information can assist the nurse in planning services for the status posthospitalized patient.

It is not uncommon for one spouse to become the caregiver for his or her partner. The nurse must assess the caregiver spouse. It is not unusual for the caregiver to feel alone, to become depressed, or to feel overwhelmed and fatigued. The nurse should help identify and guide the caregiver and his or her family to available community resources. When one spouse of an older couple dies, it is not uncommon for the adult children to become the caregivers of their remaining parent. The nurse should evaluate the ability of the patient's family to assume the caregiver role. It may be necessary to help guide the family to share in the responsibilities of care for the older patient.

Abuse or neglect can occur when the caregiver is overtaxed with responsibilities. Abuse or neglect may present with the patient having bruising or fractures, showing a lack of hygiene, or appearing malnourished. The patient may cower in fear or withdraw from the abuser. The nurse must report suspected abuse. If the patient lives alone, is unable to care for himself or herself, and presents to the health care organization with symptoms of neglect, the nurse should contact adult protective services. Adult protective services will assess the situation and protect the patient if he or she is proved to be incompetent to care for himself or herself.

Medication Forms

Listed in the vertical box is a medication. For each of the remaining boxes list the following:

Box 1: List a laboratory result you would need to monitor. Explain the significance of the laboratory test to the medication.
Box 2: List one food that may interact with the medication. Explain the significance of the food item to the medication.
Box 3: List one patient educational instruction you would give to the patient regarding the medication. Explain the significance of the instruction to the medication.

List other educational information you could provide this patient. Are there websites you can refer to? What about travel overseas and health issues? How should the medication be stored? Does the medication being administered interfere with other medications?

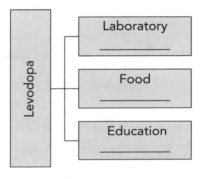

Listed in the vertical box is a medication. For each of the remaining boxes list the following:

Box 1: List a laboratory result you would need to monitor. Explain the significance of the laboratory test to the medication.
Box 2: List one food that may interact with the medication. Explain the significance of the food item to the medication.
Box 3: List one patient educational instruction you would give to the patient regarding the medication. Explain the significance of the instruction to the medication.

List other educational information you could provide this patient. Are there websites you can refer to? What about travel overseas and health issues? How should the medication be stored? Does the medication being administered interfere with other medications?

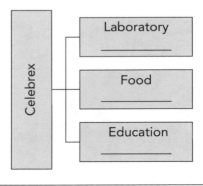

SURVEY ON ELDER CARE

Each student should interview two people of various ages, complete the following questions, and return by preconference next week.

1. At what age (number of years) is someone old?

2. At what age (number of years) is someone elderly?

3. At what age (number of years) is someone middle-aged?

4. Do you believe getting old means becoming forgetful? Explain.

5. Can you list the problems that the elderly must face?

6. What do you believe is the annual income of an elderly person?

7. Do you know anyone who is elderly?

8. Do you socialize with that person (if applicable)?

9. How do the elderly get to their doctors, the grocery store, and so on?

10. Have you thought about what will happen when you become elderly?

11. Will you have someone to help you if needed?

12. What should the elderly do if they have no family/friends?

13. Do you believe the elderly are a target for crime?

14. Do you believe the community has a responsibility to its elderly residents?

15. What would be a way to assist the elderly?

16. What is your age?

GERIATRIC CASES

ELDER CARE CASE

A 74-year-old male with Alzheimer's disease is experiencing short-term memory loss and is currently due for discharge. His wife is worried about his safety at home because she does volunteer work and still drives. The wife states that the patient "frequently wanders off and forgets where he is going or what he is doing." The patient is still able to help with decisions about his care.

What resources could you offer this patient and his wife? Write out your answers and return by preconference next week.

1. _____
2. _____
3. _____
4. _____
5. _____
6. _____

ANSWERS TO ELDER CARE CASE

1. Contact support groups at the local Alzheimer's Association website.
2. There are tracking devices available, such as GPS in shoes, in case the patient gets lost.
3. There are door alarms with movement sensors that will trigger an alarm noise if the door is opened.
4. Provide a phone with a larger key display and a larger screen text size. Use this phone to display a list of things the patient needs to do.
5. Arrange pre-trip planning, utilizing telemedicine, medication dispensers, and vital sign monitoring.
6. Arrange for a waterproof watch with wireless indoor and outdoor locator and for virtual heath records, a medical advisor, a nutritional status, a cognitive problem prognosis, home help, and a caregiver retreat plan.

WEEK 7 POSTCONFERENCE

Discuss with the students the physiological differences they may have noticed between themselves and their patients. Inquire whether any student has had the opportunity to care for an elderly relative. Discuss the elder survey with the students and instruct them to observe for older citizens when they are out conducting the survey. During preconference next week, they are to discuss the various ways the elderly perform ADL, such as ambulation, eating (including in restaurants), and driving.

The instructor will discuss mid-term evaluations with each student individually. The evaluation forms are completed by the instructor prior to Week 7. The students review the form and return the evaluation to the instructor. The instructor will then use the same form to complete the final evaluation. The student can then see how far he or she has come and what he or she has achieved. Students will be notified of areas of strengths and weaknesses. Students are strongly encouraged to focus on areas of weakness. How a student can improve can be discussed at a pre-arranged meeting with the instructor during office hours. This will eliminate the wait time of classmates and ensure that the instructor offers proper instruction to the student in need.

Chapter 11

ASSESSMENT AND TREATMENT OF MUSCULOSKELETAL SYSTEM DISORDERS

This chapter examines:

- Assessment procedures and diagnostic tests related to musculoskeletal system diseases and disorders
- The structure and function of muscles, bones, and joints
- Causes, symptoms, and treatment of osteoarthritis, osteoporosis, and other bone disorders
- Diagnosis and treatment for bone fractures and related complications

Week 8 introduces the musculoskeletal system and the various abnormalities that can occur within it. This week's focus is on understanding the various musculoskeletal system conditions that occur, how they are diagnosed, and whether they are due to injury or due to changes from within the body and the musculoskeletal system.

WEEK 8 PRECONFERENCE

Hand out:
- Musculoskeletal system exercise
- Musculoskeletal system cases
- Medication forms (Skelaxin and calcium)

Collect:
- Elder care case
- Medication forms (levodopa and Celebrex)
- Survey on elder care
- Concept maps
- Care plans
- Physical assessment form
- Journals

Instruct students that during clinical they should observe for musculoskeletal deformities; abnormal symmetry; and gait, mobility, or other musculoskeletal abnormalities in their patients. The students should be prepared to discuss their findings during postconference.

THE MUSCULOSKELETAL SYSTEM

The musculoskeletal system includes three types of muscle tissue:

1. Skeletal
2. Cardiac
3. Smooth

Muscles allow the body to maintain its posture and permit movement. The ability to move is produced by the combined function of the muscles, bones, and joints. There are several terms that describe properties that allow the muscles to assist with homeostasis:

Excitability: Muscles receive and respond to stimuli
Contractility: Muscles' ability to shorten when stimulated adequately
Elasticity: Permits muscles to return to original state
Extensibility: Permits muscle stretching

The cardiac muscle consists of striated muscle fibers and performs involuntarily. The branched, striated muscles fibers are connected by gap junctions that are located between the cells to allow for rapid electrical and chemical communication. The cardiac muscle is regulated by the sinus atrial node, which is also known as the internal pacemaker. In accordance with Starling's law, stretching the heart muscle (based on venous return) causes the muscle to contract more forcefully.

However, the autonomic nervous system responds to impulses from the baroreceptors in the carotid artery and aortic arch walls. The autonomic nervous system allows acceleratory or inhibitory actions of the cardiac muscles, based on the impulses from the baroreceptors.

The skeletal muscles are stimulated by impulses traveling on nerve fibers (axons) from the central nervous system (CNS) to permit voluntary movements. The nerve impulses reach the surface of the muscle fiber where a small gap lies. This gap (synapse) accepts the neurotransmitter (acetylcholine), which then attaches to receptors, resulting in stimulation of the muscle fibers. The enzyme cholinesterase (within the muscle membrane) breaks down the acetylcholine into acetate and choline; this action prevents the nerve impulse from further stimulation of the muscle fiber.

Energy is required for all muscle contractions. Energy can be obtained from the production of adenosine triphosphate (ATP). There are several methods used to produce ATP, including the phosphagen system (breakdown of creatine phosphate) and the glycogen–lactic acid system (breakdown of glycogen into glucose).

Smooth muscle lines the blood vessels, visceral organs, stomach, intestine, bladder, uterus, and various ducts. Contractions of smooth muscles occur in a wave over the fiber (smooth muscle cells) in response to impulses from the CNS.

The skeletal system consists of 206 bones. Bones are classified by their shapes: long, short, flat, sesamoid, and irregular bones:

- **Long bones:** Clavicle, humerus, radius, ulna, femur, tibia, fibula, metacarpals, metatarsals, and phalanges
- **Short bones:** Ankle and wrist bones
- **Flat bones:** Sternum, ribs, and skull bones
- **Sesamoid:** Knees
- **Irregular bones:** Vertebrae, pelvic and hip bones

The organic framework of bones consists of proteins (one of which is alkaline phosphatase), fibers, and collagen, which provides strength to withstand stretching and twisting. Osteoblasts are bone-forming cells. Osteocytes are the mature osteoblasts found in the bone marrow. Osteoclasts are cells that remove damaged bone cells and enable the bone to repair itself and change shape.

An articulation (joint) is the junction between two bones. Joints are classified (synarthrotic, amphiarthrotic, and diarthrotic) according to allowable movement:

- **Synarthrotic:** Immovable joints (teeth)
- **Amphiarthrotic:** Joints that allow slight movement (symphysis pubis)
- **Diarthrotic:** Freely movable joints

Diarthrotic joint categories include gliding, hinge, pivot, condyloid, saddle, and ball and socket joints:

- **Gliding joints:** Gliding movement with limitations due to ligament attachment (hands)
- **Hinge joints:** Capable of flexion and extension (knees, elbow)
- **Pivot joints:** One bone fits into bone groove of another (ulna)
- **Condyloid joints:** Permits flexion, extension, abduction, adduction, and circumduction (metacarpophalangeal)
- **Saddle joints:** Freedom of movement (thumb)
- **Ball-and-socket joints:** Ball-like head of one bone fits into socket of another (hip)

Skeletal muscles attach to the skeleton and allow action (flexion, extension). Contracting skeletal muscles, under the influence of the nervous system, exert force on bones. Composed of thin sheets of skeletal connective tissue, the fascia separates the muscle into compartments not bundles. The skeletal muscles are attached to bones by thin extensions of fascia or by tendons.

Bursae are small sacs lined with synovial fluid, acting as cushions where muscle or tendons slide across bone. Ligaments are bands of fibrous tissue that connects bones at joints and add stability during movement. Cartilage resists forces of tension and compression.

Skeletal muscle contraction occurs when a stimulus excites an individual muscle fiber. Nerve impulses release stored acetylcholine from the end of the motor neuron in the synapse. The action potential triggers contraction of the sarcomeres by releasing calcium inside the cell. A continuous flow of stimuli maintains muscle tone and the use of ATP, so muscle cells need large amounts of oxygen and glucose.

A motor unit is the motor neuron and all the skeletal fibers it supplies. Small motor units produce fine motor control, whereas large motor units will coordinate the response of large muscles. Muscles that provide propulsion are found in the walls of hollow conduits in the body; the force of this contraction applies pressure that may mix, break up, or move substances forward (gastrointestinal tract muscles, airway muscles, and smooth muscle in the arterioles). Muscles also play a role in heat production: body heat is released by sweating and vasodilatation; however, when the body is cold, heat is produced by shivering.

HEMATOPOIETIC FUNCTION OF BONES

Bones house the hematopoietic tissues used to manufacture red blood cells, platelets, and most white blood cells (WBCs). Red blood cells, platelets, and most WBCs arise in red marrow. Yellow marrow produces fat cells. Fat cells are created in the shafts of long bones. To maintain homeostasis, the body will release minerals for cellular metabolism. When calcium falls, the parathyroid hormone increases calcium movement from bone into extracellular fluids. Bone remodeling maintains calcium in the body and allows for bone repair.

ASSESSMENT OF THE MUSCULOSKELETAL SYSTEM

Begin the musculoskeletal assessment by first listing the patient's chief complaint. Also list the clinical manifestations. Assess the patient's pain. Identify the cause of the pain. Understand the patient's perception of pain and level of pain. Determine where the pain is located, its quality and duration, and ask about aggravating and alleviating factors. Joint stiffness may indicate a rheumatological disorder. Question whether there are sensory changes such as tingling or burning, and question whether there is muscle weakness. Assess for swelling, because swelling accompanies bone and muscle injury. Assess for deformity and limited range of motion (ROM). Evaluate for spasm, joint pain, crepitus, and deformities in joints or bones. Evaluate muscle masses for symmetry, involuntary movements, tenderness, tone, and strength. Assess bones, limb length, gait, mobility, posture, general joint motion, and balance. Assess for scoliosis (spine curved from side to side, shaped like an S), lordosis (inward curvature of a portion of the vertebral column, as in pregnancy), and kyphosis (forward curvature of the upper thoracic spine, a common condition).

DIAGNOSTIC TESTING

Noninvasive tests: X-ray, magnetic resonance imaging (MRI), CAT scan, DEXA scan. A DEXA scan is a radiological test performed to determine bone density (used to assess the bone's strength). Women often suffer from hypocalcemia, which in later years may increase their risk for bone fractures

Invasive tests: Arthrocentesis (needle aspiration), arthrogram (x-ray after injection), arthroscopy (surgical fiber-optic scope), electromyography (EMG) (nerve conduction test using needle electrodes placed into the nerve signal pathway)

Indium scan: Used to test for osteomyelitis (infection)

Bone scan: Used to test osteoporosis

DISORDERS OF THE MUSCULOSKELETAL SYSTEM

OSTEOARTHRITIS

Osteoarthritis is a degenerative joint disease (DJD; arthritis). Being overweight is a risk factor. Osteoarthritis can be primarily idiopathic in origin, often appearing with no history of joint disease or illness that would contribute to arthritis. Osteoarthritis is more common in women and is an incurable disorder. A secondary diagnosis of osteoarthritis is more common in men, due to trauma, DJD, and neuropathic disorders.

The definition of osteoarthritis is the process of cartilage matrix degradation, which is accompanied by the body's ineffective ability to heal, the loss of its ability to resist wear, and erosion in the superficial layer of cartilage as collagen fibers rupture.

Signs and symptoms used to diagnose osteoarthritis: Patient history, physical examination, worsening pain and limitation of movement, and asymmetrical joints. Tests are used to rule out other conditions such as gout (high uric acid), rheumatoid arthritis, bursitis, and sedimentation rate. A sedimentation rate is a laboratory test used to detect inflammation and to diagnose arthritis. Goals for patients with osteoarthritis are mobility, functional independence, and maintenance of quality of life.

Treatment may include weight-bearing exercises, weight loss, heat application, Tai Chi, topical application of capsaicin cream, herbal supplements, calcium supplements, and nonsteroidal anti-inflammatory drugs (NSAIDs). NSAIDs can cause GI bleeding, hypertension, fluid retension, and kidney and heart problems. Tylenol is the recommended drug of choice (maximum dosage 4 g/d). Cox-2 anti-inflammatories (Celebrex) may be prescribed, but they do come with significant warnings (may cause cardiac infarction and stroke). Herbal supplements used to treat osteoarthritis include: glucosamine, S-adenosylmethionine (also known as Sam-e), and chondroitin.

Surgical management may be necessary. An osteotomy involves a cut made across a bone with resection of a bone fragment to realign. An arthritic hip may cause misalignment. An osteotomy can help realign the hip. An arthrodesis is a surgical procedure in which bone ends are removed so that bone edges unite like a healing fracture to prevent grinding against each other. An example of this procedure is the fusion of two vertebrae bones. Knee replacement surgery can be an option for the patient with a severely diseased knee joint(s). An artificial joint made of metal alloys replaces the damaged knee joint and replicates the work of the natural knee. With any joint surgery, a vacuum-collection device (Hemovac or Jackson Pratt) is commonly used to collect drainage from the post-op site. These collection devices should be emptied and checked every 4 hours for excessive bleeding, because anemia is a common complication.

After a physical therapy (PT) evaluation, a continuous passive motion (CPM) machine may be used to flex and extend the knee post knee surgery to increase movement and decrease scarring. Premedicate the patient prior to application of the CPM because it will cause pain and the patient may try to remove it.

Common complications of orthopedic surgery are DVTs and pulmonary and fat embolisms. The postsurgical patient needs an anticoagulant (heparin, Lovenox, aspirin, or Coumadin) with monitoring of anticoagulation and platelet count.

Avoid positions of external hip flexion (90°). This creates an outward turn of the leg. Keep the postsurgical patient's leg straight; do not allow the leg to be rotated internally or externally. Secure in place with an abduction foam wedge or pillow. Do not turn the patient on the post-op site unless ordered.

OSTEOPOROSIS AND LOSS OF BONE MASS

Osteoporosis disorders may alter bony equilibrium (the balance of bone development and replacement) and may affect bones when there is a deficiency of estrogen (which helps to utilize calcium), a parathyroid problem, a vitamin deficiency, malabsorption, or physical inactivity/immobility.

Systemic skeletal disorders are characterized by compromised bone strength with a predisposition to an increased risk of fracture. Osteopenia is low bone mineral density condition that results in a high risk of fracture. The high risk for a fracture due to low bone density is a major health problem.

Risk factors for women include genetic factors (80% inherited), environmental factors, and perimenopausal status, which can result in loss of bone mass equal to 15% of their total body mass, with rapid bone loss once ovaries are nonfunctioning. Bone loss in men starts later in life and progresses more slowly. Osteoporosis also can be a result of other medical conditions and can be caused by medications (steroids, anticonvulsants) or thyroid abnormalities.

Signs and symptoms of osteoporosis can be compression fracture characterized by a sudden onset of severe back pain that worsens with movement. It may be relieved with rest, or can become a chronic pain or disability.

Diagnosis of osteoporosis is made by a bone scan, which is the "gold standard"; the T-score difference between the patient's score and the young adult norm; and CBC, Ca (calcium), and parathyroid and thyroid hormone (T3, T4, TSH) tests.

Prevention is the key. Prevent loss of bone mass by consuming calcium-fortified dairy products or calcium supplements. Avoid high dietary intake of sodium or coffee as they increases calcium loss. Vitamin D plays a major role in calcium absorption and bone metabolism. Sunscreen blocks absorption of vitamin D because it allows limited sunlight exposure. Efforts should be made to change lifelong behaviors. Patients should increase exercise, decrease alcohol consumption, and refrain from tobacco usage.

OTHER BONE DISORDERS

Paget's disease is an idiopathic bone disorder that presents with abnormal bone resorption and formation in one or more bones (femur, lower spine, pelvis, and cranium). It is usually diagnosed in those less than 40 years of age. Signs and symptoms of Paget's disease include skeletal deformity, deep bone pain, pathological bone fractures, and nerve compression. Diagnosed by bone scans, alkaline phosphatase tests, and presence of fractures. Treatment may include Fosamax, Actonel, NSAIDs, heat therapy, and massage.

Gout arthritis is a metabolic bone disorder that occurs when the purine (protein) metabolism is altered and uric acid accumulates. The primary cause is heredity (in 85% of cases). Men are more prone to gout than are women. Gout can lead to increased or decreased renal excretion. A secondary diagnosis is acquired from hematopoietic disorders (multiple myeloma, polycythemia), chemotherapy (from massive destruction of cells), use of aspirin (ASA) or thiazides (diuretics), alcohol consumption (ETOH), and starvation. Signs and symptoms include nighttime attacks of swelling, tenderness, and redness, and sharp pain in the patient's big toe (most common). Diagnosed by uric acid level (not reliable) or by aspirating uric acid crystals from the knee.

Osteomalacia is a condition in which the bone is abnormally soft, which can be due to low levels of vitamin D, calcium, or phosphorous. The widespread decalcification and softening of bones results in the bones becoming bent and flattened, with cyst formation. It can be caused by renal failure, anticonvulsants, and hyperthyroidism disorders. Treatment includes vitamin D, calcium, and phosphorous.

Scoliosis is a lateral curvature of spine that is distinguished as a structural curvature (does not self-correct) as opposed to a nonstructural curvature (easily corrected on forced bending). Scoliosis is an idiopathic disorder occurring most commonly in pre-adolescents and adolescents. Adult scoliosis may actually result from an undiagnosed childhood condition, There may be a progressive curvature of up to 40° to 45° (causing cardiopulmonary distress), or less than 20°.

The etiology of scoliosis is congenital or neuromuscular. Congenital scoliosis presents with a malformation of a bony vertebral segment of the spine, absence of a portion of a vertebra, or absence of normal separations between vertebrae (caused by cerebral palsy, polio, spinal muscle atrophy, or muscular dystrophy). Scoliosis is diagnosed by x-ray tests that usually include a posterior, anterior, and lateral view. Treatment includes braces, electrical stimulation (transcutaneous electrical nerve stimulation [TENS]), PT, chiropractic manipulation, or use of the Harrington rod system to stabilize the spine.

Kyphosis presents with a humpback or posterior rounding of the thoracic spine. Kyphosis is more common when metabolic disorders such as osteoporosis and osteomalacia are present. It may be accompanied by cardiopulmonary and GI dysfunction. Treatment consists of orthopedic braces to treat the spine, and exercise to strengthen the muscles.

Lordosis (swayback) is an excessive inward curvature of the lumbar spine that is seen in pregnant or obese patients. Swayback results in sagging shoulders, an exaggerated pelvic angle, and medial rotation of the legs. Treatment includes bracing or spinal fusion.

Osteomyelitis is a severely pyrogenic (fever-causing) infection of the bone and surrounding tissues. It is caused by *Staphylococcus aureus*, *Escherichia coli*, *Pseudomonas*, *Klebsiella*, *Salmonella*, and *Proteus*. Men are affected more (due to physical trauma), and incidence is also increased when IV drug use, diabetes mellitus (DM), malnutrition, ETOH abuse, or liver failure are involved. Signs and symptoms vary according to site. It may not be acute. Osteomyelitis is diagnosed by lab studies (elevated WBC and erythrocyte sedimentation rate [ESR]). Treatment includes antibiotics (Abx), surgical debridement, or hyperbaric oxygen therapy.

Septic arthritis is a closed-space infection characterized by invasion of synovial membrane by pus-forming bacteria. The most common bacterial cause is *Neisseria gonorrhoeae*, with *S. aureus* being the second-most common cause. It is usually spread hematogenously (through the blood) from a remote site. This infection reflects a failure of multiple defense mechanisms in the body. The affected synovial membrane fills with neutrophils that release proteolytic enzymes that destroy cartilage, bone, and capsule and will cause an effusion within 3 to 24 hours. Signs and symptoms are diagnosed by CBC, ESR, antinuclear antibodies (ANA), renal failure, or aspiration. Treatment includes antibiotics, decompression of the infected joints (needle aspiration), debridement, ROM exercises, immobilizers, splints, CPM, and pain medications.

A bone tumor may be malignant or benign. When a tumor is benign, there are no signs or symptoms. Malignant bone tumors may go undiagnosed. A malignant bone tumor is diagnosed via ultrasound or x-ray. Tumors are rare in bone cells (osteosarcoma being the most common), and they present as bone pain (night), fracture, or lesion at the site. Bone tumors may be caused by exposure to carcinogens such as asbestos, dioxin, or radium. Bone tumors are more prevalent with sarcomas that spread primary carcinomas from sites in the breasts, lungs, or kidneys that may metastasize to the bone via the lymphatic system. Treatment includes chemotherapy, radiation, and surgery (a bone graft from a cadaver). Treatment goals may be palliative if patient is in remission.

TREATMENT OF BONE FRACTURES

Fractures are a break in the bone. There are various types of fractures include (not all inclusive) complete, incomplete, comminuted, greenstick, simple, compound, transverse, spiral, and avulsion. One of the most serious fractures is the compound fracture, where a fractured bone breaks the skin and is exposed to the air, causing a risk for infection. Causes of fractures can include (not all inclusive): a trauma fall, osteoporosis (pathological), multiple myeloma, tumors, osteomyelitis, therapy (including chemotherapy, radiation therapy, or proton pump inhibitors for ulcers), and aging. Assessment findings should include pain, pain on movement, tenderness, loss of function, edema, ecchymosis, or deformity. Patients diagnosed with a fracture not only must be treated but also must deal with loss of wages, medical expenses, and potential disability. Fractures are diagnosed by x-rays. Some fractures may result in the need for traction. Traction options include Buck's traction (skin traction) or skeletal traction requiring surgical insertion of pins into the bone. When traction is used, the weights should hang free and should not be resting on the floor or dragging on the bed. A fracture is accompanied by a high risk for deep vein thrombosis or pulmonary or fat emboli. As is discussed later, a fracture injury may result in compartment syndrome (CS).

Another form of traction is the application of a cast. The materials of the cast may be plaster or fiberglass. The cast is applied to prevent movement of the joints, thereby stabilizing the injury and allowing the fracture to heal. The cast will be wet when it is applied. The cast should be allowed to dry thoroughly. The cast must be handled carefully for 48 hours (until dry) and must only be handled with the palms, not the fingers. The patient should be advised not to put any object into the cast. Elevate the

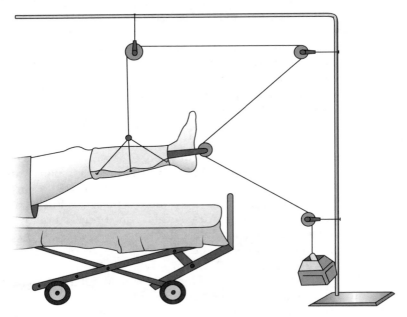

FIGURE 11-1 BUCK'S TRACTION A sleeve is secured around the lower leg. Cords are attached to the sleeve. The cords are threaded around pulleys and then attached to a weight. The weight provides traction to maintain bone alignment and prevent muscle spasms.

cast above the level of the heart, if possible, to aid in circulation and decrease edema. Once dry, cast edges should be examined to ensure no sharp or jagged areas are present that may irritate the patient's skin. Do not get the cast wet; but once it is dry, individuals can decorate the cast. The cast should be examined to ensure the cast is not too tight. A tight cast may limit blood flow and cause necrosis, and may need to be bi-halved (cut in half). The nurse must assess the skin distal to the cast (color, sensation, movement, temperature, and pulses).

If the patient requires an external fixation device, the patient will have metal pins inserted into the bone. The metal pins are attached to metal rods that will stabilize the bones during healing. External fixation devices are used when the patient has suffered complex injuries. This device is often used in an effort to prevent amputation in cases where the limb has sustained multiple fractures of varying severity. Pin care using aseptic technique, as directed by the physician, will be required to help lessen the risk of osteomyelitis and infection of tissue.

Fracture injuries can also result in CS. CS occurs when extreme pressure (from edema) occurs within the extremity. The intense pressure causes reduced blood flow, and ischemia occurs. Signs and symptoms include poor capillary refill, paresthesia, pain, pallor, and paralysis. Without surgical intervention, the extremity can develop loss of muscles, nerves, and functionality. A fasciotomy must be performed to decompress the extremities. The wound remains open to prevent further compromise.

The nurse should monitor fracture injuries for pallor, pain, and pressure. If the skin color is pale, it could be a sign of decreased perfusion. Pain can be expected from the injury, but intense, unrelenting pain not in proportion to the type of injury is a sign that the injury is worsening. The extremity's skin will look extremely tight and taut, and may appear shiny. This is a medical emergency. The doctor must be notified immediately.

Pelvic fractures can happen in motor vehicle crashes (MVCs) or be caused by a fall. An open-book pelvic fracture occurs in traumatic injuries when the bones of the pelvis are forced open (such as when a pedestrian is struck by an automobile). A pelvic sling must be applied in efforts to keep the pelvis aligned. Patients that sustain open-book pelvic fractures are at great risk for injuring other organs, and therefore should not be moved unless ordered by the physician. Hemorrhaging is of great concern because the fracture may cause intra-abdominal injuries (sharp bone edges of the pelvis may injure the bladder or the colon). Infection and risk of deep vein thrombosis are of great concern.

If the patient sustains a closed-book pelvic fracture, the severity of the fracture will determine the medical treatment. Stable closed-book fractures may only require bed rest. More severe cases may require a hip spica cast, external fixation devices, or skeletal traction.

A hip fracture can occur from a fall or a trauma. The patient presents with pain and a shortening of the extremity. The limb is usually externally rotated. The patient requires open reduction and internal fixation (ORIF) surgery to repair the hip. Until surgery can be performed, the patient is placed in Buck's traction to align the bones and reduce muscle spasms. After surgery, an abduction pillow will be used to keep the hip from dislodgement and internal rotation.

Facial fractures can occur from injury or physical altercations. The nurse's main objective is to ensure a patent airway. If the injuries are severe, teeth or blood can occlude the airway. Even if the fractures do not involve the airway, the nurse may need to monitor for swelling that can impend circulation. For example, orbital fractures may jeopardize the eye. Mandibular fractures may need immobilization (the patient's jaw is wired). A tracheostomy tray and wire cutters need to be at the bedside. With facial fractures, never insert a tube, such as a nasal endotracheal or nasogastric tube, into the nose. Depending on the type of facial fracture, a tracheostomy may be required to maintain the airway.

A cervical fracture will require stabilization and immobilization of the spine. Halo or Crutchfield tongs will be secured by pins attached to the skull or by surgical intervention.

AMPUTATIONS

Unfortunately, there are some injuries that require amputation. The physician must determine whether blood flow is sufficient and will order vascular studies. The limb will be assessed for the type of surgery required. The amputation will be performed to create a stump for future weight bearing. The patient should be informed that phantom limb pain may be experienced. Phantom pain is very real to the patient even though the limb has been amputated. The patient needs to be reassured, and pain medications as well as alternative therapies should be administered. Whether the patient receives a below-the-knee or above-the-knee amputation, the nurse should ensure that there are no pillows placed below the remaining leg. Elevating the remaining leg can result in flexion contractures.

ADDITIONAL MUSCULOSKELETAL SYSTEM INJURIES

Additional injuries can occur in the musculoskeletal system. (Note that this discussion is not all inclusive.) A sprain is an injury to the ligaments surrounding a joint. When a patient experiences a sprain, the injury is diagnosed by the various levels of damage that occur. A sprain at Level 1 is a mild injury, involving minor tearing of ligaments that usually will heal without medical intervention. The patient only needs to rest and prevent further aggravation to the site. A sprain at Level 2 results in partial tearing of the ligament, with additional swelling and increased pain, and may require surgical intervention. A third-degree sprain involves the total tearing of the ligament and requires surgical intervention. There are many nerve endings at the joint areas, accounting for the tremendous amount of pain experienced when a sprain occurs. A cervical sprain in the neck from trauma caused by acceleration and deceleration (whiplash) will affect the patient's ability to maintain normal neck movement. The muscles and ligaments may become so weak that the patient may experience further injury. A cervical collar may be required.

A strain occurs when a muscle is overstretched. The levels of injury related to strains are similar to those of sprains. A strain at Level 1 is a mildly "pulled" or tight muscle. A strain at Level 2 reveals a moderate muscle tear. A strain at Level 3 means that the muscle is severely torn. Again, the degree of injury determines the need for medical intervention.

A dislocation is the total displacement of the bone from its socket. It is an orthopedic emergency. When the bone is forced free of its socket (usually from trauma), there is a high risk of necrosis that can occur from the disruption of normal vascular blood flow. The bones must be realigned. The surgical procedure to realign the bone with its joint is called a closed reduction. Postsurgery, the affected extremity must be immobilized to allow healing. A subluxation is the partial dislocation of the bone from its socket and it places the patient at the same risk as a total dislocation.

Carpal tunnel syndrome occurs when the median nerve is compressed, resulting in a compression neuropathy. The causes of carpal tunnel syndrome include trauma, arthritis, a ganglia cyst, or inflammation. This condition is often seen in patients whose profession requires repetitive motion of the wrist (assembly-line workers, seamstresses, and typists). Symptoms that present are weakness, numbness, pain, and decreased sensation. A positive Phalen's test produces a tingling or numbness when the wrist is held for a full minute.

Rotator cuff injuries may occur due to aging, overuse (baseball pitcher), or trauma. A rotator cuff injury presents with a decreased ability to perform ROM exercises, weakness, and pain. The rotator cuff injury can be diagnosed by an MRI test. If the injury is severe, surgery is necessary.

Meniscus injury is common among athletes. The stress placed on the knee during athletics can cause a tear in the meniscus. The McMurray test is performed (the knee is flexed, internally rotated, and then extended). The patient may state that the knee feels unstable. Surgical intervention is a choice if the limitations of the knee affect the patient's occupation or cause physical limitations and pain.

Bursitis is the inflammation of the small fluid-fill sac that decreases the friction between bones and tissue. An injury (joggers) or disease process (rheumatoid arthritis, gout, or infection) can cause the bursa to become inflamed. The inflammation causes

Medication Forms

Listed in the vertical box is a medication. For each of the remaining boxes list the following:

Box 1: List a laboratory result you would need to monitor. Explain the significance of the laboratory test to the medication.
Box 2: List one food that may interact with the medication. Explain the significance of the food item to the medication.
Box 3: List one patient educational instruction you would give to the patient regarding the medication. Explain the significance of the instruction to the medication.

List other educational information you could provide this patient. Are there websites you can refer to? What about travel overseas and health issues? How should the medication be stored? Does the medication being administered interfere with other medications?

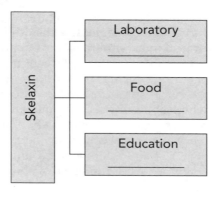

Listed in the vertical box is a medication. For each of the remaining boxes list the following:

Box 1: List a laboratory result you would need to monitor. Explain the significance of the laboratory test to the medication.
Box 2: List one food that may interact with the medication. Explain the significance of the food item to the medication.
Box 3: List one patient educational instruction you would give to the patient regarding the medication. Explain the significance of the instruction to the medication.

List other educational information you could provide this patient. Are there websites you can refer to? What about travel overseas and health issues? How should the medication be stored? Does the medication being administered interfere with other medications?

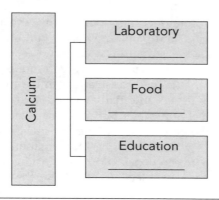

decreased function and pain. Treatment (ice pack, immobilization, and elevation) is geared toward reducing the inflammation. NSAIDs are used for pain and inflammation.

MUSCULOSKELETAL SYSTEM EXERCISE

Choose an athlete who participates in an outdoor sport. Write about the muscles involved when your chosen athlete performs his or her sport. The report should include what each muscle is doing (flexion, extension), what muscle groups it may work with, whether strength or endurance are involved, and what muscles may be antagonistic. Note which muscles are more prone to sports-related injuries and be sure to include the heart muscle in this assignment. This assignment is due by the next clinical preconference.

MUSCULOSKELETAL SYSTEM CASES

Read the following cases and answer the questions. Return by preconference next week.

CASE #1

A 24-year-old female suffered a compound fracture of her right humerus and right radius 8 months ago. Her right arm was placed initially in an external fixator device. She now complains of a severe burning sensation and pain in her right arm complicated by muscle wasting. She has also noticed temperature changes between her arms with a change in color. She was diagnosed with complex regional pain syndrome (CRPS or reflex sympathetic dystrophy).

1. What is CRPS?
2. What causes CRPS?
3. How is it diagnosed?
4. What and where are the signs and symptoms?
5. What is the treatment for this condition?
6. What nursing treatment modalities need to be addressed with this patient?

ANSWERS TO CASE #1

1. CRPS is a painful dysfunction and disuse syndrome characterized by abnormal pain and swelling of the affected extremity. The injury produces overactivity of the sympathetic nervous system. There are different types of CRPS that may involve nerve damage and may become chronic.

2. Some of the causes include trauma, surgery, stroke, shingles, and heart disease.

3. Sympathetic nervous system tests, MRI, and bone scan.

4. Severe burning sensation and pain in patient's right arm, muscle wasting, temperature changes, thickened skin, and contractures.

5. Spinal cord stimulators, nerve blocks, steroids, antiseizure and antidepressant medications, and PT.

6. Nursing treatment modalities that need to be addressed with this patient are:

- Pain
- Body image

- Tissue perfusion
- Emotional support
- Mobility
- Patient teaching about the disease

CASE #2

A 56-year-old female had not been seen for 2 days. When her family investigated, she was found on her left side. She had suffered a stroke to her left temporal hemorrhagic subdural without midline shift on CT scan. She has a past medical history of congestive heart disease, chronic obstructive pulmonary disease, deep vein thrombosis, and atrial fibrillation. On admission, she has right-sided weakness and edema to her right-side extremities. Urine is decreased and dark red. Patient has been diagnosed with rhabdomyolysis in addition to her stroke. The creatine kinase (CPK) is 30,000 mcg/mL, myoglobin 1,500 ng/mL, and potassium 5.6. One day later, the nurse has noticed blanching of the right arm, capillary refill greater than 3 seconds, and radial pulse of 1+. The physician was notified immediately, and the patient was diagnosed with CS.

1. What is rhabdomyolysis?
2. What is the significance of this leakage of these proteins and enzymes?
3. What causes rhabdomyolysis?
4. What are the signs and symptoms?
5. How is rhabdomyolysis diagnosed?
6. What treatment should be done?
7. What is compartment syndrome and why is it an emergency?
8. Why is the potassium elevated?

ANSWERS TO CASE #2

1. Rhabdomyolysis is the rapid destruction of the myoglobin protein in the urine. CPK, which assists with chemical reactions in the cells, is also released. Since tissue is damaged, the tissue will release potassium from cells, causing hyperkalemia.

2. These enzymes will clog the filtering tubules in the kidneys, causing renal failure.

3. The more common causes are: muscle trauma, burns, infection, immobility, drug intoxication (especially cocaine), myopathies, myxedema coma, statins, psychiatric drugs, hypothermia, and hyperthermia.

4. Signs and symptoms include stiffness and weakness, dark urine, nausea, and confusion.

5. Rhabdomyolysis is diagnosed with lab studies: complete blood count, complete metabolic panel, liver function tests, urinalysis, and CPK.

6. Stop the offending drug, hydration, and treatment with sodium bicarbonate and Mannitol (osmotic diuretic).

7. Compartment syndrome is a condition in which damage to an area causes edema and increased pressure, which in turn causes compromised tissue circulation and function. Irreversible changes can occur in hours and may require surgical intervention (fasciotomy).

8. The potassium may be elevated because of dehydration but also may be elevated because of potassium being released from the muscle tissue because of the injury.

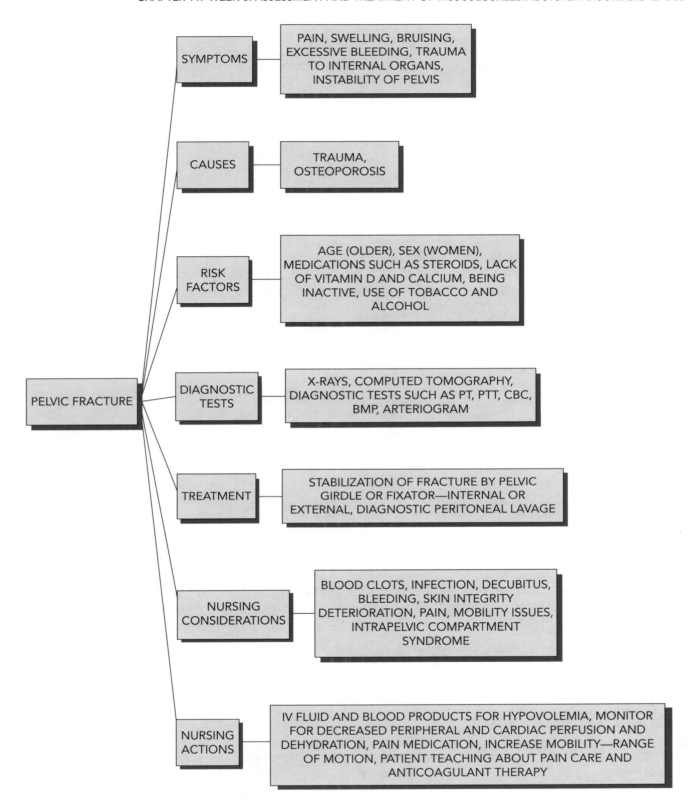

FIGURE 11-2 Example of a concept map.

WEEK 8 POSTCONFERENCE

Encourage students to discuss the abnormalities of their patients' musculoskeletal systems. Inquire whether the students noticed their own musculoskeletal systems while they were bending, lifting, or walking. Inquire whether the students understand the need to use appropriate ergonomics. For example, are they arranging the bed or performing tasks and using equipment in a safe and efficient manner, such as lifting with their legs and not with their back? Ask students to include in their discussion how ergonomics affect their profession.

Chapter 12

PHARMACOLOGY, PATIENT SAFETY, AND LABORATORY TESTS

This chapter examines:

- Pharmacology and patient safety
- Importance of lab work in understanding specific patient responses to medications
- Potential for drug interactions and toxicities
- Safe medication administration

Week 9 discusses pharmacology and the important relationship of laboratory tests to administering medications. It is important to stress the need for patient safety when administering medications. Students should be able to successfully verbalize the "five rights" of medication administration.

Discussing the ways that errors can occur will help the students to understand how easily mistakes can happen. Stress that the bedside nurse is on the front line of patient safety and is the last safety check before any and all medications are given. It is the bedside nurse's responsibility to ensure that the right medication and right dosage reach the right patient at the right time, via the right route. Students should be encouraged to research the process that takes place when a medication error occurs.

WEEK 9 PRECONFERENCE

Hand out:
- Pharmacology exercise
- Medication forms (oxycodone and aspirin)
- Medication survey

Collect:
- Musculoskeletal exercise
- Musculoskeletal cases
- Medication forms (Skelaxin and calcium)
- Care plans
- Physical assessment form
- Journals

Instruct students that they must discretely observe other nurses as they pass medications. Students will be expected to discuss in postconference the manner in which the medications were obtained and how the nurse identified the patient. Did the nurse explain the medications to the patient? Did the nurse assess appropriate lab work or vital signs before administration? Was sterile technique used with IV fluid administration? Did the students observe any actions that may be considered unsafe?

MEDICATION ADMINISTRATION AND SAFETY

Patients today are rarely treated without the use of pharmacological interventions. It is therefore necessary to understand how drugs work. The body must process medications for the medications to be effective. Medications travel throughout the body and undergo various processes in order to be useful to the patient. The medication is administered and must then reach the intended cell sites to be effective.

Medications come in many forms and they offer the opportunity to be administered via different routes. It is important to note that medications affect different people in different ways. How people absorb medications may depend on many factors, including age, lifestyles, weight, and route of medication administration.

Oral medications, once swallowed, are dissolved in gastric fluid (bile). The medication is then absorbed into the bloodstream system via the small intestine. The absorption of some medications may be affected if they are taken with food. Acidic foods or beverages may destroy the medication, rendering it useless. The absorption of certain medications (e.g., acetaminophen and Dilantin) is reduced when taken with food. Vitamins, as well, can reduce the effectiveness of certain medications if they are taken together.

Medications administered via intramuscular injection (IM) are absorbed quickly and more effectively than are oral medications. The IM medication reaches the bloodstream more rapidly. Intravascular (IV) medications also reach the target cells quickly because the medication is administered directly into the bloodstream. Most medications bind to target receptors, although there are some medications that do not act on target cell receptors. Medications that change gastric pH are used to neutralize gastric acid. Chelating drugs bind with heavy metals (lead) to promote excretion.

Dose and frequency are medication variables that determine the patient's response to a medication. Patients who are fearful of becoming "addicted" to a narcotic may not take the prescribed dosage of the narcotic and may not take it at the prescribed frequency. The patient's decision to limit intake of the prescribed medication will cause an ineffective result, because the dose is too low.

On the other hand, a patient may take larger-than-prescribed doses of the medication. The "more is better" rationale for a continuously or chronically used medication can result in toxicity. Although all medications come with a warning label, the recommended medication dosages are only guidelines.

Some medications should be taken 1 hour before or 2 hours after a meal, and others may need to be taken on an empty stomach to ensure adequate absorption. Nurses should be aware of any potential food and drug interactions. Patient education should be given if a prescribed medication has a probability of a food and drug interaction. Patients should be encouraged to make efforts to ensure that medication and food interactions do not occur.

Patients prescribed Coumadin should be told to avoid dark green leafy vegetables. Dark green leafy vegetables contain vitamin K. Vitamin K is the antagonist to Coumadin. Taking monoamine oxidase inhibitors (MAOIs) when consuming cheese or wine, which both contain tyramine, results in a release of norepinephrine that renders the MAOI ineffective and may place the patient in grave danger by elevating the blood pressure. Grapefruit, when consumed as a food or a beverage, prevents the metabolism of certain medications (statins).

Some medications can interfere with other medications. One medication may either hinder or potentiate the effectiveness of another medication. For example, a patient using a prescribed narcotic may consume a glass of wine or beer. The alcohol potentiates the effect of the narcotic, resulting in a sedative effect. This can and often does cause respiratory depression.

A patient may be prescribed a topical medication (lidocaine patch) to be used along with a prescribed narcotic medication. This synergistic effect allows better pain management. This blend reduces the need to increase the dosage of the narcotic and thus provides greater patient safety. Some topical medications, such as nitro paste ointment, are changed every 6 hours for therapeutic effect. The nurse must be mindful of where the topical medication is applied so that it can be changed with the next dose, or taken off in emergencies such as defibrillation or the need to remove a patch due to hypotension.

There are circumstances, because of disease processes, when medications are given through a gastrectomy or nasal gastric tube. Medications that need to be crushed are administered via a gastrectomy or nasal gastric tube. Ensure that the medication is not Enteric coated. Enteric coated medications should never be crushed. Students should be instructed that any medications that are combined for administration are compatible. This will prevent clogging of the tube, medication interactions, wasting of medications, and so on. Many students will observe during clinical that the pills to be administered are frequently placed together and then crushed. This is a topic for discussion, and the instructor should ensure proper administration of the drugs. Each medication should be crushed individually and then mixed in 10 mL of water, then 10 mL of water is given to flush the tube to ensure patency. Keep an accurate measurement of the fluid given so that it can be included in the patient's intake total. Sometimes tube feedings must be withheld for 2 hours both before and after administration of a drug such as Dilantin suspension, because the tube feedings will decrease the absorption of the drug. In cases like this where tube feedings are withheld, the dietary team has to be informed so that they can properly assess the patient's nutritional needs.

As people age, their ability to process medications may decline. The older adult has a reduced amount of metabolizing enzymes in the liver. This physiological change can result in an accumulation of medications in their system. Many older adults are polypharmaceutical users, meaning they use an increased number of medications. This increases the risk of medication-to-medication interaction, potentiation, or overdose.

It is prudent for the nurse to be aware of the antidote for each medication administered, if applicable. The following table is a list (not all inclusive) of antidotes to various medications.

Medication	Antidote
Acetaminophen	Acetylcysteine (Mucomyst)
Anticholinergics	Physostigmine
Benzodiazepines	Flumazenil (Romazicon)
Beta blocker toxicity	Glucagon
Calcium channel blocker toxicity	Calcium gluconate
Digoxin	Digoxin immune Fab (Digibind)
Heparin	Protamine sulfate
Magnesium	Calcium gluconate
Opioids	Naloxone (Narcan)
Thrombolytics	Aminocaproic acid (Amicar)
Tricyclics	Sodium bicarbonate
Warfarin (Coumadin)	Phytonadione (vitamin K), fresh frozen plasma
Oral toxins (check with poison control)	Activated charcoal with sorbitol

IMPORTANT FACTS CONCERNING ORAL MEDICATIONS

Oral medications should be taken with or without food, as directed, to enhance therapeutic absorption. Enteric-coated medications should *never* be chewed, crushed, or halved for easier swallowing. Extended-release medications should *never* be crushed. Crushing extended-release or long-acting medications (such as extended-release medication in a capsule), can result in consumption of a toxic dose. If the time-released medication is contained within a capsule, never open and administer the contents. Some time-released medications such as potassium chloride (KCL) can be mixed with a small amount of water and then be administered as a "slurry." Other medications in a capsule that are not time-released medications can be taken out of the capsule form and administered, but always consult with the pharmacist first.

HERBAL REMEDIES

Patients may not even consider the herbal remedies they take as medications, but herbal remedies often do have medication properties. The nurse should inquire whether the patient uses herbal remedies. Herbal remedies are not usually monitored by the Food and Drug Administration (FDA) and they often have unknown ingredients (especially metals) or properties that increase coagulopathy. Herbal remedies are also marketed as being safe for use for various conditions, and this may delay the patient from seeking appropriate health care advice. Herbs will increase the risk of bleeding if used in conjunction with anticoagulation medications such as aspirin or warfarin. Herbs that stimulate the immune system may counteract medications used in preventing transplant rejection, may exacerbate a pre-existing autoimmune disease, or may precipitate an autoimmune disease in people genetically predisposed to such disorders.

Patients taking immunosuppressant drugs such as cyclosporine, corticosteroids, prednisone, or methotrexate should be educated not to take the herbs alfalfa, astragalus, echinacea, ginseng, or licorice root, or the mineral zinc.

Many herbal and dietary supplements claim to be effective in treating various conditions; however, appropriate studies often do not support the labeled claims. For example, ginger has been "said" to treat nausea. Although ginger may work as well as a piece of candy in treating nausea, ginger in fact increases coagulopathy and increases the risk of miscarriages. It is therefore advisable to thoroughly research herbal medications prior to consuming them. The website for the National Center for Complementary and Alternative Medicine (NCCAM; www.nccam.nih.gov) is a great place to find accurate information on herbal medicines.

RECOGNIZING DRUG TOXICITIES AND PREVENTING ADVERSE REACTIONS

The effects of medications on the body may be good or bad. It is important to understand how the medications work, their actions, desired effects, and contraindications. Medications are usually excreted or "cleared" by the liver (hepatic) or kidneys (renal). It is therefore important to determine the patient's ability to excrete medications. Evaluate blood urea nitrogen (BUN), creatinine (CR), and liver function tests (LFTs).

Drug toxicities are usually caused by a high dose of a particular medication in the system. High levels can occur from increased ingestion (chronic usage), larger dose ingestion (the "more is better" rationale or a suicide attempt), or impaired excretion. High levels of various medications may present with "signs" such as the patient complaining of "ringing in the ears" (tinnitus) from medications such as aspirin, antibiotics (-mycins), and diuretics (Lasix).

Patients should be educated on monitoring for signs of toxicity. Patients should also be informed not to abruptly stop any medication without first consulting with their primary care physician (PCP). Patients should be notified that routine laboratory testing may be required to verify that adequate excretion of prescribed medications is occurring.

The aging individual may have decreased gastric absorption, decreased hepatic clearance, and reduced renal drug excretion ability, as well as less body water and fat. The aging individual must be monitored more closely for toxicity.

Medication	Adverse Reaction	Drug-to-Drug Interaction	Laboratory Tests
Gentamicin	Nephrotoxicity	Acyclovir, amphotericin B, cephalosporins, and vancomycin	BUN, creatinine, gentamicin level
Amoxicillin, penicillin (PCN)	Anaphylactic reaction	Hormonal contraceptives	WBC, H/H, K, BUN, creatinine
Ancef	Seizures, anaphylactic reaction	Aminoglycosides	ALT, AST
Bactrim	Hepatic jaundice	Cyclosporine	BUN and creatinine
Acyclovir	Acute renal failure	Interferon	BUN and creatinine
Atenolol	Heart failure	NSAIDs and oral antidiabetic medications	BUN and creatinine
Mevacor	Rhabdomyolysis	Antifungals (Azole)	ALT, AST, and CK
Oxycodone	Respiratory depression	Anticoagulants and alcohol	Amylase, lipase
Dilantin	Toxic hepatitis	Amiodarone and antihistamines	Dilantin
Robinul	Anaphylactic reaction	Zantac and antihistamines	None
Zofran	Arrhythmias	Cimetidine, phenobarbital, and rifampin	ALT, AST, BUN, CR
Decadron	Acute adrenal insufficiency	Antidiabetics, NSAIDs	Glucose
Progesterone	Pulmonary embolism	Antiseizure medications	Hepatic profile
Aldactone	Hyperkalemia	ACE inhibitors	BUN, potassium
Coumadin	Hepatitis	Acetaminophen	ALT, AST, INR, PT, PTT
Allopurinol	Renal failure, hepatitis	Amoxicillin, anticoagulants	ALT, AST

Note: Many of the medications listed require monitoring of renal and hepatic functioning to ensure toxicity does not occur.

The nurse should monitor every patient for toxicity. A baseline laboratory level should be drawn on admission to determine the patient's renal and hepatic functions. Baseline lab work should always be done prior to initiation of medications such as heparin, Coumadin, and streptokinase. Medications such as Tylenol and antibiotics are withheld until the blood cultures are obtained. Many medications have therapeutic levels and the physician should be reminded to order laboratory baseline levels of these medications on admission. For example, lithium can become toxic if the level is greater than 2 mmol/L. If the patient must be NPO (nothing by mouth), dehydration may increase the patient's level. The following table lists a variety of medications (not all inclusive) and their adverse reactions, drug-to-drug interactions, and laboratory tests.

SAFE DRUG ADMINISTRATION

Administering medication is an important and vital step in the recovery of patients. It is necessary to provide safe drug administration. To ensure safe drug administration, it is important to ensure patient safety during each step of the drug administration process.

The nurse should not expect the doctor or pharmacist to be solely responsible to prevent incorrect dosages of medications. Errors occur in transcription, translation, and dispensing. The nurse must ensure that the order is for a safe and correct dose. There are many medications on the market. Many of the medications have very similar names. It is prudent to double check the original order to ensure the medication is the intended prescribed medication.

The nurse is responsible for knowing the peak and duration of each drug. For example, metoprolol 25 mg should be ordered every 6 hours for a myocardial infarction. The duration of the drug is 6 hours and the peak is usually 3.5 hours. The physician may order this drug as "QID" (four times a day) thinking that it means the same as "every 6 hours," which is inaccurate. The pharmacy will transcribe the order as QID, which according to their schedule is usually 8:00 a.m., noon, 4:00 p.m., and 8:00 p.m. This will result in overdosage of the medication, because the drug was supposed to be administered at 6:00 a.m., noon, 6:00 p.m., and midnight. This will result in a wide variance of effects on the patient. TID (three times a day) and QID orders must be carefully screened, depending on the type of drug being administered.

Abbreviations have also caused problems with medication administration. A list of do-not-use abbreviations has been developed to ensure patient safety:

- U, u (unit); write out "UNIT"
- IU (international unit); write out "INTERNATIONAL UNIT"
- QD, qd, Q.D., q.d. (each day); write out "DAILY"
- QOD, qod, Q.O.D., qod (every other day); write out "EVERY OTHER DAY"
- MS (morphine sulfate); write out morphine sulfate
- Mg (magnesium); write out magnesium
- 5.0 mg; do not use a trailing zero; write 5 mg
- .5mg; needs a leading zero; write 0.5 mg

Each hospital develops a list of abbreviations that are not to be used and have the potential to increase the risk of medication error.

Abbreviated medication names can also be misinterpreted. Physicians should write out the full name of all medications ordered to ensure safety. High-risk medications use capital letters for look-alike drug names that are often confused, such as oxyCODONE and OxyCONTIN. Remember the five rights of drug administration: Ensure the right patient, the right medication, the right drug, the right route, and the right time.

Electronic medical records require the nurse to scan the patient's identification band as well as the medication ordered prior to administration. Nurses may get a false sense of security from this practice. The nurse is still responsible to ensure the medication is the actual medication ordered, at the right dose, the right time, the right route, and most importantly, is being administered to the right patient. Critical thinking must also be utilized with this process, and medications can be withheld if there are contraindications. The doctor should be informed of any withholding or refusal of medication.

PHARMACOLOGY EXERCISE

Answer the following questions and return by preconference next week.

1. What would the nurse monitor for in order to assess for signs or symptoms of nephrotoxicity and ototoxicity?
2. Are there nursing actions that can prevent nephrotoxicity? If so, explain.
3. List the laboratory values that should be monitored when a drug is metabolized.
4. List the most serious and adverse effect that can occur with antibiotics.
5. List what may be considered as reactions to an administered medication. What is the difference between a side effect and an adverse reaction?
6. At what times should antibiotic medication be given?
7. List the five rights of medication administration.

ANSWERS TO PHARMACOLOGY EXERCISE

1. Changes in renal function (BUN and creatinine) and changes in hearing (detectable with audiometry only).
2. Adequate hydration, lower dose of medication, and longer duration of frequency.

3. Liver function tests.
4. Anaphylactic reaction.
5. Skin rash, urticaria, difficulty in breathing, seizures, and anaphylactic reaction. A side effect is a symptom found after taking a medication that is a natural consequence of the drug. An adverse reaction is a side effect that is of a serious nature and may be life threatening for the patient.
6. Some antibiotics should not be consumed with certain foods and drinks. Others should not be taken with food in your stomach—these would normally be taken about an hour before meals, or two hours after.
7. Right patient, right medication, right dosage, right route, and right time.

Medication Forms

Listed in the vertical box is a medication. For each of the remaining boxes, list the following:

Box 1: List a laboratory result you would need to monitor. Explain the significance of the laboratory test to the medication.
Box 2: List one food that may interact with the medication. Explain the significance of the food item to the medication.
Box 3: List one patient educational instruction you would give to the patient regarding the medication. Explain the significance of the instruction to the medication.

List other educational information you could provide this patient. Are there websites you can refer to? What about travel overseas and health issues? How should the medication be stored?

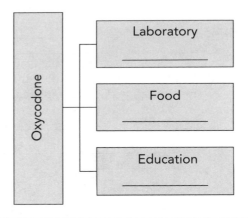

Listed in the vertical box is a medication. For each of the remaining boxes, list the following:

Box 1: List a laboratory result you would need to monitor. Explain the significance of the laboratory test to the medication.
Box 2: List one food that may interact with the medication. Explain the significance of the food item to the medication.
Box 3: List one patient educational instruction you would give to the patient regarding the medication. Explain the significance of the instruction to the medication.

List other educational information you could provide this patient. Are there websites you can refer to? What about travel overseas and health issues? How should the medication be stored?

Aspirin	Laboratory _____
	Food _____
	Education _____

MEDICATION SURVEY

Answer the following questions and return by preconference next week.

1. Take a walk to your neighborhood pharmacy, or look at the drugs in your medicine cabinet. List at least six of the various medications available over the counter (OTC).

_____
_____
_____
_____
_____
_____.

2. Read the labels of several of the medications (paying special attention to the respiratory and leg cramp medications). Do any of the OTC medications contain what normally would be a prescription medication? If so, list those medications.

_____
_____
_____
_____
_____.

WEEK 9 POSTCONFERENCE

Inquire whether the students were able to observe the administration of medications. Were there any actions or behaviors that seemed inappropriate? Students should be informed that learning can be from positive as well as negative examples. Inquire whether students saw nurses systematically using the principles discussed in this chapter to ensure patient safety while administering medications. Discuss what each student believes is the most challenging part of medication administration. Discuss each response.

Inform students that pharmacology is one of the areas that can be the most critical to a patient. Patients require safe and timely medication administration. Patients trust the nurse to know what medications have been ordered, the rationale for the medication, the safe dosage for the patient, adverse reactions, and incompatibilities. The nurse holds a great trust and should continue to uphold that trust by practicing medication safety.

Chapter 13

CRITICAL CARE NURSING

This chapter examines:

- Anatomy, physiology, and electrophysiology of the heart
- Assessment of heart function diagnosis and treatment of irregular heart conditions
- Respiratory system, brain, and renal system

Week 10 will briefly touch on key topics (not all inclusive) that arise in critical care nursing. The potential for any hospitalized patient to deteriorate is great. Although there are usually certain warning signs that present prior to the patient becoming severely ill, the medical–surgical nurse may not be adequately trained or skilled to observe those signs. When a patient requires more intensive monitoring and care, the patient is transported from the medical–surgical unit to the critical care or intensive care unit. The critical care nurse must be skilled in the necessary observations and interventions to care for the critically ill patient.

Critical care nursing is often a challenge to teach because it requires the nurse learning to make rapid assessments and then determine nursing interventions based on those findings. The nurse's skill in observation and determining interventions often prevents further deterioration of the patient, or could provide lifesaving action.

Discuss what the students discovered last week when observing the nurses passing medications. Were there divergences from the five rights? Did the students observe the nurses comparing the patient's information with the medication administrative record? Were there any interesting discoveries?

WEEK 10 PRECONFERENCE

Hand out:

- Anatomy exercise
- Medication forms (metoprolol and nitroglycerin)
- Critical thinking exercise

Collect:

- Medication forms (oxycodone and aspirin)
- Pharmacology exercise
- Medication survey form
- Care plans
- Physical assessment form
- Journals

Inform the students that this week focuses on critically ill patients and the nursing skills required to care for those patients. The instructor may need to obtain permission to allow the students to take a guided tour of the intensive care or critical care units. If the students will tour the critical care units, inform them that they will be required to list all the various kinds of equipment and then discuss the differences between their assigned units and the critical care area.

ANATOMY AND PHYSIOLOGY OF THE HEART

To become proficient in critical care nursing, the nurse must understand the basic anatomy and physiology of the heart.

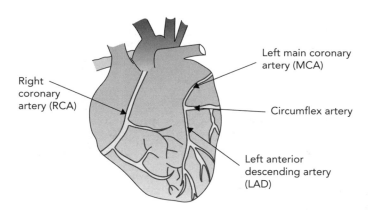

When the anatomy is learned, it is easy to understand what cardiac tissue can be affected when an occlusion occurs. Originating from the aorta, the right coronary artery (RCA) is located between the right atrium and ventricle. The RCA supplies blood to the right side of the heart and supplies the Bundle of His (the muscle that connects the atria with the ventricles) and the atrioventricular (AV) node (fibers located at the base of the interatrial septum that transmit the cardiac impulses from the sinoatrial [SA] node).

The left main coronary artery (MCA) branches into the left anterior descending artery (LAD) and the circumflex artery, which supply blood to the left side of the heart. The LAD supplies the anterior wall of the left ventricle, right bundle branch, and walls of the left ventricle.

The left circumflex artery supplies the lateral walls of left ventricle, left atrium, and 50% of the SA node. Blood leaves through the left ventricle into the aorta. The aorta is the main trunk of the systemic artery system that carries blood from the left ventricle, where it branches off into the two main coronary arteries that supply the entire heart muscle.

There is an opening in the aorta above the aortic valve, called the coronary ostium, that feeds blood to the coronary arteries. When the left ventricle is pumping blood through the aorta, the aortic valve is open and the coronary ostium is partly covered.

The inferior vena cava and superior vena cava carry deoxygenated blood from the body into the right atrium. The pulmonary artery (PA) carries blood away from the right ventricle, where it splits into the right and left pulmonary arteries, which carry blood into the right and left lungs. The four pulmonary veins, two on the right and two on the left, carry oxygenated blood from the right and left lungs into the left atrium.

View the diagram above. Note that occlusion of the left main coronary artery is known as the "widow maker." It is justly labeled so, because the myocardium (heart muscle) would be deprived of oxygen and nutrients if the LAD and the circumflex artery were denied blood flow. When the myocardium becomes ischemic, this results in injury to the cardiac muscle (ischemia) or tissue death (infarction).

KEY NOTE: The heart is the only muscle in the body that never rests. It is consistently working.

ELECTROPHYSIOLOGY OF THE HEART

To continue with the anatomy of the heart, the electrophysiology of the heart should be explained.

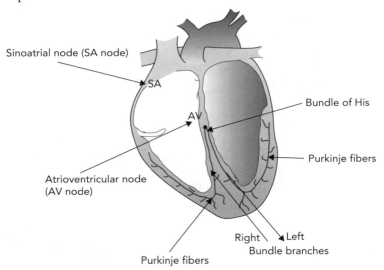

Each heartbeat begins with an electrical impulse. The electrical impulse is initiated in the SA node located in the right atria. The electrical impulse spreads throughout the atrial musculature and stimulates atrial contraction. The electrical impulse continues to the AV node and continues to the Bundle of His. The electrical impulse travels down the left and right bundles, reaching the Purkinje fibers and resulting in ventricular contraction.

KEY NOTE: Cardiac cells have an inherent characteristic of being able to assume the role of pacemaker in the event that the SA node is unable to or fails to act as the pacemaker, or when an abnormality occurs.

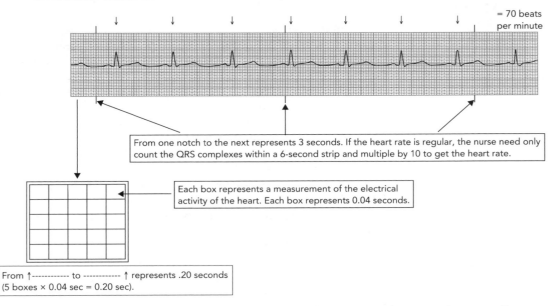

Each electrical impulse in the heart can be measured on an electrocardiogram (ECG, also known as EKG). The EKG is used to assess the electrical functions of the heart, heart disease, pacemaker integrity, and medication effectiveness. An EKG can also be used to gain baseline patient information or as a prescreening tool for surgical patients.

> **KEY NOTE:** To obtain an EKG, electrodes (stickers with conductive gel) are applied to specific areas of the body. The predetermined areas for the electrodes allow for various "electrical" pictures to be taken of the heart. The EKG uses 12 leads (different angles) to view the heart. The precordial leads are V1 through V6. The limb leads are placed on the arms and legs. Be aware that an EKG is usually a left-sided EKG, but a right-sided EKG, can also be done to evaluate the right ventricle. An EKG machine will usually determine the rhythm with measurements, but the nurse still needs to assess the EKG rhythm.

Critical care areas use continuous cardiac monitoring. Critical care monitors demonstrate one or two lead views with some monitors offering the capability of providing a 12-lead view. For the purpose of discussion, this book discusses continuous cardiac monitors and cardiac rhythms (not all inclusive). Electrocardiogram basics follow below.

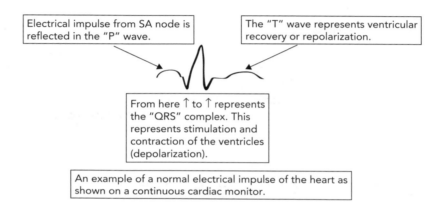

Electrical impulse from SA node is reflected in the "P" wave.

The "T" wave represents ventricular recovery or repolarization.

From here ↑ to ↑ represents the "QRS" complex. This represents stimulation and contraction of the ventricles (depolarization).

An example of a normal electrical impulse of the heart as shown on a continuous cardiac monitor.

CARDIAC IRREGULARITIES AND TREATMENT

Learning the normal electrical activity of the heart allows the nurse to recognize when the heart is demonstrating an irregularity. Here is an easy way to remember the "waves": For the "P-wave," think "P" as in "power"; this is where the electrical stimulation occurs. For the "QRS," think of "Q" as in "quest," that is, a quest to travel to the far reaches of the Purkinje fibers. For the "T" wave, think of "T" as in "tired." The heart is tired and needs to recuperate or repolarize. "QT" represents the time for both ventricular depolarization and repolarization to occur, and normal QT intervals are less than 0.44 seconds. Prolonged QT could be due to a genetic defect or to effects of drugs such as statins, antipsychotics, and cardiac medications such as beta blockers, antibiotics, and so on. It is important to measure these intervals to prevent life-threatening cardiac arrhythmias. A new formula that evaluates prolongation is the "QTc." If prolongation lasts more than 500 milliseconds the patient is placed at risk for life-threatening arrhythmias.

A regular or normal sinus rhythm indicates that the SA node initiates the electrical impulse and the electrical activity of the heart is discharged at a rate of 60 to 100 beats per minute (see rhythm strip on previous page).

When the SA node sends electrical signals at a rate of greater than 100 per minute, this rhythm is called sinus tachycardia. The heart rate may be elevated due to several causes, including exercise, elevated temperature, or anxiety. An elevated heart rate results in extra work of the heart. The extra workload of the heart requires greater oxygen consumption. This could pose a problem for a patient who is sensitive to ischemia (angina or myocardial infarction [MI]).

When the SA node sends electrical signals at a rate of less than 60 per minute, this rhythm is called sinus bradycardia. A slow heart rate may cause a decrease in cardiac output (CO). The patient may present with complaints of chest pain, symptoms of dizziness, or syncope due to reduced perfusion to the heart or the brain. It is wise to have atropine IV nearby in the event the patient becomes symptomatic. The patient may require a pacemaker if the heart rate remains too low.

When the atria receive chaotic electrical signals at a rate of 250 to 400 per minute, the atrium beats rapidly. However, the AV node blocks most of those impulses, resulting in multiple flutter waves (a series of 1 to 4 flutter waves) followed by a ventricular beat. The rhythm appears "sawtooth"-like. A patient who presents with symptomatic atrial flutter should be synchronized cardioverted. (Cardioversion is discussed later in this chapter.) Digoxin is the drug of choice to use in atrial flutter. The doctor will order Digoxin IV in several doses sufficient to achieve a controlled rate, a process called digitalization.

When an ectopic focus in the atrium sends electrical signals at a rate greater than 400 per minute, the atrial musculature cannot maintain that high rate. Unable to recover from the previous electrical response, the atrial contractions are erratic. The AV node cannot receive and respond to 400 beats per minute, and therefore, only a small portion of those electrical impulses activate the ventricles. The EKG strip may demonstrate frequent "f" waves with irregular ventricular contractions. This rhythm is called atrial fibrillation. The heart rate may be normal or may be accelerated. When the rate is extremely high, this is called "atrial fibrillation with a rapid ventricular response." Digoxin is the drug of choice for atrial fibrillation, but the patient's potassium level must also be addressed at this time. Synchronized cardioversion may also be used.

> **KEY NOTE:** Because the blood-rich ventricles are awaiting the signal from the erratic atrial musculature to pump blood into the system, clots can form in the pooled ventricular blood (loss of "atrial kick"). Patients with atrial fibrillation are placed on a blood thinner to prevent potential clots from causing cerebral embolic strokes, pulmonary emboli, or MIs. Coumadin is the drug of choice. Blood levels must be drawn to ensure that the PT and INR coagulation levels are at therapeutic range and, once at therapeutic level, every 3 months afterward. Patient education should be given regarding dietary considerations (avoid foods high in vitamin K).

Heart blocks resulting from AV conduction delays may be caused by pharmacological means or from tissue injury or ischemia at the AV node. Electrical conduction delays result in a lengthened PR interval (which is from the beginning of atrial contraction to the beginning of the ventricular contraction). If the PR interval measures greater than 0.20 on the EKG rhythm strip, this rhythm is considered a first-degree heart block. If the patient is asymptomatic, the only necessary measure is monitoring the patient's cardiac electrical activity to ensure the first-degree block does not progress to a second- or third-degree block.

The second-degree heart block has two classifications; Mobitz I and Mobitz II. In Mobitz II, the SA node sends out repetitive signals to the AV node. The AV node blocks most of the signals. What presents on the EKG monitor is a "P" wave that appears faithfully before each QRS complex; however, there are additional "P" waves accompanying each heartbeat. The number of impulses that reach the QRS complex will determine the number of "P" waves, being labeled as a 2:1, 3:1, or 4:1 block. This block is more often caused by ischemia to the AV node.

Another second-degree heart block, known as the Wenckebach block or Mobitz I, presents with the SA node sending signals to the AV node. The AV node irregularly blocks the electrical impulses, resulting in an EKG strip that shows the "P" wave before the consecutive ventricular complexes becoming wider and wider, until a ventricular complex drops and the cycle begins again.

KEY NOTE: Patients with a second-degree heart block are at a greater risk for progression to a third-degree heart block. It is wise to have a transvenous pacemaker nearby.

A third-degree heart block occurs when the AV node blocks all electrical activity from the SA node. The atrial musculature and the ventricles beat independently of each other (regularly).

KEY NOTE: The ventricles have an underlying rate of 40 beats per minute. Perfusion is the potential problem. The rate may be too slow to perfuse the body and the brain adequately. A permanent pacemaker is needed.

Junctional arrhythmias are impulses coming from a source in the area of the AV node with a rate of 40 to 60 beats per minute. This rhythm produces a narrow QRS complex and absent P waves. The junctional arrhythmia may be due to digitalis toxicity, which is treated with administration of atropine and Digibind.

Ventricular fibrillation occurs when the electrical impulses are erratic. The ventricles do not contract but instead quiver. This is a life-threatening condition. If a code is not called, or if intervention is not initiated immediately, the patient will die. Torsades de Pointes ("twisting of the point") is a distinctive type of ventricular tachycardia that can be caused by electrolyte imbalances, especially magnesium- and drug-induced QT prolongation.

Ventricular tachycardia can be baffling. It can present with a pulse or without a pulse. The underlying cause is usually MI. There are also various underlying diseases that may cause ventricular tachycardia. If the patient has a pulse, treat the underlying cause. If the patient is pulseless, call a code.

Asystole is the absence of any electrical activity. This condition is life-threatening. Assess the patient quickly before calling a code. The cardiac lead may have come loose, resulting in what appears as asystole on the cardiac monitor. As an old saying goes, "treat the patient and not the machine." If the patient is pulseless, call a code.

Pulseless electrical activity occurs when there is a rhythmic electrical activity of the heart but there is an absence of heart contractions. In other words, the telemetry (cardiac monitoring) will show a heart rhythm but the patient will not have a pulse and will be unresponsive. Always feel for a pulse—do not just rely on the telemetry. This is a life-threatening condition and can be due to many causes. The prognosis is poor unless the underlying cause is found and corrected. Among the many causes of pulseless electrical activity are acidosis, hypovolemia, tension pneumothorax, toxins (drug overdose), hypoxia, electrolyte imbalance, emboli (coronary or pulmonary), and cardiac tamponade.

It is important to understand the various physiological conditions that may present with the various cardiac rhythms. A patient diagnosed with acute coronary syndrome (ACS) may actually have one of several conditions that are listed under the heading of ACS. ACS may also be known as "acute ischemic coronary syndrome." ACS occurs when a coronary artery becomes blocked. Remember, the coronary arteries provide the heart with oxygen and nutrients.

When the coronary artery becomes blocked, the myocardium becomes ischemic, resulting in injury to the cardiac muscle (ischemia) or tissue death (infarction). Acute coronary syndrome may result in angina, non-ST segment elevation MI (NSTEMI), ST elevation MI (STEMI), or sudden cardiac death. ST elevation is the increase in millivolts reflective of an enlarging ST segment (end of ventricular contraction and beginning of the resting or repolarization phase) on the EKG or cardiac monitor. This evidenced by

1 mm (electrical measurement of the EKG strip) in limb leads and 2 mm in precordial leads. As plaques build within the lumen of the coronary arteries, the risk increases for blockage.

When the cardiac musculature does not receive enough oxygen, a symptom known as angina pectoris (chest pain) occurs. The classic chest pain symptoms occur at the mid- or left chest, epigastric area, radiate down the arm, and radiate up to the jaw, left shoulder, or shoulder blades. The pain *does not* increase with deep inspirations or movement. Apply oxygen in case the chest pain has an underlying ischemic cause. Nitroglycerin SL (a vasodilator) is given for pain. "MONA" is a pneumonic to help remember treatment: morphine, oxygen, nitroglycerin, and aspirin.

Myocardial infarction occurs when the heart does not get the blood or oxygen it needs. If the underlying cause is a blockage, the treatment is to open up the blocked vessel. The nurse should apply oxygen and anticipate the administration of a fibrinolytic (also known as a clot buster). The doctor may want to perform a coronary angioplasty on an emergency basis. A coronary angioplasty is a procedure in which a catheter is inserted into a blood vessel (the femoral artery and, more recently, the radial artery). A small balloon is at the end tip of the catheter. Under fluoroscopy, the doctor threads the catheter to the area of blockage and slowly inflates the balloon. The balloon opens the blood vessel to allow blood flow.

A stent may be placed to maintain this patency. Pre- and postprocedure, patient teaching is essential. If the patient is a diabetic and taking Glucophage, the contrast dye can cause kidney failure. Therefore, the medication must be held for 2 days before and after having an x-ray procedure (such as an angiogram) or starting on a renal buffer such as Mucomyst or sodium bicarbonate. Prior to the procedure, the patient pedal pulses need to be marked, the patient must be screened for allergies, and labs must be done for coagulation and electrolytes. Post-op care would involve monitoring vital signs, peripheral pulses, and for arrhythmias as well as checking the groin puncture site for hematoma or bruit. Hydration should be given to prevent renal complications. Do not let the head of the patient's bed be elevated more than 30 degrees, and the patient must keep the leg straight for at least 6 hours. To prevent aspiration, the bed can be put in the reverse Trendelenburg.

If the patient is too unstable (hypotensive or irregular cardiac rhythms), the doctor may choose to perform a coronary artery bypass graft (CABG). A CABG is a procedure in which the sternum is opened, a donor vein is harvested from the patient's leg, and then the occluded coronary arteries are replaced with the harvested vein. Pre-op care may consist of lab work, two-dimentional Echo, functional and psychosocial assessments, type and cross match of blood, nutritional assessment and education, fluid balance, intake-output, height, weight, and peripheral edema assessment. Post-op care would involve a ventilator, chest tubes, arterial line, EKG monitoring, Swan-Ganz monitoring for CO, and assessing for potential complications such as cardiac tamponade, bleeding, and myocardial and renal failure.

When the cardiac valves do not work properly, the patient is diagnosed with valvular heart disease. Valvular heart disease may be caused by valvular stenosis or valvular insufficiency. Valvular stenosis occurs when the valves become rigid and the blood flow is reduced. Valvular insufficiency, also known as regurgitation, occurs when the heart valve does not close completely. This incomplete closure allows for the backward flow of blood. A murmur may be heard on auscultation. Depending on the severity of the regurgitation, treatment will depend on the symptoms that may present (pulmonary hypertension, pulmonary edema, or chronic heart failure [CHF] symptoms). Surgery may be required and pre- and postoperative treatment will be the same as for a CABG. If a metal valve is placed, a "click" will be heard when assessing the patient, and anticoagulation is required.

Elevation of the blood pressure is known as hypertension. Diagnosed early, the patient can make lifestyle changes to correct this health issue. When the blood pressure is severely high, organs within the body (heart and kidneys) can become damaged, resulting in end-stage renal or cardiac disease, where "end-stage" means "end of life."

An aortic aneurysm is an enlargement or outpouching of the vessel wall in the aorta. The aorta is a major artery that supplies the majority of blood throughout the body. The aorta is located in the midline trunk of the body and continues to the heart. Often an aortic aneurysm goes unnoticed. When the aneurysm develops large enough, the patient may notice several health issues that cause concern and that will lead the patient to the doctor: abdominal pulsations (close to the navel), back pain, or a constant abdominal pain that the patient describes as "a deep pain." When the nurse is assessing the patient, a soft blowing bruit may be detected. In addition, there may a significant difference of blood pressure readings between arms.

Aortic aneurysms are more common in the abdomen, but they do occur in the aortic arch. When the aortic aneurysm is located in the abdomen, it may be called an "AAA" (abdominal aortic aneurysm). Treatment of an AAA varies based on its size and rate of growth. Treatment may be to monitor the aneurysm or it may be to surgically repair the aneurysm. Unfortunately, an undiagnosed aortic aneurysm may require emergency surgery if the aneurysm ruptures.

There are several factors that may contribute to the development of an aneurysm: smoking, atherosclerosis, syphilis, trauma, diabetes mellitus, hypertension, age, and gender (occurring in men more often than in women). When an aneurysm dissects (tears occurring in the aortic walls), bleeding occurs and this situation becomes life-threatening. The patient may experience sudden onset of intense abdominal or back pain, shock-like symptoms (clammy, dizzy, N/V, low blood pressure), tachycardia, difficulty in breathing, and a change in level of consciousness. Aneurysms can be diagnosed by TEE (transesophageal echocardiography), CT scans, and EKG. Treatment includes bed rest, preventing straining, preventing crossing of legs, a calm environment, beta blockers, and antihypertensives.

When surgery is performed on an AAA, a graft is placed in the aorta to prevent rupture of the blood vessel. The graft is made of material that allows stretching in response to blood pressure or movement, but protects the weakened areas of the aorta (the aneurysm) from excessive pressure. Risks from surgery include: MI, arrhythmias, infection, bowel and limb ischemia, bleeding, embolism, and lung and spinal cord injury. After surgery, assess for leakage from the graft site, decreased Hgb and Hct, increasing abdominal girth, weak peripheral pulses, hypotension, decreased urinary output, and hypovolemic shock. Post-op treatment includes maintaining tissue perfusion and motor and sensory function.

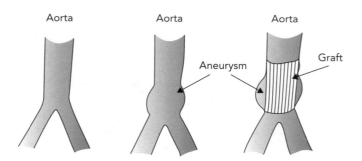

The pericardium is the sac enclosure surrounding the heart. There are approximately 15 to 50 mL of a protein-rich fluid within the pericardium that surrounds the heart. When the pericardium is injured or diseased, fluid accumulation can occur, resulting in a pericardial effusion. If the amount of fluid accumulation is too great (amount varies in each individual), the heart is restricted in movement and results in poor CO. Undiagnosed or untreated, the pericardial effusion can result in death.

A pericardial effusion can develop slowly over time, offering no symptoms. However, when symptomatic, the patient can present with shortness of breath, dyspnea, orthopnea, and a chronic cough. Patients usually seek medical attention when the symptoms become severe or chest pain occurs. If the pericardial effusion restricts the heart from performing (pumping), this condition is called tamponade. Beck's triad is a sign of cardiac tamponade characterized by muffled heart sounds, narrowing pulse pressure, and jugular venous distention (JVD). Pulsus paradoxus is the negative pressure created in the thorax during normal inspiration that limits cardiac filling, decreases CO, and causes a weaker pulse. So when you listen to a manual blood pressure (BP), you will not hear the BP sounds for 10 mmHg or more, which is a significant sign for cardiac tamponade. If the tamponade is left untreated, death can and usually occurs.

Treatment for the pericardial effusion is a pericardiocentesis. A pericardiocentesis allows the aspiration of the excess pericardial fluid from the pericardial sac (pericardium). Once the fluid is aspirated, it should be sent to the laboratory for analysis. The pericardial fluid may have collected because of infection or cancer. Lupus, an autoimmune disease, may also be the cause of a pericardial effusion. The fluid accumulation may require a long-term solution. The patient may need a pericardial window. A pericardial window is the removal of a small section of the pericardium to allow drainage. A chest tube is placed to collect the pericardial fluid. Pacing wires may also be placed in case a temporary pacemaker is required. These wires, if not placed in a pacemaker, must be in a protective cover because microshocks can occur to the patient's heart if they are handled without gloves or are exposed to static electricity.

Cardioversion is a procedure performed by chemical (medications) or electrical stimulation. Synchronized cardioversion is electrical simulation that is synchronized with the "R" wave in the QRS complex at lower voltage. It may convert the electrical impulse of the heart to a normal, regular rhythm. Electrical cardioversion is performed by placing electrical gel pads on the patient. The patient will require conscious sedation, and an anesthesiologist needs to be present. A code cart should be readily available, and the patient placed on continuous monitoring. Digoxin should be withheld for 48 hours prior to the procedure to avoid arrhythmias.

Adenosine is the drug of choice for chemical cardioversion. Adenosine is given rapidly in an initial dose of 6 mg, followed by 12 mg given intravenously. Adenosine causes a temporary asystole rhythm of short duration. The heart basically restores itself to a normal, regular rhythm.

In the intensive care or critical care unit, patients with an underlying cardiac disease or health issue may require hemodynamic monitoring. The goal of hemodynamic monitoring is to monitor the patient for adequate tissue perfusion. To adequately evaluate hemodynamic monitoring, certain invasive equipment has to be inserted to provide a clear picture of systemic, pulmonary arterial, and venous pressures, and CO. This will help the clinician to evaluate the effects of drug modalities to improve perfusion. It can also assist the clinician to determine what interventions may be needed (medications, pacemaker, diuretic, etc.). Hemodynamic monitoring allows the nurse to monitor central venous pressures (CVP), pulmonary artery pressures (PAP), CO, cardiac index (CI), and will include arterial blood pressures. A Swan-Ganz catheter is used to assess the hemodynamic response to medication therapies and management of hemodynamic instability after cardiac surgery.

A Swan-Ganz catheter (also known as the pulmonary artery catheter) is a thermodilutional catheter that is inserted into the patient's pulmonary artery to indirectly measure the pressures of the left atrium. At the tip of the catheter is a small balloon that can be inflated by the nurse. The balloon allows the catheter to "wedge" into the pulmonary artery, offering pressure measurements of the left atria. It is also used to measure preload and afterload blood flow.

The Swan-Ganz catheter has multiple lumens in order to allow infusion of medications as well as to measure another area of the heart. The CVP can be measured via one lumen in the Swan-Ganz. The CVP can measure the pressure in the right atrium (preload) and indirectly measures pressures in the left heart (afterload). The CVP pressure (2–8 mmHg) is in close correlation to the pulmonary wedge pressure (8–12 mmHg). If the Swan-Ganz catheter does not "wedge," or in the absence of a pulmonary artery catheter, a central venous catheter can be set up to monitor the CVP, offering an indirect measure of the left heart. For students considering a career in critical care nursing, a critical care course would offer more in-depth and detailed knowledge. Complications of a Swan-Ganz catheter include infection, air emboli, thrombosis, PA infarction, PA rupture, and balloon rupture.

An arterial line is a catheter inserted into the patient's radial, brachial, or femoral artery. This allows a more accurate measurement of the patient's blood pressure and allows blood sampling. This measurement is very critical to septic patients or those patients who may be hemodynamically unstable. The major complications associated with the arterial line are bleeding, infection, and rarely, a lack of blood flow to the tissue supplied by the artery. The arterial line is considered more accurate, so there will be a blood pressure variance between radial and manual BP. An Allen's test must be performed prior to insertion. The Allen's test evaluates the ulnar and radial pulses and evaluates collateral circulation. To perform an Allen's test, elevate the hand above the heart and make a fist. Apply pressure to both the radial and ulnar pulses, and then release the ulnar pulse while still occluding the radial pulse. Normal color should return to the hand within 3 to 7 seconds. If prolonged after 7 seconds, then the hand does not have a dual blood supply and that radial artery should not be utilized.

Critical care nurses care for patients who may present with complex disease processes. Complex disease processes are diseases caused by lifestyle, environmental, and often, genetic factors (or a combination of several factors) with unknown etiology. Examples of complex disease processes are Alzheimer's, asthma, multiple sclerosis, renal failure, and autoimmune diseases.

THE RESPIRATORY SYSTEM

The primary purpose of the respiratory system is gas exchange, which involves the transfer of oxygen and carbon dioxide between the atmosphere and the blood. When a serious incident occurs that will affect the intake of O_2 from the lungs, tissue hypoxia will occur.

Diseases of the lungs and pulmonary system affect this delicate gas exchange and impact the amount of oxygen circulating in the body. Surfactant is a lipoprotein produced by the alveolar surface that lowers the surface tension in the alveoli. CO determines the amount of O_2 delivered to the body.

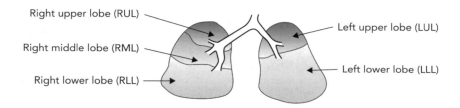

Right upper lobe (RUL)

Right middle lobe (RML)

Right lower lobe (RLL)

Left upper lobe (LUL)

Left lower lobe (LLL)

ANATOMY OF THE LUNGS

The main stem bronchi bifurcate into right and left bronchi, which is important because aspiration is more likely to occur in the right bronchi versus the left bronchi. The bronchioles are encircled by smooth muscle that will constrict and relax in response to certain stimuli. The smallest tubes (bronchioles) are only millimeters wide and anything that makes them contract, such as asthma or an anaphylactic reaction, will narrow the passages.

No exchange of oxygen or carbon dioxide takes place until the air enters the respiratory tract. The anatomic dead space is the area of the respiratory tract from the nose to the respiratory bronchioles. This area serves as an anatomic dead air space that holds about 150 ml of air (it does contribute to the warming of inspired oxygen). A normal tidal volume is the volume of the air exchanged with each breath. Alveoli are interconnected, which allows movement of air from alveolus to alveolus. These cells are open and more vulnerable to bacteria. Alveoli are close to capillaries, which allow easy passage or exchange of O_2 and CO_2.

In conditions such as pulmonary edema, excess fluid fills the interstitial space and alveoli, reducing gas exchange. This will cause a ventilation perfusion mismatch. This basically means that the patient is breathing (ventilation), but because of fluid or tissue enlargement the alveoli cannot exchange oxygen, which then does not perfuse the tissues. Surfactant is produced by the alveoli. Surfactant decreases the tendency of the alveoli to collapse and also protects the lungs. If insufficient surfactant is present, the alveoli will collapse, causing atelectasis. A reduction in surfactant is present in cystic fibrosis, chronic obstructive lung disease, and acute respiratory distress syndrome.

KEY NOTE: The lungs provide oxygenation to the body and other organs. Maintaining an appropriate level of oxygen will ensure better health and recovery.

Assessing, monitoring, maintaining, and improving health are actions that are taken frequently by the critical care nurse. Patients who are unable to support their oxygenation requirements may need intubation. Intubation is the insertion of a hollow tube through the vocal cords and remains above the carina to provide oxygen exchange. The inserted tube is called an endotracheal tube and is attached to a machine (ventilator) that regulates breath rate, respiratory depth (tidal volume), inspirational pressures, and positive end expiratory pressures. Numerous medical diseases and conditions may require ventilation, such as status asthmaticus, severe atelectasis (collapsed alveoli), pulmonary infiltrates (a density in the lung, often pneumonia, edema, or cancer), and those with acute respiratory distress syndrome.

Ventilator alarms that need immediate attention are:

- **High pressure**: peaked alarm, water in tubing, biting tube, patient restless
- **Low pressure**: leaking cuff, extubation
- **Complications**: barotraumas (pneumothorax), decreased BP
- **Interventions**: to prevent ventilator-associated pneumonia, good mouth care
- **Cuff leak**: if the patient can talk, the cuff is deflated

Different ventilator modes support ventilation in situations when the airway system is compromised. Different modes are used depending on the ability of the patient to assist with spontaneous respirations:

- Assist control
- SIMV (synchronized intermittent mandatory ventilation)
- Pressure support and CPAP (continuous positive airway pressure)
- Pressure-controlled ventilation
- PEEP (positive end expiratory airway pressure), usually positive 5 to 10 cmH$_2$O. PEEP can cause pneumothorax because it can rupture an emphysematous bleb or fragile tissue. Subcutaneous emphysema is the leakage of air into the tissues, which can cause airway obstruction. Oxygen should not be kept on 100%, because at that concentration it destroys the alveoli.

Flail segment occurs when a part of the rib cage no longer has a bony connection with the rest of the rib cage and it floats independently during ventilation. This is caused by trauma. Paradoxical respiration results in respirations that cause "sucked in" ribs (broken bones that have no security) with inspiration that are "blown out" during expiration.

THE BRAIN

The brain is a sensitive organ that needs a continuous supply of oxygen, glucose, and nutrients for energy. Cerebral blood flow meets metabolic demands by pressure autoregulation. Ischemia occurs when there is a deficit of oxygen and nutrients or an obstruction. The body will then switch to anaerobic metabolism, causing lactate accumulation. Lactate does not cross the blood brain barrier but does cause cerebral acidosis, which results in vasodilation.

The Monroe-Kellie hypothesis describes the process that maintains the balance in the fluid volume of brain, blood, and cerebral spinal fluid (CSF). An increase in one will cause a decrease in another to maintain a balance. Increased vasodilation due to anaerobic metabolism can create problems of fluid balance in the brain, such as increased intracranial pressure (ICP).

Intracranial monitoring can be ordered to monitor for ICP. A catheter is inserted into the brain to provide continuous pressure monitoring. Normal ICP pressures are

0 to 15 mmHg. Dynamic changes in ICP measurements can occur with increased respiratory rate, misaligned body positioning, suctioning, or pain.

CPP (cerebral perfusion pressure) depends on cerebral blood flow and ICP. To calculate the CPP: CPP (80–100) = MAP – ICP. It is crucial to have a CPP over 70 to ensure adequate cerebral oxygenation. Reducing ICP may require stimulating the body to rid itself of or gain fluids by stimulating the renal system.

THE RENAL SYSTEM

The renal system will assist in maintaining the balance of fluid by promoting either fluid retention or fluid elimination. The urinary system anatomy contains two kidneys, two ureters, one urinary bladder, and a urethra. The nephron is the functional unit of the kidney. It is composed of glomerulus, tubular apparatus, and collecting duct. Surrounding each glomerulus is Bowman's capsule. The primary function of the Bowman's capsule is to filter the waste products from the blood as it flows through the kidneys.

When the patient presents with renal failure, fluids and toxins accumulate in the body. The patient may experience congestive heart failure, hypertension, neurological changes, or pulmonary edema. The patient may have been admitted with one health issue, but it can progress to a complex health care situation. Complex health issues can occur slowly (chronic) or suddenly (acute). Sudden onset or emergent health changes are frightening for the patient and their family. Sudden onset can occur in a pre-existing condition, in a newly diagnosed condition, with etiology unknown, or by trauma.

CRITICAL CARE SITUATIONS

Trauma patients are also part of the ICU population. Whether the trauma occurred from an accident (fall from a ladder), a motor vehicle crash (MVC), assault (stabbing), gunshot wound (GSW), or self-inflicted (suicide attempt), the critical care nurse must be sufficiently knowledgeable and skilled to care for each.

Critical care situations can occur in a matter of seconds. The following are a set of examples (not all inclusive) of ICU situations and interventions.

Problem	Intervention	Expected outcome
Hypotensive	Fluid bolus(es), 5% albumin, 25% albumin, blood transfusion (if anemic); may need to initiate vasopressors (volume resuscitate before vasopressors).	Improved blood pressure
Hypertensive	Administer IV antihypertensive. May need to initiate IV drip of Nipride.	Improved blood pressure
Low heart rate	Determine underlying cause. If symptomatic, atropine IVP. May need transvenous pacemaker, or permanent pacemaker.	Improved heart rate
High heart rate	Determine underlying cause. Administer metoprolol IV. May need to perform synchronized cardioversion	Improved heart rate
Increased respiratory rate	Determine underlying cause. May need to administer Lasix for fluid overload. For CO_2 retention, may need to administer Diamox and antianxiety medication. May require intubation.	Improved respiratory rate
Decreased respiratory rate	Determine underlying cause. May need Narcan (opiate antidote) or Romazicon (benzodiazepine antidote) for over-sedation. May require intubation.	Improved respiratory rate

(continued)

Problem	Intervention	Expected outcome
No or decreased urinary output	Determine underlying cause. Fluid bolus. Monitor laboratory values (electrolytes, BUN, and creatinine). May require dialysis.	Improved renal function
Excessive urinary output	Determine underlying cause. May require demopressin or vasopressin in diabetes insipidus or a response to a diuretic.	Normal renal output
Agitated or extremely restless	Determine underlying cause. May be ETOH withdrawal, electrolyte imbalance, dementia, psychosis, increased ICP, cerebrovascular accident (CVA), etc.	Improve mental status
Unresponsive	Determine underlying cause. May be over-sedated, elevated CO_2 levels, low blood sugar, or having a neurological event (CVA). Obtain a CT scan. Call a code if the patient has no respirations or pulse.	Improve mental status

The list is lengthy when discussing the various conditions that can bring a patient to the critical care unit. A solid knowledge foundation in anatomy and physiology will help in understanding the various disease processes. Aging can cause deterioration of health. The critical care nurse must ensure the patient is provided every intervention to assist with recovery unless the patient has specifically documented otherwise.

A do-not-resuscitate order offers guidance to the health care team by ensuring that the patient's final wishes are known. Unless specified otherwise, the critical care nurse will provide all interventions, including advanced cardiac life support measures. Patients who document that they do not wish for extraordinary measures will be afforded comfort care interventions.

ANATOMY EXERCISE

Label the coronary arteries of the heart and return by preconference next week. Label the artery that is considered the "widow maker."

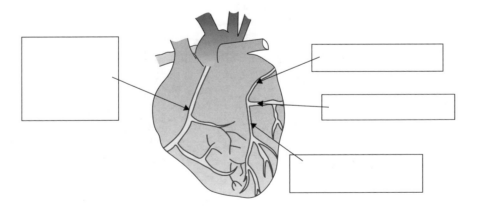

Medication Forms

Listed in the vertical box is a medication. For each of the remaining boxes, list the following:

Box 1: List a laboratory result you would need to monitor. Explain the significance of the laboratory test to the medication.

Box 2: List one food that may interact with the medication. Explain the significance of the food item to the medication.

Box 3: List one patient educational instruction you would give to the patient regarding the medication. Explain the significance of the instruction to the medication.

List other educational information you could provide this patient. Are there websites you can refer? What about travel overseas and health issues? How should the medication be stored?

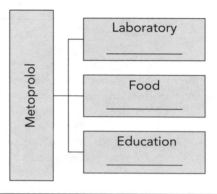

Listed in the vertical box is a medication. For each of the remaining boxes, list the following:

Box 1: List a laboratory result you would need to monitor. Explain the significance of the laboratory test to the medication.

Box 2: List one food that may interact with the medication. Explain the significance of the food item to the medication.

Box 3: List one patient educational instruction you would give to the patient regarding the medication. Explain the significance of the instruction to the medication.

List other educational information you could provide this patient. Are there websites you can refer? What about travel overseas and health issues? How should the medication be stored?

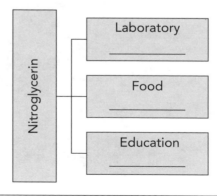

CRITICAL THINKING EXERCISE

Match the lettered critical care situations in the boxes to the appropriate interventions listed below. Return by preconference next week.

A. Low B/P	B. Low heart rate	C. Low urinary output
D. High B/P	E. High heart rate	F. High urinary output
G. Low respiratory rate	H. High respiratory rate	I. Unresponsive

Consider a pacemaker _____
Consider a fluid bolus _____
Consider Narcan _____
Consider DDAVP _____
Consider Diamox _____
Consider Nipride _____
Consider a CT scan _____
Consider vasopressors _____
Consider cardioversion _____

ANSWERS TO CRITICAL THINKING EXERCISE

Match the lettered critical care situations in the boxes to the appropriate interventions listed below.

A. Low B/P	B. Low heart rate	C. Low urinary output
D. High B/P	E. High heart rate	F. High urinary output
G. Low respiratory rate	H. High respiratory rate	I. Unresponsive

Consider a pacemaker <u>B</u>
Consider a fluid bolus <u>C</u>
Consider Narcan <u>G</u>
Consider DDAVP <u>F</u>
Consider Diamox <u>H</u>
Consider Nipride <u>D</u>
Consider a CT scan <u>I</u>
Consider vasopressors <u>A</u>
Consider cardioversion <u>E</u>

WEEK 10 POSTCONFERENCE

Discuss with students the equipment seen in the critical care areas (if applicable). If unable to tour the critical care areas, inquire what equipment and types of patients may be in the critical care areas. Ask students to list the various types of specialty units available in the hospitals.

Inform students that many areas in nursing currently require a specialty certification. Medical–surgical and critical care are two of those areas that do have specialty certification.

Discuss with students how they believe the critical care nurses become so skilled and knowledgeable.

Remind students there are only 4 additional weeks left in clinical. Any student that may need to make up missed clinical days or assignments should make arrangements to do so now.

Chapter 14

EMERGENCY NURSING

This chapter examines:

- Assessment, treatment, and decision-making skills
- Emergency levels and triage decisions
- Emergent nursing situations
- Illicit and illegal drug emergencies

Week 11 continues the discussion of advanced nursing skills with a focus on emergency nursing. Nurses need to be aware of the various types of situations that may occur and the assessment and treatment resources available for interventions.

WEEK 11 PRECONFERENCE

Hand out:
- Medication forms (atropine and Isuprel)
- Emergency nursing exercise
- Crash cart exercise
- Emergency cases
- Emergency prioritizing case

Collect:
- Medication forms (metoprolol and nitroglycerin)
- Anatomy exercise
- Critical thinking exercise
- Concept maps
- Care plans
- Physical assessment form
- Journals

Inform students that emergency situations occur each day. Instruct students to stay alert for "codes" or "rapid response" calls via the overhead pager system. Students must have permission to participate in code or rapid response calls and basic life support (BLS) certification. The instructor should arrange for a guided tour of the emergency room and trauma bay and should ask the rapid response nurse to speak at postconference.

EMERGENCY NURSING

Emergency nursing can mean several things. Emergency nursing may refer to the nurses who work in the emergency department. Emergency nursing can also refer to the nurse who must provide care and interventions during an emergency situation. An emergency nurse is a nurse with specialized diagnostic and treatment skills in emergency nursing. This nurse has to be able to handle life-threatening emergencies and must be aware of a wide range of illnesses, injuries, treatments, medications, and complications. The nurse must also be knowledgeable in advanced monitoring and treatment equipment.

The emergency nurse will be exposed to a variety of patients of all ages, both sexes, and many nationalities. When a patient arrives, there is no diagnosis, and the nurse must appropriately triage the patient until the patient can be seen by a physician. Triage evaluates a patient and, based on those findings, matches the patient to guidelines based on the patient acuity level. Patient emergency levels are labeled as Priority Levels I, II, III, or IV based on their medical, psychological, community, and substance-abuse requirements. The nurse must be able to remain calm amid numerous emergencies. The emergency nurse may also be required to work in a fast-track section of the ER that deals specifically with low-acuity patients.

ILLICIT AND ILLEGAL DRUG EMERGENCIES

There may be patients who are admitted to the emergency room under the influence of illicit and illegal drugs. Drug screening should be done if there appears to be any changes in the patient's mental status or trauma or injury. The following discussion surveys the most frequently abused illicit and illegal drugs, their signs and symptoms, and the appropriate emergency nursing interventions and treatments.

Heroin: A drug made from morphine. Heroin can be injected, smoked, or snorted. Health risks of heroin use involve miscarriages, heart infections (endocarditis), and infectious diseases, including HIV/AIDS and hepatitis. Use of heroin will lead to tolerance.

Signs and symptoms of withdrawal include restlessness, muscle and bone pain, diarrhea, vomiting, and cold flashes. Withdrawal symptoms will begin within 12 hours of the last dose, peak in intensity after 2 or 3 days, and last for a week or longer.

Treatment: Methadone, naltrexone, or buprenorphine, as an opiate substitution medication; cognitive behavioral therapy, psychotherapy, and supportive rehabilitation treatment

Cocaine: A frequently abused major stimulant with powerful psychological addiction properties. Cocaine is often used with alcohol and sedatives such as Valium, Ativan, or heroin (a common polydrug abuse problem). Cocaine is used for surgery, nosebleeds, and as a local anesthetic for cuts in children. The breakdown products of cocaine will be excreted and can be detected in the urine for 24 to 72 hours. For chronic users, it can be detected for up to 2 weeks.

Causes: Cocaine addictive disease is believed to be caused by genetics and environment. Repeated exposure to cocaine will cause alterations in dopamine levels, which is associated with cocaine's pleasurable "rush"; this prevents re-uptake of norepinephrine at the neurotransmitters.

Signs and symptoms: Hyperactivity, constricted pupils, nausea, vomiting, headache, vertigo, emotional instability, apprehension, cold sweats, tremors, twitching of small muscles, hallucinations, cocaine psychosis, schizophrenia, high blood pressure, perforated nasal septum, and angina (vasospasm will also cause the abnormal rhythms). Those rhythms may be ventricular tachycardia and ventricular fibrillation. "Body packers" are people who smuggle drugs by swallowing plastic bags of drugs, holding them until eliminated. These individuals may have various diagnoses depending on whether the packets remain intact or whether they leak, which may lead to massive cocaine intoxication.

Treatment: Activated charcoal may be used initially to absorb any drug that has leaked. Treat any symptoms that are caused by the use of cocaine. Instruct patients not to reuse or share needles.

Central nervous system (CNS) stimulants: Caffeine, amphetamines, and anorexiants (Didrex, Sanorex, and Ritalin). Used for weight reduction, attention deficit hyperactivity disorder (ADHD), narcolepsy, and euphoria.

Signs and symptoms: Stimulate CNS, "rush," tachycardia, increased activity and rapid speech, blocks rapid eye movement (REM) sleep, dilated pupils, paranoid psychosis, belligerence, hallucinations, palpitations, arrhythmias, hyperthermia, shock.

Treatment: Reduce stimulation and fever, supportive care, induce vomiting, and treat with antipsychotics

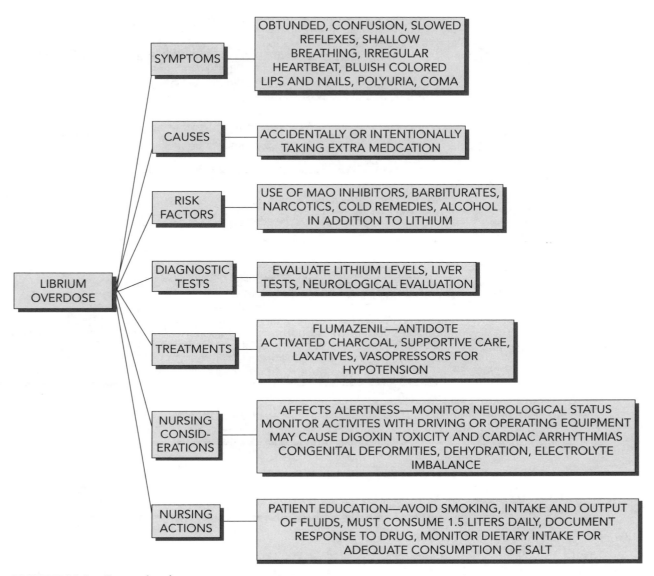

FIGURE 14-1 Example of a concept map.

Barbiturates: Drugs that depress the CNS such as Amytal, Nembutal, phenobarbital, and secobarbital oral or IV

Sedative–hypnotics: Librium, Valium, and Equanil oral or IV

Indications: sedation, seizures, antiemetic, anti-anxiety

Signs and symptoms: Slowed body functions, fixed and dilated pupils, physical dependence, anorexia, and impaired judgment; accelerates the rate of metabolism of many drugs; effects increased with ETOH

Treatment: Activated charcoal, supportive measures, hypothermia, hypotension, respiratory depression, Narcan

Glue sniffing: Will cause euphoria and increased sensory awareness

Signs and symptoms: Slurred speech; impulsive, destructive behavior; tremors; resembles alcohol intoxication; tinnitus; and muscle and joint pain

Treatment: Supportive respiratory and cardiac treatment

Hallucinogens: LSD, psilocybin, mescaline, PCP, and tetrahydrocannabinol (THC; also known as marijuana)

Signs and symptoms: Central autonomic hyperactivity, pupil dilation and hypertension (HTN), rapid mood swings, seizures, coma, paranoia, delusions, and flashbacks

Treatment: Avoid tranquilizers, support airway, quiet environment

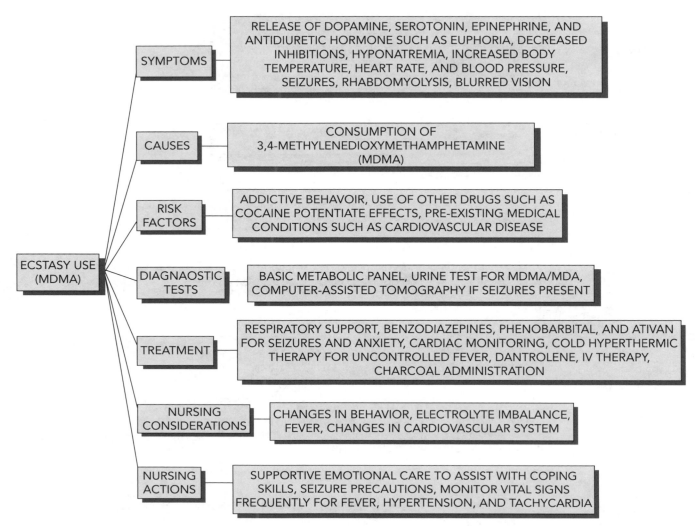

FIGURE 14-2 Example of a concept map.

Marijuana (Cannabis, THC): Inhalation, oral; peaks within 30 minutes, subsides within 2 to 4 hours; strong psychological dependence, but no physical dependence. Approved medical uses of marijuana include treating glaucoma, as an anticonvulsant, and to increase appetite of cancer patients.

Signs and symptoms: Impaired judgment, time disorientation, increased appetite and awareness, feelings of loss of control, psychosis, overdose, nausea, dizziness, and vomiting

Treatment: Supportive psychological interventions, medications to counteract the effects of tachycardia, hypotension, avoid activities that require concentration

Narcotics: Demerol, morphine, or heroin taken IV, oral, or smoked

Ecstasy: stimulant with amphetamine and hallucinogen properties. Even though ecstasy enhances pleasurable effects, the negative side effects include hyperthermia, tachycardia, HTN, seizures, and diaphoresis. This can lead to severe dehydration, rhabdomyolysis, and cardiovascular failure.

KEY NOTE: Large pupils suggest anticholinergic effects or adrenergic drugs (cocaine, amphetamines). Small pupils suggest opioids, alcohol, benzodiazepines, and lithium.

EMERGENCY LEVELS

Priority I emergencies are those emergencies that require immediate attention, such as injuries that will affect respiratory, cardiac, abdominal, or spinal organs; excessive bleeding; and comatose or unconscious patients. Certain medical conditions such as diabetic ketoacidosis would fit into this category.

Priority II emergencies are those patients who require treatment within 30 minutes, but there is no threat to the patient's life. Examples would include lacerations and injuries for which the bleeding is controlled.

Priority III patients are in an even less serious condition that needs treatment but is not a life-threatening situation.

Priority IV patients have minor conditions such as a sore throat.

Patients may also be classified as emergent, urgent, and non-urgent, or they may be color coded. Color coded is usually used in mass casualty situations where there is a huge influx of patients at one time.

1. **Red**: Immediate treatment necessary: unstable, such as occluded airway or actively bleeding; must be evaluated first. Injuries are life-threatening—but survivable with minimal intervention—such as hemothorax, tension pneumothorax, unstable chest and abdominal wounds, amputations, open fractures of long bones, and second- and third-degree burns covering 15% to 40% of total body surface.
2. **Yellow:** stable, can wait up to an hour for treatment. For example, second-degree burns. Injuries are significant and require medical care but can wait hours without threat to life or limb. This will also include stable abdomen wounds without evidence of hemorrhage; fractures requiring open reduction, debridement, and external fixation; and most eye and CNS injuries.
3. **Green:** stable, can wait even longer to be seen, "walking wounded." Minimal: Injuries are minor and treatment can be delayed to hours or days. Individuals in this group should be moved away from the main triage area. Examples are upper extremity fractures, minor burns, sprains, minor lacerations, and behavior disorders.

EMERGENT SITUATIONS

Emergency nurses must be prepared to recognize and treat any number of emergent situations, some of which are discussed in this section. A common scenario is that a patient can seem comfortable and improving, and then suddenly an emergent situation occurs. One such emergent situation occurs when a patient complains that he or she can't breathe. Dyspnea is often subjective for the patient. The patient may complain of having trouble breathing, yet may not appear to be in any distress.

Patients may have trouble breathing when experiencing infections, pulmonary infarctions, malignancies, rheumatoid arthritis, and lupus erythematosus. The underlying cause of difficulty in breathing may be pleural effusions (a collection of fluid in the pleural cavity), infiltrates, direct infection of the pleural space from bacterial pneumonia, the rupture of a lung abscess, subdiaphragmatic infection, or trauma.

HEMOTHORAX

Patients who have experienced a traumatic event may be experiencing a hemothorax (blood in the pleural cavity) or a rupture of a great blood vessel. A moderate-to-large hemothorax requires immediate drainage and volume replacement. The hemothorax may cause lung compression. The signs and symptoms of a hemothorax include respiratory difficulty. Fluid movement into the pleural space may cause lung compression.

PNEUMOTHORAX

A pneumothorax (air in pleural cavity) can be either a partial or a complete collapse. The pneumothorax can be slow to develop or spontaneous. The cause of a pneumothorax can be the rupture of an air-filled bleb on the lung surface that allows air to enter pleural space or it can be due to a medical procedure, such as central line placement.

Primary spontaneous pneumothoraxes are typically seen in tall, thin males who are smokers. A secondary spontaneous pneumothorax can be seen in persons with underlying lung disease with air trapping (such as emphysema, asthma, tuberculosis, or carcinomas). A traumatic pneumothorax is usually secondary to fractured ribs that penetrate the pleura, or it can result from positive pressure ventilation. Additional causes may include an injury of the trachea or bronchus, or rupture of the esophagus.

When the lung collapses, the patient experiences a sudden, sharp pain. The patient presents with asymmetrical chest wall movement, respiratory distress, and absent breath sounds on the affected side. The patient may become hypoxic, dyspneic, and cyanotic. Tachycardia (compensatory) occurs to assist with oxygenation, but may also occur because of pain and anxiety. There is chest rigidity on the affected side. If air leaks into the tissue (crepitus or emphysema), a crackling can be felt beneath the skin when palpated.

When a tension pneumothorax occurs, there are a decrease in cardiac output, distended neck veins, and subcutaneous emphysema. Hypotension occurs. The patient appears anxious, pale, and weak. There is greater tension within the lungs and the mediastinum will cause tracheal deviation to the unaffected side. A chest tube must be established to reestablish negative pressure in the lung. A thoracotomy tray, thoracic catheter suction, suture material, and chest drainage set will be required. The chest tube has to be connected to a chest tube drainage set that the nurse will set up. The chest drainage set will provide 10 to 20 cm suction. The drainage systems must be kept lower than the insertion site, the patient's tubing must not be kinked, and the nurse also needs to monitor for air leaks.

Complications of a chest tube insertion can be excessive bleeding, infection, or subcutaneous emphysema. It is essential both to perform a comprehensive pulmonary assessment and to avoid tube dislodgement. The most important intervention goal is to improve oxygenation.

CHRONIC INFLAMMATORY AIRWAY DISEASE

Chronic inflammatory airway disease produces recurrent episodes of airway obstruction. The chronic inflammatory airway disease presents with wheezing, breathlessness, chest tightness, and cough. There are two types of triggers or stimuli: bronchospastic (i.e., cold air, exercise, emotional upset, or exposure to bronchial irritants) and inflammatory.

An acute episode of this disease occurs when a patient is exposed to an inhaled antigen or irritant, resulting in a severe bronchospasm. This condition may be reversed by bronchodilators, but corticosteroids are of little effect.

A delayed (late) response presents with inflammation and the bronchoconstriction can last for days or weeks. This condition may respond to cholinergic mediators.

A common sign of chronic hypoxia is clubbing, which is the selective, bulbous, and painless enlargement of the fingers. It is associated with diseases that interfere with oxygenation.

PULMONARY HYPERTENSION

Pulmonary HTN is indicated by pulmonary artery pressures (PAPs) above 25 mmHg (normal is 10–20 mmHg). Causes can be mitral stenosis resulting in pulmonary HTN with chronic hypoxia, acidosis, or both.

There are several types pulmonary HTN that selectively affect the pulmonary arterial tree, including those that affect venous circulation, and those that alter pulmonary function or structure.

- **Idiopathic:** Primary; occurs in the absence of disease; in women, more associated with sleep disorder
- **Familial:** Secondary, associated with genetic mutation, rare

Clinical manifestations:
- Dyspnea
- Fatigue
- Chest pain (CP)
- Palpitations
- Muscular weakness
- Elevated PAP

Outcome management:
- Supportive oxygen
- Anticoagulants
- Vasodilator therapy: Prostacyclin (reduces right ventricular dilation, prevents tricuspid regurgitation [TR], and has antithrombotic properties on platelets); Viagra has also been used for pulmonary HTN
- Heart–lung transplantation

INFLUENZA

Influenza is an acute viral infection of the respiratory tract. Parainfluenza viruses typically produce lower respiratory symptoms initially and then affect upper airways with reinfections.

Signs and symptoms: Fever, myalgia (muscle pain), and cough. The difference from a cold is that influenza is a sudden onset infection and has widespread occurrence.
Treatment: Depends on manifestations. Vitamin C and E supplements, hand washing
Note: Side effects of decongestants may be harmful to persons with HTN, heart disease, hyperthyroidism, or diabetes.

> **KEY NOTE:** No flu vaccine is allowed for those with Guillain–Barré syndrome or for those who are less than 6 months of age.

BRONCHIECTASIS

Bronchiectasis is a type of obstructive bronchitis that causes abnormal dilation and distortion of the bronchi and bronchioles. This disease causes chronic inflammatory changes. Some causes are congenital: cystic fibrosis, sinusitis, dextrocardia (heart on right side).

The medical treatment for this disease is the same as for chronic obstructive pulmonary disease (COPD) (see COPD discussion below).

PULMONARY EMBOLISM

A pulmonary embolism is a thrombus that travels to the lung. Most emboli develop in the deep calf, femoral, popliteal, or iliac veins; they can also develop from fat or septic or amniotic fluid; or because of major operations such as hip, knee, abdominal, and pelvic procedures, as well as immobility for long periods.

Pathophysiology: Ventilation perfusion (VQ) mismatch; vasoconstriction; platelet degradation; and release of histamine, serotonin, catecholamines, and prostaglandins. A VQ mismatch means that even though the patient is breathing, there is interference with either the ability to ventilate (which could be due to trauma or a neurological disorder) or a problem with perfusion that occurs at the alveoli exchange of the oxygen and carbon dioxide, which could be caused by pneumonia, fluid, or an autoimmune disorder.

Clinical manifestations: Tachycardia, dyspnea, anxiety, CP, hypoxemia.
Diagnostic findings:

- ABGs: low PaO_2, and low $PaCo_2$
- V/Q scan: IV injection of albumin/iodine
- Spiral computed tomography (CT)
- Pulmonary angiography: injected into right atrium
- D-dimer: may be elevated with pulmonary embolus, myocardial infarction, sepsis, and other conditions

Medical and surgical management:

- Stabilizing the cardiopulmonary system: O_2, fluids, and inotropic agents such as digoxin, dopamine, and milrinone. Inotropic agents alter the force or energy of muscular contractions. Positively inotropic agents increase the strength of muscular contractions.
- Anticoagulant therapy: heparin (does not break up existing clots) drug therapy initiated, and then Coumadin until INR level is two and a half to three times normal level; takes 2 to 3 days to achieve effect; patient needs to be on Coumadin for 3 to 6 months.
- Fibrinolytic therapy: for massive PE, thrombolytic therapy (TPA, streptokinase)
- Pulmonary embolectomy
- Vena cava filter

Nursing management:

- Assess vital signs and lung sounds
- Monitor for hypoxemia and distress
- Auscultate heart sounds (right-sided heart failure, S3, S4)
- Assess for edema, liver engorgement
- Elevate the head of the bed
- Alleviate fears and anxiety
- Monitor labs (PTT, PT, D-dimer, routine labs)
- Treat pain (morphine)

VENOUS AIR EMBOLISM

A venous air embolism (VAE) is air trapped inside the venous system that can be caused by removal of a central venous catheter, a craniotomy, pelvic operations in the Trendelenburg position, or gas insufflations in laparoscopy.

Signs and symptoms: dyspnea, CP, mill wheel murmur (loud churning, machinery-like murmur), decreased level of consciousness.

Make sure to prime all tubing, and secure all connections in the central line tubing. If VAE is suspected, place patient in the Trendelenburg position and rotate toward the left lateral decubitus position (this will trap air in apex of right ventricle).

ASTHMA

Asthma is the inflammatory and hyperresponsiveness of airways. There is a release of histamine, prostaglandin, and leukotriene. Bronchial tubes are infiltrated by neutrophils, eosinophils, and lymphocytes, adding to the congestion. Bronchial spasms, increased vascular permeability, edema, thick tenacious mucus, impaired mucociliary function, thickening of the airway walls, and increased contractile response of the bronchial smooth muscle result in a compromised airway.

CHRONIC OBSTRUCTIVE PULMONARY DISEASE

COPD presents with inflammation and fibrosis of bronchial walls, hypersecretion of mucus, and loss of elastic lung fibers and alveolar tissue. The fibrosis and loss of elastic lung fibers result in decreased surface area for gas exchange and alveolar collapse.

Permanent enlargement of gas-exchange airways and destruction of alveolar walls result in the loss of elastic recoil, causing a decreased expiratory flow rate and increased residual volume. The lungs become hyperinflated with little ability to expel gases trapped within the lungs.

If the patient is unable to breath, the nurse needs to call a code. Implementation of CPR quickly will lessen the morbidity. In the event the patient is experiencing a cardiac event, a "code heart" should be called.

ACUTE RESPIRATORY DISTRESS SYNDROME

Acute respiratory distress syndrome (ARDS) is a sudden, progressive form of respiratory failure characterized by severe dyspnea, hypoxemia, and diffuse bilateral infiltrates. This can be due to acute hypoxic injury caused by a direct or indirect pulmonary injury. Direct injury such as aspiration, pulmonary infection, near drowning, thoracic trauma, or toxic inhalation. Indirect injury would be due to shock, sepsis, hypothermia, disseminated intravascular coagulation (DIC), multiple transfusions, eclampsia, pancreatitis, and burns. Treatment consists of treating the source. Complications will include pulmonary fibrosis or pneumothorax, emboli, or cognitive impairments.

BASIC LIFE SUPPORT GUIDELINES

All health care workers are required to attain their BLS credentials. BLS guidelines instruct the health care worker to assess whether the patient is responsive and able to breathe, and whether there is a pulse. Guideline interventions are taught for each situation. If the patient is having difficulty breathing, the airway must be assessed and opened, and respiration or oxygen should be initiated. A pulse oximetry sensor should be placed on the patient to provide continuous monitoring.

If the patient has no pulse, call for help and begin chest compressions. The patient's outcome is in the hands of the nurse. Immediate and appropriate interventions may save the patient's life. Students should research where the "crash cart" is located on their unit. The instructor can arrange for the students to see an open crash cart. Learning the various types of equipment housed on the cart as well as the readily available medications will help the students to understand what equipment and medications may be used in an emergent situation.

The nurse should attempt to diagnose the underlying cause of the problem. It is often the fast and accurate diagnosis of the underlying cause that prevents the patient from dying. The patient will be transferred to the critical care area if the patient requires continuous monitoring. If the patient has an underlying heart disease and is presenting with difficulty in breathing, the patient may only require a dose of Lasix. If the underlying cause is fluid overload, a stat chest x-ray, oxygen, a small dose of morphine (anxiety), and Lasix can prevent the patient from being transported to the critical care area.

SHOCK

To understand the process of cardiogenic shock, the nurse must first understand the physiological factors involved: the heart (pump), the veins and arteries (plumbing), and the blood (fluid). The cardiovascular system is a closed system that works effectively and efficiently. If one part of the cardiovascular system fails, the remaining parts attempt to compensate. The nurse must pick up on subtle clues and intervene to prevent further deterioration.

Assess the patient's level of consciousness. If the level of consciousness has declined or deteriorated from the patient's baseline neurological assessment, this may be a clue to impending shock. The patient may exhibit restlessness or confusion when hypoxic. Monitor for changes in behavior that differ from the patient's baseline.

Vital signs will also provide clues to impending shock. The heart rate will increase (tachycardia) and the pulse pressure will narrow. The respiratory rate will initially increase (tachypnea). Blood backs up in the system and fluid enters the lungs. The patient becomes cyanotic. Crackles and rhonchi can be heard when the lungs are auscultated.

The patient's skin will become pale, cool, and clammy. Cardiac output decreases, resulting in decreased urine output.

When there is a dysfunction of the heart (myocardial infarction or cardiomyopathy), the cardiac output is compromised. The heart is unable to pump blood through the systemic vascular system due to a weakened or damaged myocardium. As the systemic vascular resistance increases, the workload of the heart increases, which results in increasing myocardial oxygen consumption.

As the shock state continues, the sympathetic nervous system causes an increased heart rate and further vasoconstriction. This response is to help maintain perfusion to vital organs. With increased vasoconstriction, there is a further decrease in the cardiac output. The decreasing cardiac output results in a narrowing pulse pressure and decreasing urinary output. Troponin levels, an EKG, and a chest x-ray may be used to diagnose cardiogenic shock, and angioplasty or a coronary artery bypass graft (CABG) may be used to treat the shock.

Hypovolemic shock occurs when the body loses a significant amount of blood volume (approximately 15%) from trauma or gastrointestinal bleeding. The body attempts to compensate by causing vasoconstriction of the vasculature. Fluid shifts from interstitial areas to the vasculature can initially mask the impending shock. Cardiac output then decreases, resulting in decreased urinary output. The respiratory rate will initially increase (tachypnea) to "blow off" elevating CO_2 and then progress to shallow breaths. Anxiety and confusion occur. Patient safety is a priority. Blood and fluid must be administered to maintain the blood pressure. Correct the underlying cause and monitor hemoglobin and hematocrit.

Neurogenic shock can occur when there is a spinal cord injury at the thoracic vertebra (T5) level and above or when spinal anesthesia is administered. Onset of the neurogenic shock is 30 minutes, with a duration of weeks. The patient becomes hemodynamically unstable as the body fails to elicit the sympathetic nervous system response. The body undergoes a complete vasodilation process. This occurrence causes blood pooling in the vasculature, resulting in hypoperfusion of the tissues, hypotension, bradycardia, and hypothermia.

Anaphylactic shock is a life-threatening allergic reaction. The symptoms occur with sudden onset. The patient suffers vasodilation with increased capillary permeability. Fluid leaks from the vasculature into the interstitial space. Difficulty in breathing, angioedema, and pruritus are only a few of the symptoms that occur. The nurse must administer epinephrine (via an EpiPen or IV) and Benadryl to prevent further deterioration. If the patient's airway is compromised, intubation is required.

Septic shock is an inflammatory process in response to a pathogen. Septic shock presents with hypotension even though fluid resuscitation has been implemented. The coagulation processes and inflammatory processes of the body increase. The body is responding to an antigen with an overly exaggerated effort. Hyperventilation occurs, resulting in respiratory alkalosis. Eventually the body weakens and respiratory failure ensues. Acute respiratory distress syndrome develops, placing the patient in a constantly escalating critical state.

The prudent nurse will monitor more closely those patients who have an underlying condition that can trigger shock or a shock-like state. Anticipating the likelihood of the patient developing shock will keep the nurse ahead of the situation and will provide the safest care for the patient.

Medication Forms

Listed in the vertical box is a medication. For each of the remaining boxes, list the following:

Box 1: List a laboratory result you would need to monitor. Explain the significance of the laboratory test to the medication.
Box 1: List one food that may interact with the medication. Explain the significance of the food item to the medication.
Box 1: List one patient educational instruction you would give to the patient regarding the medication. Explain the significance of the instruction to the medication.

List other educational information you could provide this patient. Are there websites you can refer to? What about travel overseas and health issues? How should the medication be stored? Does the medication being administered interfere with other medications?

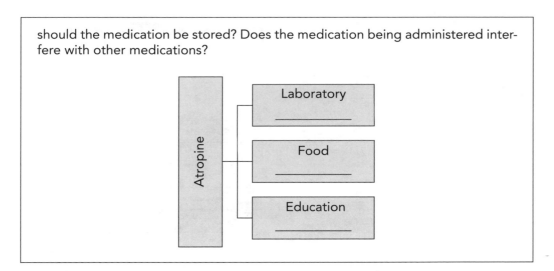

Listed in the vertical box is a medication. For each of the remaining boxes, list the following:

Box 1: List a laboratory result you would need to monitor. Explain the significance of the laboratory test to the medication.

Box 2: List one food that may interact with the medication. Explain the significance of the food item to the medication.

Box 3: List one patient educational instruction you would give to the patient regarding the medication. Explain the significance of the instruction to the medication.

List other educational information you could provide this patient. Are there websites you can refer to? What about travel overseas and health issues? How should the medication be stored? Does the medication being administered interfere with other medications?

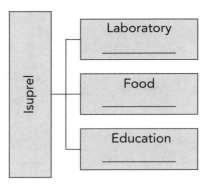

EMERGENCY NURSING EXERCISE

Describe what might be an emergent situation. List the interventions that should be implemented for the condition you described. Discuss your chosen emergent situation and compare it to a "rapid response" situation (a condition that can be treated without transport to the critical care unit). Return by preconference next week.

_____
_____
_____
_____
_____
_____
_____
_____
_____
_____
_____
_____
_____

CRASH CART EXERCISE

List the equipment you would find in a "crash cart." Briefly explain what the equipment is and what it is used for. Return by preconference next week.

_____
_____
_____
_____
_____
_____
_____
_____
_____
_____
_____
_____
_____
_____
_____
_____
_____

EMERGENCY CASES

CASE #1

Mr. Smith is a 78-year-old African American male who was admitted 2 days ago for uncontrolled HTN. On admission, Mr. Smith's vital signs were BP 187/101, HR 102, RR 28, T 98.8°F, and O_2 saturation 93%. Mr. Smith was given 100 mg of Spironolactone PO, one- time, 1-inch dose of nitroglycerin ointment, O_2 at 4 L/min per NC, and 2 mg morphine intravenously pushed (IVP) for chest pain. One hour after admission, his vital signs were BP 153/88, HR 92, and O_2 saturation 95%. The physician then started the patient on Capoten 50 mg orally twice daily in addition to the Spironolactone 50 mg twice daily. To prevent deep vein thrombosis (DVT), the physician ordered Lovenox 80 mg SC daily and 81 mg aspirin daily.

Mr. Smith was told he would be discharged in the morning because his blood pressure was controlled. You notice Mr. Smith's call bell is on. On arrival to his room, you see Mr. Smith on the floor but he is responding to commands. The patient care technician (PCT) is taking a set of vital signs that are BP 82/35, HR 167, RR 38, and O_2 saturation 88%. A rapid response is called.

Answer the following questions and return by preconference next week.

1. Based on the information presented, what "could" be the underlying problems?
2. What interventions would you implement for the underlying problems?

ANSWERS TO CASE #1

1. There may be many reasons.

   a. BP has dropped to 82/sys. The extra medication that was ordered may have been too much because of his age, or there could be a neurological event such as a stroke.
   b. Hyperkalemia
   c. Retroperitoneal bleed, because Lovenox can cause retroperitoneal bleeds.
   d. The patients pulse oxygen is low, so there may be a respiratory problem present.

2. There may be many interventions.

   a. The patient's BP should be assessed frequently, BP meds should be withheld, and nitropaste (NTP) removed from patient. If there is no contraindication, give a fluid bolus of isotonic fluids.
   b. Hyperkalemia: Draw an electrolyte panel. The results will determine whether the patient is experiencing hyperkalemia. Spironolactone can cause hyperkalemia. If the patient is experiencing hyperkalemia, give the patient 10% calcium gluconate one amp IVP slowly. This will help to reduce the high potassium level.
   c. If the patient is experiencing a bleed: The patient should be typed and cross-matched for blood. A CT scan may need to be completed when the patient is more stable.
   d. The low pulse should be evaluated by chest x-ray, arterial blood gases, continuous O_2 saturation, and application of oxygen. Evaluate for bilateral breath sounds; the patient may need a VQ scan to evaluate for pulmonary emboli.

   The patient should be transferred to the critical care unit for each of these potential problems.

CASE #2

Have students evaluate the following scenarios and prioritize which patients should be seen first. Answers are to be returned by preconference next week.

The nurse has been assigned to six patients. Which two patients would need to be assessed immediately?

Patient 1: A 20-year-old asthmatic patient with respiratory rate of 24 and O_2 saturation 98%; patient is wheezing and awaiting discharge
Patient 2: A 48-year-old, overweight, uncontrolled diabetic patient complaining of dull epigastric pain
Patient 3: A 30-year-old male who has suffered first-degree burns on the posterior surface of his left arm
Patient 4: A 24-year-old with a spiral fracture of right tibia
Patient 5: A 30-year-old female who has mild smoke inhalation, respiratory rate of 20, O_2 saturation 95, and in no acute distress
Patient 6: A 20-year-old complaining of fibromyalgia

ANSWERS TO CASE #2

The patients should be prioritized as listed here:

Patients 2 and 5: The diabetic patient needs to be evaluated because the epigastric pain may be an impending heart attack. Diabetics may have minimal symptoms because of their neuropathy and undetected coronary artery disease. Anyone with smoke inhalation also needs to be evaluated because there will continued inflammation and edema from the smoke irritant that may impede the airway

Patient 3: The first-degree burn is the least serious of burns and is not extensive

Patients 6 and 4: The patient with fibromyalgia and the patient with a fractured tibia need intervention but do not need immediate treatment

Patient 1: Even though the first patient has asthma, she has been stabilized and is ready to be discharged

> **KEY NOTE:** When prioritizing patients, always assess for airway, breathing, and circulation problems that will be a threat to the patient's safety or that need immediate intervention.

WEEK 11 POSTCONFERENCE

Allow the invited rapid response nurse to discuss how the rapid response system works. Inquire as to the types of patients who are frequently in need of the rapid response nurse. Also ask about the responsibilities of the rapid response nurse and how a typical rapid response situation is handled from beginning to end. Inquire about the skills and knowledge required of the rapid response nurses. Discuss those areas within the hospital to which the rapid response nurses are assigned and how that determination came to be.

Discuss with the students the various types of patients they believe would benefit from nursing interventions by the rapid response nurse. Discuss the benefits of treating the patient at the patient's current location rather than transporting the patient to a critical care unit and then treating the patient. Discuss with the students what they believe would be the benefits of the rapid response nurse program.

Inquire whether the students were able to "hear" any code blue or rapid response pages. Discuss what the students believe are the differences between a code blue and a rapid response.

Chapter 15

HEMATOLOGY, THE ENDOCRINE SYSTEM, AND RELATED DISORDERS

This chapter examines:

- Hematology and the endocrine system
- Autoimmune disorders and diseases
- Diabetes mellitus
- Blood transfusions and infectious diseases

The endocrine system plays a key role in many bodily functions. Students should become familiar with the functions of the endocrine system and the hormones associated with each endocrine gland.

Hormones related to the sex organs will be examined in Chapter 16, which discusses the reproductive system.

WEEK 12 PRECONFERENCE

Hand out:
- Medication forms (Benadryl and prednisone)
- Hematology exercise
- Critical thinking exercises
- Endocrine matching exercise

Collect:
- Medication forms (Isuprel and atropine)
- Emergency nursing exercise
- Crash cart exercise
- Emergency cases
- Concept maps
- Care plans
- Physical assessment form
- Journals

Inform the students that this week's topics are the endocrine system and hematology. Each student should be assigned a patient with diabetes melltius to aid in postconference discussions.

Medication Forms

Listed in the vertical box is a medication. For each of the remaining boxes, list the following:

Box 1: List a laboratory result you would need to monitor. Explain the significance of the laboratory test to the medication.
Box 2: List one food that may interact with the medication. Explain the significance of the food item to the medication.
Box 3: List one patient educational instruction you would give to the patient regarding the medication. Explain the significance of the instruction to the medication.

List other educational information you could provide this patient. Are there websites you can refer to? What about travel overseas and health issues? How should the medication be stored? Does the medication being administered interfere with other medications?

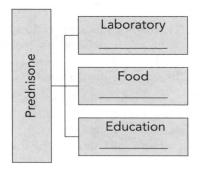

Listed in the vertical box is a medication. For each of the remaining boxes, list the following:

Box 1: List a laboratory result you would need to monitor. Explain the significance of the laboratory test to the medication.
Box 2: List one food that may interact with the medication. Explain the significance of the food item to the medication.
Box 3: List one patient educational instruction you would give to the patient regarding the medication. Explain the significance of the instruction to the medication.

List other educational information you could provide this patient. Are there websites you can refer to? What about travel overseas and health issues? How should the medication be stored? Does the medication being administered interfere with other medications?

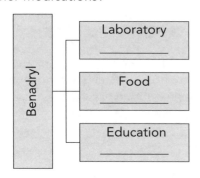

HEMATOLOGY

Hematology refers to the study of how blood is formed (i.e., how the cells are produced and the tissues involved). To understand hematology, the student must recognize the various blood cells and the purpose of these cells. The erythrocytes (red blood cells [RBCs]) are the largest group of blood cells. The RBCs are responsible for transporting oxygen throughout the body. Leukocytes (white blood cells [WBCs]) and lymphocytes are the body's defenders against infection. Platelets (PLTs) provide the blood with the ability to coagulate (clot). Analysis of mean corpuscular volume will help differentiate the different types of anemia. Low mean corpuscular volume (MCV) is indicative of iron deficiency and thalassemia anemias (hemolytic disease and sickle cell disease). A high MCV may be indicative of pernicious anemia or folic deficiency.

The production of red blood cells is dependent on adequate nutrition (vitamins). The kidneys secrete erythropoietin in conditions of low oxygen levels to stimulate RBC production. Low oxygen levels can occur in disease processes, anemia, or high altitudes.

The WBC can be further broken down into different cells. Neutrophils assist in the inflammatory process and destroy microorganisms by ingestion; that is, they are phagocytes. Basophils produce inflammatory mediators and stimulate the inflammatory response. Lymphocytes provide immunity. Eosinophils participate in the inflammatory response and react to allergens. Monocytes and macrophages provide phagocytic capability, but they also secret a colony-stimulating factor (CSF) that is required to grow macrophages and granulocytes in the bone marrow.

Hematopoiesis is the development or formation of blood cells. This process occurs in the bone marrow. Blood composition changes little over the life span. Blood cell production may decrease or be delayed in anemic conditions. The elderly patient may have a reduced response to infection, and the adhesiveness of PLTs increases with age, which will make the blood more prone to clot.

The body's ability to prevent blood loss is called hemostasis. To protect the body from blood loss, the body triggers a sequence of events. For example, the blood vessels (vasculature) narrow (vasoconstriction) to prevent blood loss when an injury occurs. The injury causes PLTs to collect (aggregate) at the injury site. When PLTs react to injured tissue, they release substances that stimulate coagulation.

The spleen assists the body by breaking down old or damaged red blood cells. The spleen recycles some portions (iron) of the destroyed red blood cells and also serves to store excess PLTs.

The liver serves the body in the roles of filtration and storage. The liver stores iron and plays a key role in iron regulation. The liver's parenchymal cells play an important role in hemostasis because they produce most of the coagulation factors needed (factors XII, IX, and X).

BLOOD DISORDERS

Neutropenia is a decrease in neutrophils. Patients diagnosed with neutropenia are at great risk for infection and sepsis. When infection is present, the patient may not present with typical signs and symptoms of infection because neutropenia will mask the symptoms. Neutropenia may be drug induced or the result of an autoimmune disease process. There is an impairment in the phagocytic mechanism that places the patient at greater risk for infection. The patient would require a bone marrow aspiration or biopsy to diagnose the cell morphology. Treatment is aimed at identifying the underlying cause. The etiology can be medications (chemotherapy drugs) or autoimmune disease (arthritis or lupus). The doctor may prescribe Neupogen to stimulate cell growth.

Thrombocytopenia is a reduction in the amount of PLTs. Low PLT counts increase the risk of bleeding in the patient. Spontaneous bleeding can occur, as well as petechiae (red or purple pinpoint spots under the skin), ecchymosis (can occur from the pressure of a blood pressure cuff), and bleeding gums (from brushing teeth). Thrombocytopenia can develop from disease processes (aplastic anemia or cancer) or from an acquired condition (medications or alcoholism). Causes of thrombocytopenia include bone marrow suppression by a disease process, or it can be medication induced or due to excessive PLT usage. Medications that can cause thrombocytopenia include chemotherapy drugs and heparin. Heparin-induced thrombocytopenia can cause thrombosis, which can result in strokes or hemorrhage. Treatment for thrombocytopenia includes replacing PLTs (transfusion) or discontinuing all forms of heparin (subcutaneous, intravenous [IV] drips, or hep-lock flushes). Argatroban should be used in place of heparin drips if the patient requires anticoagulant dosing.

Idiopathic thrombocytopenic purpura causes blood clots to form throughout the body, causing injury to all the organs and resulting in decreased PLTs. Bleeding, petechiae, and purpura, as well as symptoms of organ damage, will be present. Treatment consists of fresh frozen plasma, corticosteroids, and plasmapheresis.

Hemophilia is a genetic disorder presenting with a deficit of factor VII. Hemophilia A is more common than hemophilia B (which is characterized by a lack of the Von Willebrand coagulation protein). Hemophilia presents with prolonged bleeding or inability to clot when small lacerations or minor injuries occur. This patient is at great risk for hemorrhagic shock or death. Severe bleeding can occur when the injury or assault is more prominent, such as gastric bleed (ulcers), a punch in the nose (altercation or fight), or splenic rupture (motor vehicular crash). Bleeding can occur without injury (menorrhagia), resulting in the need for an antifibrinolytic (plasminogen activator inhibitors).

Hemophilia symptoms present with cyanotic tissue. The ischemia leads to necrosis, respiratory distress, and cardiovascular changes. Treatment is individualized based on presenting signs and symptoms. Interventions are aimed at both prevention and the replacement of needed clotting factors. The patient should wear a medical-alert bracelet that notifies medical staff that the patient lacks the ability to clot, resulting in continuous bleeding. Recurrent bleeding will be a lifelong threat.

Disseminated intravascular coagulation (DIC) is a complicated hemorrhagic and clotting disorder that presents with a physiological response that produces a bleeding and clotting event. The condition is triggered by sepsis, shock, malignancy, or tissue damage. When bleeding occurs, the body responds by clotting. This clotting intervention depletes the body's clotting factors. The excessive clotting actives the fibrinolytic system, which in turn breaks down clots. When the body begins to break up clots (lysis), it results in the release of fibrin split products that further adds anticoagulant properties. There is a systemic occurrence of clotting and hemorrhaging. Symptoms present with cyanotic tissue. The ischemia leads to necrosis, respiratory distress, and cardiovascular changes. To correct DIC, the underlying cause must be diagnosed (shock, trauma, or anaphylaxis). Treatment is individualized based on presenting signs and symptoms. Treatment involves replacing PLTs and treating with an anticoagulant to halt thrombosis formations.

Anemia is a decrease in red blood cells. The cause of anemia can be due to disease processes, blood loss, or the body's inability to produce red blood cells. Decreased red blood cell levels can also occur because of insufficient supplies of iron and cobalamin (vitamin B_{12}), or folic acid deficiencies, or decreased erythropoietin production. Clinical manifestations or symptoms of anemia often present as the body's response to hypoxia. Additional symptoms may be tarry stools (gastrointestinal bleed) or pallor.

Mild to severe anemia can present at rest or with activity. The body often compensates to maintain homeostasis by increasing respirations and heart rate, decreasing urine output, and changes in blood pressure. To compensate for low hemoglobin, the heart rate increases to move the oxygen-rich blood throughout the body. With decreased oxygen levels, this increases the workload of the heart and can result in chest pain or a myocardial infarction.

Treatment for anemia is aimed at correcting the underlying cause. If the anemia is caused by blood loss, the intervention is a blood transfusion. If the anemia is caused by an iron, vitamin B_{12}, or folic acid deficiency, the intervention would be vitamin replacement. Erythropoietin (Epogen or Procrit) is the intervention used when the body fails to produce an adequate number of red blood cells.

Iron deficiency anemia is usually caused by poor dietary intake or blood loss (menstruation or gastrointestinal bleed). Supplemental iron is the intervention or treatment.

> **KEY NOTE:** Iron absorption is enhanced when taken with vitamin C.

Pernicious anemia occurs when the body fails to secret the protein (intrinsic factor) required to absorb vitamin B_{12} from foods. Underlying causes may be a vegetarian diet, gastric surgery, or overgrowth of gastric bacteria. Pernicious anemia is common among people of Caucasian descent. Signs and symptoms include nerve damage, digestive tract problems, fatigue, a smooth red tongue, and anemia.

Tests for pernicious anemia include a complete blood count (CBC), vitamin B_{12} level, and homocysteine level. A Shilling's test is performed to determine the patient's absorption of B_{12}. Treatment consists of administration of vitamin B_{12} supplements; dietary changes to increase consumption of liver, poultry, and eggs; and discontinuation of offending medications.

Megaloblastic anemia is caused by a folic acid deficiency. Folic acid deficiency is a result of poor diet, celiac disease, alcohol abuse, and certain medications (Dilantin and metformin). Treatment is oral doses of folic acid, which may need to be administered intravenously if gastric absorption is unlikely.

Aplastic anemia presents with pancytopenia (reductions in RBC, WBC, and PLT). The causes (not all inclusive) of aplastic anemia are infections (bacterial and viral) and certain medications (including antiseizure medications). Symptoms present as shortness of breath, dyspnea, or fatigue. Treatment is aimed at removing the underlying cause.

Thalassemia is an inherited blood disorder that forms abnormal red blood cells, which leads to excessive destruction of red blood cells, causing anemia. The severity depends on the genes affected. This disease is frequently seen in individuals of Mediterranean, Asian, and African American descent. This type of blood disorder causes anemia, stillbirth, genetic defects, heart failure, and endocrine and liver problems. Genetic counseling is essential.

Sickle cell anemia is a genetically inherited disorder. The sickle cell episode can be caused by infection, dehydration, stress, blood loss, or etiology unknown. The sickle red blood cell is crescent shaped with decreased flexibility. The decreased flexibility results in the red blood cell having difficulty moving through the small veins and capillaries. Occlusions can occur that cause tissue ischemia, pain, and injury. The sickle cell clumping causes decreased blood flow and thrombi and can lead to shock. Sickle cells can cause an occlusion in any area of the body, resulting in stroke (brain), pulmonary emboli (lungs), and renal failure (kidneys). The sickle cells that continue to circulate are hemolyzed, which further increases the anemic state.

Polycythemia vera is a genetically inherited disorder of unknown etiology that produces too many red blood cells, which may cause clotting.

Leukemia is a malignant disorder that affects bone marrow and results in the production of dysfunctional cells. Treatment is aimed at producing a remission. Causative factors are genetic or environmentally related. Types of leukemia include acute myelogenous leukemia (AML), acute lymphocytic leukemia (ALL), chronic myelogenous leukemia, and chronic lymphocytic leukemia. An acute diagnosis reflects rapid growth or onset. A chronic diagnosis reflects slow growth or slower onset.

AML is a cancer that presents with flulike symptoms. Etiology is an abnormal production of blood cells within the bone marrow that prevents the development of normal blood cells. AML causes may include exposure to radiation, benzene exposure (chemical or smoking), and chemotherapy drugs. Treatment options are chemotherapy or a bone marrow transplant.

ALL is a cancer that presents with an overgrowth of abnormal WBCs within the bone marrow that prevents the development of red blood cells, normal WBCs, and PLTs. Symptoms vary based on the degree of abnormal growth or normal cell production. The patient may present with fatigue, shortness of breath, petechiae, frequent infections, and bone pain. Treatment options are chemotherapy or a bone marrow transplant.

Lymphomas are neoplasms originating in the bone marrow. Hodgkin's lymphoma or Hodgkin's disease presents with proliferation of abnormal or large cells (Reed–Sternberg cells) within the lymphatic system (nodes). The patient presents with lymph node enlargement. The patient may complain of fatigue, weight loss, or night sweats. The Epstein–Barr virus or environmental toxins are causative factors in the development of lymphomas.

Treatment is based on the causative factor and the progress of the disease. Chemotherapy begins in the early stages and continues to be administered in the intermittent and advanced stages of lymphoma as well.

Non-Hodgkin's lymphoma is a malignancy affecting the B cells. The patient presents with enlarged lymph nodes. Etiology has not been determined. Treatment is chemotherapy or radiation therapy.

The patient may require a bone biopsy or a lymph node biopsy to confirm an underlying hematological disorder. Often these tests are performed to validate a diagnosis when standard methods, such as blood slides or physical examination, cannot.

Hemochromatosis is a common genetic blood disorder that presents with a buildup of too much iron in the body. The body absorbs only about 10% of the iron in the food, but in this disease, more iron is absorbed and the body is unable to eliminate the extra iron. Extra iron is stored in the liver, heart, and pancreas, which can cause diabetes mellitus, hypothyroidism, liver cancer, and heart disease. The treatment consists of therapeutic phlebotomy. Early diagnosis and treatment of hemochromatosis is essential and may prevent and reverse complications of the disease.

HEMATOLOGY EXERCISE

Answer the following questions and return by preconference next week.

1. Which blood cells are responsible for transporting oxygen?
2. What is the defender of the body against infection?
3. What cells are involved in the blood's ability to coagulate?
4. What nutritional component is needed for production of RBCs?
5. What organ secretes erythropoietin under conditions of low oxygen levels?
6. Which WBCs destroy microorganisms by ingestion (phagocytes)?
7. What type of granulocyte stimulates the inflammatory response (a mediator)?
8. What type of WBC housed in the immune system provides immunity?

9. In which organ are excess PLTs stored?
10. What is the term used to describe the development or formation of blood cells?

Enter "T" for "True" or "F" for "False" after the following statements:

11. Blood cell production increases in anemic conditions. _____
12. The elderly patient has built up an immune response to infections. _____
13. Neutropenic patients are at great risk for infections. _____
14. Neutropenia is caused solely by an autoimmune disease. _____
15. Thrombocytopenia is an excess amount of PLTs. _____
16. Alcoholism can improve thrombocytopenia. _____
17. Polyuria is a symptom of DIC. _____
18. Hemophilia is the development of blood cells. _____

ANSWERS TO HEMATOLOGY EXERCISE

1. Red blood cells
2. White blood cells
3. Platelets
4. Adequate nutrition (vitamins)
5. Kidneys
6. Neutrophils
7. Basophils
8. Lymphocytes
9. Spleen
10. Hematopoiesis
11. Blood cell production increases in anemic conditions. _F_
12. The elderly patient has built up an immune response to infections. _F_
13. Neutropenic patients are at great risk for infections. _T_
14. Neutropenia is caused solely by an autoimmune disease. _F_
15. Thrombocytopenia is an excess amount of PLTs. _F_
16. Alcoholism can improve thrombocytopenia. _F_
17. Polyuria is a symptom of DIC. _F_
18. Hemophilia is the development of blood cells. _F_

CRITICAL THINKING EXERCISE #1

A 24-year-old African American female is admitted with sickle cell crisis. The patient is complaining of substernal chest pain 5/10, her skin is cool to touch, she is slightly diaphoretic, her HR is 120, BP 92/62, and O_2 Saturation 92% on room air. Stat basic metabolic panel, magnesium, phosphorous, arterial blood gas, complete blood count, troponin, and creatine phosphokinase-MB (CPK-MB). Type and screen and transfuse 2 units of leukoreduced split-pack red blood cells. Patient's blood type is O positive. Patient has had a mild febrile reaction in prior transfusions and is to receive Tylenol 650 mg and Benadryl 25 mg po 30 minutes before transfusion.

Answer the following questions and return by preconference next week.

1. What is sickle cell disease?
2. What are the complications of sickle cell disease?
3. How long will red blood cells last?
4. Why would the sickle cell patient be more susceptible to infection?
5. What are the risks of blood transfusions?
6. For how long is a type and cross match good before it expires?
7. What types of blood can be transfused to this patient?
8. What is a febrile nonhemolytic reaction?
9. What is the time limit for a unit of blood to be transfused?
10. What is a split pack? What is leukoreduced blood?

ANSWERS TO CRITICAL THINKING EXERCISE #1

1. Sickle cell disease is an autoimmune disease that causes the red blood cells to become adhesive and abnormally shaped, which causes blockage of blood vessels and extreme pain. This disease is common among individuals of Mediterranean, African American, and Hispanic descent.

2. Complications include: acute chest syndrome, stroke, pulmonary hypertension (HTN), blindness, skin ulcers, and gallstones.

3. Red blood cells last 120 days, but in sickle cell anemia the RBCs only last 10 to 20 days.

4. The spleen, which helps with immunity, is usually damaged in sickle cell anemia.

5. The risks of blood transfusions include transfusion reaction, hepatitis B and C, HIV, bacterial contamination, malaria, and Lyme disease.

6. A type and crossmatch is good for only 72 hours.

7. This patient can only receive O positive and O negative blood.

8. A febrile nonhemolytic reaction is exhibited by a fever, chills, and a headache. It is caused antigens on PLTs, lymphocytes, and granulocytes.

9. A unit of blood must be transfused within 4 hours.

10. A split pack is a unit of blood divided into two units. A normal unit of blood may be 300 to 400 mL, so the pack will be split into two. Since sickle cell patients may have trouble with large amounts of fluid, split packs are used to prevent volume overload. Leukoreduced means that there was a removal of WBCs from the blood components to reduce an allergic response.

CRITICAL THINKING EXERCISE #2

A 28-year-old Caucasian male is admitted with complaints of numerous spontaneous ecchymotic bruises. Patient complains of dyspnea, weight loss, and bone pain. Diagnostic tests reveal enlargement of the liver and lymph nodes, anemia, and elevated WBC. A bone marrow aspiration from the pelvic bone was performed. Conscious sedation was performed for the procedure. The bone marrow reveals a diagnosis of acute lymphoblastic leukemia (ALL).

Answer the following questions and return by preconference next week:

1. What is acute lymphoblastic leukemia (ALL)?
2. What are the complications of ALL?
3. What is the prognosis for ALL?
4. What are the treatments for this condition?
5. What is conscious sedation?

ANSWERS TO CRITICAL THINKING EXERCISE #2

1. Acute lymphoblastic leukemia (ALL) is cancer of the blood and bone marrow, causing immature WBCs.

2. ALL can spread to all the organs, causing extensive damage.

3. ALL usually occurs in children, especially those with Down syndrome, and in older adults, but it can occur at any age. The prognosis depends on when the cancer was detected, whether it is acute or chronic, and the age of the patient.

4. Chemotherapy, stem cell transplantation, radiation, and alternative therapies.

5. Conscious sedation occurs when a patient is given a combination of drugs in small doses to help the patient to relax and not feel pain, but still remain able to respond throughout the procedure. The patient will be monitored with frequent vital signs and pulse oximetry to prevent complications. The patient should have someone to drive him home after the procedure and monitor him until fully awake.

BLOOD TRANSFUSION REACTIONS

Blood transfusion reactions can occur with immediate onset or may be delayed until hours or weeks after the blood has been infused. An acute hemolytic reaction occurs when incompatible blood is transfused. Incompatible antigens cause the patient's antibodies to react and cause cell agglutination. The agglutination process causes occlusion in the veins. The breakdown of red blood cells can occlude the renal tubules and result in renal failure. A urine specimen will reflect free hemoglobin indicative of a hemolytic reaction. There are many precautions necessary to prevent an acute hemolytic reaction. Before initiating any blood transfusion, the nurse must check the order, must have a signed blood transfusion consent, and must check the prescribed blood at the bedside with a second nurse. Both nurses must state and check the numbers on the patient's blood band and armband against the patient information and confirmation numbers on the blood product's (unit to be transfused) paperwork.

Transfusions are volume expanders (they increase pressure in the vasculature). Transfusions administered to patients with an underlying heart failure or renal disease can result in fluid overload. Care should be taken to monitor more closely those patients who are susceptible to fluid volume pressures.

Nurses who initiate a blood transfusion must be aware of the risk of transfusion-related acute lung injury (TRALI). TRALI presents with sudden onset of pulmonary edema resulting in acute lung injury. It should be noted that patients who receive mass blood transfusions can develop citrate toxicity (citrate is a blood preservative), hypocalcemia, and hyperkalemia. Treatment is for citrate toxicity is to administer calcium (calcium binds with citrate).

INFECTIOUS DISEASES

There are many diseases and infectious processes that can occur. One such disease process is methicillin-resistant *Staphylococcus aureus* (MRSA). MRSA is a resistant strain of bacteria attributed to the over- and unnecessary use of antibiotics. Bacterial infections require antibiotic treatment. Pathogens or bacterial microorganisms build up a resistance to antibiotics, resulting in infections that resist current treatment modalities. When a patient enters the hospital, the illnesses that the patient already has places that patient in a vulnerable position. Often the patient is weak and the patient's immune system is compromised. Everyday activities of the hospital may place that patient at risk for developing MRSA (e.g., by IV catheter insertion or surgical procedures).

MRSA testing is performed on the patient with a nasal swab. A culture (swab) is placed within the patient's naris, approximately ½ inch to 1 inch. The culture should touch the inner surface of the naris. One method is to "paint" the inner naris with the swab. The swab should be immediately placed in a sterile container and sent to the laboratory. It may take up to 48 hours for the test results. Patients who are positive for MRSA should be isolated to prevent transference of the resistant organism.

MRSA is resistant to multiple antibiotics. Upon positive diagnosis, blood cultures are usually drawn to determine to which antibiotics the MRSA may be susceptible. Treatment includes antibiotics, isolation, and strict hand washing.

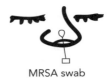

MRSA swab

FIGURE 15.1   A MRSA swab culturette is inserted into the patient's naris.

KEY NOTE: MRSA can enter the bloodstream, placing the patient at greater risk for infection throughout the body.

Vancomycin-resistant enterococci (VRE) is also a resistant organism. Bacteria within the colon are called enterococci (*Escherichia coli*). *E. coli* has been known to cause infections when it moves outside the colon. Urinary tract infections are often caused by *E. coli*. Vancomycin antibiotic treatment will usually resolve the urinary tract infection; however, when the patient has VRE, the patient will require a different antibiotic to treat the infection. VRE can be transferred from contaminated items or objects to the patient or to the health care worker's hands. IV catheters and central venous catheters have been sites for VRE entry into the bloodstream. Blood cultures can be obtained to determine whether the patient has been exposed to VRE and to which antibiotic the pathogen may be susceptible.

Many resistant organisms have developed immunity or found ways to disable many antibiotics' chemical compositions. Extended-spectrum antibiotics are antibiotics that have been modified to combat additional bacteria. It is necessary to keep modifying antibiotics because pathogens or resistant organisms continue to become more complex, making treatment more difficult.

Extended-spectrum beta-lactamase (ESBL)–producing organisms are capable of disabling an antibiotic by breaking down the antibiotic's chemical compound through a process called hydrolysis. Once hydrolysis occurs, the antibiotic is rendered ineffective. ESBL is rapidly multiplying in the patient care population and has been associated with *E. coli* and *Klebsiella pneumoniae*. Although beta-lactamase inhibitors have been developed, they too are often ineffective. The resistant organism produces the beta-lactamase enzyme, which is resistant to both gram negative and gram positive antibiotics. The carbapenems are a group of antibiotics that have been used successfully on ESBL infections. However, infectious disease personal have recently recognized the development of a species that is currently resistant to the carbapenem antibiotic group.

Infection control nurses must be vigilant in their quest to maintain adequate infection control precautions to assist in the reduction of infection transmissions. Staff must be reminded to follow the isolation guidelines, and strict hand washing is a must to prevent additional resistant strains. Nursing instructors must educate nursing students on the proper techniques of hand washing, isolation equipment, and personal protective equipment.

In order to provide for the most effective protection, the nurse must determine the appropriate personal protection equipment necessary for the required task.

TRANSMISSION PRECAUTIONS

Airborne precautions prevent transmission of extremely small particles of evaporated droplets (smaller than 5 μ) that can stay suspended in the air for long periods of time. The patient needs to be placed in a negative pressure isolation room with 6 to 12 air exchanges/hr. The room must be kept closed at all times. Hospital personnel and visitors must wear the N95 TB respirator. Patients in airborne isolation must remain in their room except for essential studies only.

Droplet precautions (for droplets greater than 5 μ in size) are used with a susceptible disease or carrier of a specific organism. These droplets are generated during sneezing, coughing, talking, and during certain procedures such as suctioning or bronchoscopy. Large droplets travel only short distances and do not remain suspended in the air. Close contact (usually 3 feet or less) with the infectious person is required for transmission of the disease. Examples of these diseases include scarlet fever, diphtheria, influenza, pertussis, meningitis, mumps, and H-influenza disease. Gowns, gloves, and masks are required.

Contact precautions are used when there is direct contact or indirect contact with contaminated secretions, skin-to-skin contact, or contact with a contaminated intermediate object from the patient's environment. Illnesses for which contact precautions are used include multidrug-resistant bacteria (MRSA, VRE, etc.); enteric infections, such as *Clostridium difficile*; and skin infections that are highly contagious such as scabies, major abscesses, and impetigo. Hospital personnel and visitors must wear gloves and gowns. Disinfection of nondisposable, reusable patient equipment must be performed before leaving the contact isolation room and before reuse with another patient. When possible, dedicate equipment solely to the contact isolation room. Proper hand washing is required with *C. difficile* since this is a spore-forming disease. Use soap and water instead of antibacterial soap or bleach wipes.

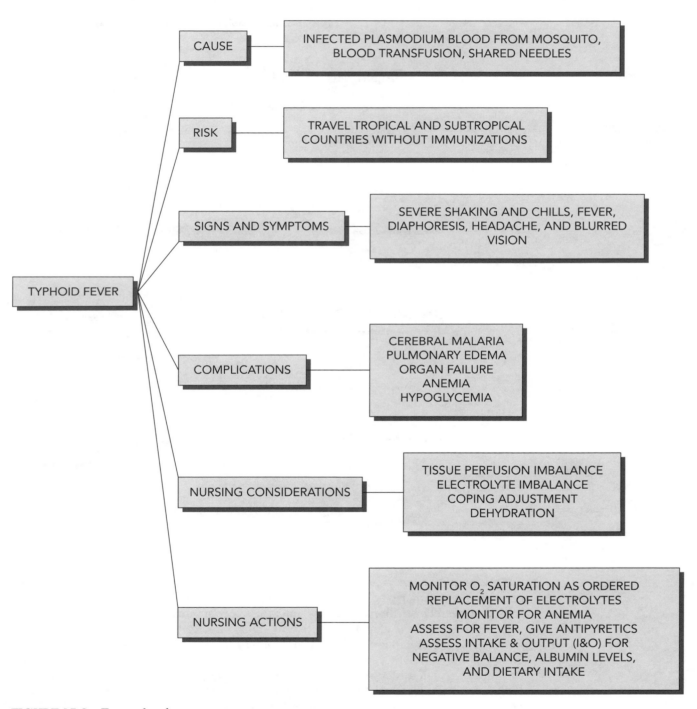

FIGURE 15.2 Example of a concept map.

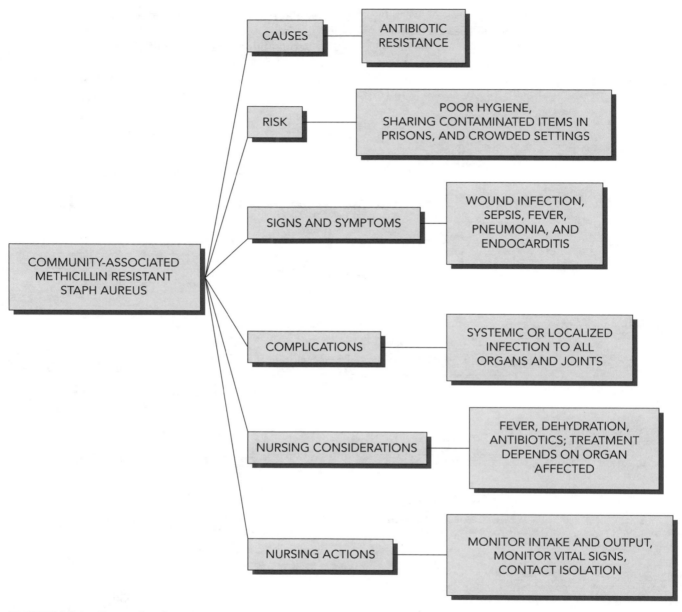

FIGURE 15.3 Example of a concept map.

ENDOCRINE SYSTEM

The endocrine system is a collection of glands—such as pineal, hypothalamus, thyroid, parathyroid, pituitary, adrenal, testes, ovaries, and thymus gland—with specialized cells that secrete hormones directly into the bloodstream. Elements of the exocrine system, including the salivary glands; the liver; pancreas; and prostrate, gastric, and sweat glands, secrete via a glandular duct. Hormones are chemicals that are produced and secreted to convey certain communications to specified target cells. The endocrine system is regulated by a negative feedback or loop system. When the body's sensory cells detects a decrease in the hormone level, they stimulate an increase in the production of that specific hormone. If there is too much of a certain hormone in the body, the sensory cells stimulate a decrease in the production of that hormone.

The hypothalamus, known as the "master" gland, helps to maintain homeostasis, is involved in the limbic (emotional) responses, and inhibits or stimulates the hormones that regulate the anterior pituitary and posterior pituitary gland.

The anterior pituitary gland secretes numerous hormones, such as the growth hormone (GH), thyroid-stimulating hormone (TSH), follicle-stimulating hormone, luteinizing hormone, adrenocorticotropic hormone (ACTH), and prolactin. Melanocyte-stimulating hormone is produced in the intermediate lobe of the pituitary gland, which is involved in appetite and sexual arousal. The posterior pituitary is responsible for the release of oxytocin and antidiuretic hormone. Any damage, abnormalities, or diseases of the pituitary gland will affect the depletion or abundance of these hormones.

ABNORMALITIES OF THE ENDOCRINE SYSTEM

The hypothalamus of the brain produces GH-releasing hormone, which stimulates the pituitary gland to produce human GH. This hormone is converted in the liver, which stimulates the fat cells to break down triglycerides and other tissues to produce insulin-like growth factor 1, which stimulates bone cells to reproduce and also produces muscle growth.

GIGANTISM

Hypersecretion of the GH in childhood before the long bone closes results in the condition known as gigantism. Diagnostic testing would consist of measuring blood levels of GH before and periodically after a preparation of glucose. Glucose normally causes GH levels to fall, but they will remain high if a tumor is present. Magnetic resonance imaging (MRI) also will confirm the diagnosis. Symptoms include enlarged organs, barrel chest, acromegaly, and an enlarged tongue. Administration of Sandostatin or octreotide, which are synthetic versions of the brain hormone somatostatin (GH release–inhibiting hormone), will block the pituitary gland's excess production. Hypersecretion of the GH is usually due to a benign pituitary tumor that can be extracted surgically.

ACHONDROPLASIA (DWARFISM)

GH deficiency, or hyposecretion of the GH, can result in achondroplasia (dwarfism). There are different types of dwarfism causing different abnormalities. Achondroplasia is exhibited by individuals with a short stature and with a relatively long trunk and shortened upper parts of their arms and legs, and is defined as an adult height of 4 feet 10 inches or less. Proportionate dwarfism results from medical conditions present at birth or during early childhood that limit an individual's overall growth and development, but the body parts are proportional. Turner syndrome is a disorder that results in short stature and impaired sexual maturation in females. There is a delay in motor skills development, such as sitting up, crawling, and walking.

Signs and symptoms of all forms of dwarfism include sleep apnea, excess fluid around the brain (hydrocephalus) that may require a shunt to drain, progressive severe hunching (kyphosis) or the forward curvature (lordosis) of the back, lumbosacral spinal stenosis resulting in pressure on the spinal cord and subsequent pain or numbness in the legs, and respiratory problems.

ADRENAL GLAND DISORDERS

The adrenal glands (located superior to the kidneys) each have two parts. The outer part (adrenal cortex) produces corticosteroids. Corticosteroids are hormones that regulate metabolism, body fluids, and the immune system. The medial part of the adrenal gland is called the adrenal medulla. The adrenal medulla produces catecholamines. Catecholamines, such as epinephrine and norepinephrine, assist the body in coping with emotional and physical stress.

The adrenal cortex produces mineralocorticoid (aldosterone) to assist the body in maintaining blood pressure by regulating sodium, potassium, and water in the renal tubules. Glucocorticoids (cortisol) stimulate the process of glycogenolysis (breakdown of glycogen into glucose by the liver) to provide energy. Cortisol (aldosterone) responds to stress, regulates blood pressure and cardiovascular function, slows inflammatory response, and helps to control sodium and water.

ADDISON'S DISEASE

Addison's disease is primarily a cortisol insufficiency due to hypofunction of the adrenal cortex, or it may be secondary due to genetic defects or removal of adrenal glands. One memory aid is to "Think Addison's disease: not enough cortisol (need to *add*)."

- **Causes:** AIDS, TB, fungal infections, adrenal cancer, and dysfunction of the pituitary, or it may be secondary due to medication changes such as sudden withdrawal of steroids
- **Diagnosis:** Addison's disease is diagnosed by low cortisol, glucose, and sodium levels; a high ACTH (adrenocorticotropic) concentration detected by an ACTH stimulation test; hyperkalemia; and a computed tomography scan of the adrenals and pituitary gland; chronic adrenal insufficiency produces insufficient steroid hormones such as glucocorticoids and mineralocorticoids; lifelong, continuous treatment with steroid replacement therapy is required
- **Signs and symptoms:** Fatigue, vertigo, muscle weakness, fever, weight loss, marked cravings for salt or salty foods due to the urinary losses of sodium, hypotension, decreased blood volume, hyperkalemia, hypoglycemia, bronze-colored skin, decreased resistance to stress, fractures, alopecia, weight loss, and gastrointestinal (GI) distress
- **Treatment:** Replace cortisol (hydrocortisone tablets, or prednisone); instruct the patient to wear a medical alert bracelet; increase medication during periods of stress or mild upper respiratory infections; immediate medical attention is needed when severe infections, vomiting, or diarrhea occur

ADDISONIAN CRISIS

"Addisonian crisis" or "adrenal crisis" indicates severe adrenal insufficiency. The signs and symptoms depend on the degree of hormone deficiency and electrolyte imbalance. Onset may occur due to stress, abrupt withdrawal of corticosteroids, or lack of cortisol. Initial signs of acute adrenal crisis are profound weakness, severe hypotension, decreased blood sugar, sexual dysfunction, abdominal and back pain, hyperpyrexia followed by a low temp, severe hypotension, and coma. Treatment includes hydration (to restore fluid balance) with normal saline, monitor and prevent hyperkalemia, correct hyperkalemia with Kayexalate, correct hypoglycemia with IV glucose, administer steroid replacement (patient will take steroids his or her entire life), and monitor glucose levels frequently (minimum Q2H).

CUSHING'S DISEASE

When a pituitary tumor stimulates the adrenal glands (ACTH), it will cause the adrenal glands to produce an excess amount of cortisol, which results in Cushing's disease.

- **Signs and symptoms:** This autoimmune disorder will exhibit classic physical characteristics: a moon face, truncal obesity, and hirsutism; other symptoms will include thin extremities, changes in mood and mental state, hypernatremia, hypokalemia, rapid weight gain, HTN (due to cortisol's enhancement of epinephrine's vasoconstrictive effect), and insulin resistance that causes diabetes mellitus, muscle wasting, and weakness
- **Diagnosis:** Diagnosis of Cushing's disease includes the ACTH test and a CT scan of the adrenal glands to detect tumors that may produce too much cortisol (ACTH) or to detect excessive levels of cortisol in the blood caused by taking glucocorticoid drugs. Lab tests will show low potassium, high sodium, and high blood sugar. A cortisone suppression test will be administered. After taking a dose of dexamethasone, cortisol levels stay abnormally high in people who have Cushing's syndrome.

- **Treatment:** If condition is due to steroids, gradually decrease them to avoid adrenal crisis. Ketoconazole, the initial drug of choice, is administered at initial doses of 200 mg (two to three times daily) with dose adjustments based on 24-hour, urinary-free cortisol levels. Radiation may also be used to destroy the tissue causing the underlying problem. If an adrenal adenoma is identified, the tumor will be removed by surgery (adrenalectomy or hypophysectomy) but lifelong steroids and mineralocorticoid replacement are required after surgery.
- **Nursing care:** Rest; low-sodium, low-caloric, low-cholesterol, high-potassium, and high-protein diet; frequent vital signs; weight daily; monitor blood sugar every 4 hours; monitor for depression; and monitor for safety.

AUTOIMMUNE DISORDERS

The immune system is composed of specialized glands, tissues, and cells throughout the body that are able to distinguish normal cells from foreign intruders. The lymphoid system consists of the lymph nodes, spleen, thymus, bone marrow, and tonsils. It helps to fight infection. Immunity can be both natural and acquired. A person is born with a natural immunity that helps to keep pathogens out and that protects against colonization by preventing pathogen adherence. Acquired immunity is developed from vaccinations or by contacting the infection or disease. From acquired immunity, the immune system will develop memory cells to attack the same antigen if exposed again. All immune cells start as immature stem cells in the bone marrow, but they respond to other chemicals such as cytokines to develop into T and B cells. The T and B cells are type of lymphocytes that will attack a particular antigen. The T cells (thymus cells) mature in the thymus and migrate elsewhere. B lymphocytes mature into plasma cells and will release antibodies. The lymphatic system monitors the body for pathogens. The nervous system will stimulate the adrenal system in response to stress by releasing hormones that may hurt the effects of immunity. The body will defend itself by the skin barrier, digestive system, and respiratory system.

Allergic reactions occur when the immune system responds to a normally harmless substance such as mold. Immunoglobulin E (IgE) is an antibody that will respond to hypersensitivity and allergic diseases.

The immune system is able to detect antigens (foreign bodies) and mount a response (antibodies) to eliminate the pathogens, but it may not recognize cancer cells. When the immune system is defective, it will attack the body's own cells, causing abnormal growth and change in the organ function, allergic diseases, and a wide range of other diseases.

A person with an autoimmune disorder will usually have a complement of other autoimmune disorders. Women of childbearing age are usually affected and autoimmune disorders occur within families. Some of the causes are unknown, but it may be linked to chemicals and to viral and bacterial infections.

Immune complex diseases are groups of antibodies and antigens that frequently become trapped in an organ's tissues, which leads to inflammation and organ damage. Immune deficiency disorders can be inherited or acquired or can be side effects from drugs used for cancer treatment or transplants. Depression of the immune system can also be caused by surgery, smoking, stress, and malnutrition.

To avoid rejection of the new transplanted organ, the immune system has to be muted. This is accomplished by administration of immunosuppressive drugs such as cyclosporine.

The thyroid gland (a butterfly-shaped gland located inferior to the larynx) will secrete thyroxine (T4) and triiodothyronine (T3). The hormones of the thyroid stimulate the systems in the body (metabolism). The thyroid gland needs iodine to synthesize and secrete the thyroid hormones T3, T4, and thyrocalcitonin (calcitonin).

The thyroid gland contains mainly two types of cells: thyroid follicular cells and C cells (also called parafollicular cells). The follicular cells use iodine from the blood to make thyroid hormones, which help to regulate a person's metabolism. The pituitary gland produces a substance called TSH to stimulate the thyroid. The parathyroid glands (glands attached to the thyroid) produce parathyroid hormone (PTH), which balances calcium and phosphorous levels.

Hypothyroidism (myxedema) is a deficiency of thyroid hormone that slows down the physical and mental functions, causing sensitivity to cold, dry skin and hair, dysphagia, respiratory difficulty, hypotension, and sinus bradycardia. Hypothyroidism may also cause cholesterol to rise because hypothyroidism decreases blood flow to the liver. If a woman is pregnant, hypothyroidism will cause birth defects such as a cleft lip. It may also cause a goiter, which is an enlargement of the thyroid gland. If the goiter becomes excessively large, it can result in breathing problems or difficult in swallowing. When the patient's airway is compromised by the goiter, the only solution is to have the goiter surgically removed. A goiter may also be caused by a diet low in iodine; faulty iodine metabolism; pituitary gland or hypothalamus injury or disease; iodine-131, which is used to treat thyroid cancer; surgical removal of the thyroid; lithium mood stabilizers; or ingestion of nutritional goitrogens (cabbage, soybeans, spinach, or medicines such as glucosteroids) that will inhibit thyroxine (T4). This disease will affect more females than males. Risk factors are sex, age, heredity, and other autoimmune disorders. Treatment consists of taking a thyroid supplement such as Synthroid for the rest of the patient's life. The patient must take the medicine first thing in the morning. It is not to be taken with iron, calcium, and antacids. Hypothyroidism is diagnosed by analyzing antithyroid microsomal antibodies, Total T3 and Total T4 (decreased), TSH increased, serum cholesterol increased, and anemia.

Myxedema coma is a state of decompensated life-threatening hypothyroidism that is precipitated by infection, medication, or environmental exposure. Primary symptoms of myxedema coma are altered mental status and severe hypothermia "cold shock," hypoglycemia, hypotension, hyponatremia, bradycardia, and hypoventilation. Treatment for myxedema coma is replacement of thyroid hormone and aggressive resuscitation.

Hashimoto's thyroiditis is the most common form of underactive thyroid and has a slow progression. Its symptoms and treatment are the same as for hypothyroidism.

Graves' disease is called hyperthyroidism (too much thyroid hormone) and it causes a rapid heartbeat, trouble sleeping, nervousness, hunger, weight loss, and intolerance to warmth. It also causes bulging of the eyes (exophthalmos) and causes thickened red skin, especially on the top of the feet (dermopathy). It will also affect the cardiac system by causing HTN; tachycardia, such as atrial fibrillation; congestive heart failure; and resistance to the effects of some drug such as digoxin and Coumadin. Graves' disease may also cause renal calculi and may compress the recurrent laryngeal nerve, producing vocal cord paralysis and respiratory stridor. Lab values will show a low TSH but a high T3 and T4. It is the most common cause of hyperthyroidism in children and adolescents and has a hereditary component. The thyroid hormones have to be suppressed, so antithyroid medication such as Tapazole and radioactive iodine therapy will be administered. Beta-blockers will be given to control the cardiovascular symptoms but will not affect the thyroid hormones.

Thyroid storm (thyrotoxicosis) occurs when the thyroid hormone levels become very high. Thyroid storm may be caused by illness, medications such as amiodarone, noncompliance with antithyroid medication regimens, diabetic ketoacidosis (DKA), and thyroid surgery.

One major distinction of thyroid storm is a marked elevation of body temperature (105°F–106°F) with tachycardia, delirium, dehydration, and HTN. T3 and T4 will be increased. There are no laboratory tests to confirm a clinical diagnosis. Treatment will consist of vigorous resuscitation; beta-blockers, which will inhibit the sympathetic nervous system; antithyroid treatments such as Tapazole, potassium iodide oral solution (SSKI), Lugol's, propylthiouracil, and corticosteroids; and subtotal thyroidectomy. Monitor vital signs and have both an available intubation tray and ampules of calcium gluconate present in the room. Place the patient in a semi-Fowler's position and prevent neck flexion and hyperextension.

Complications of thyroid surgery include vocal cord paralysis, hypocalcemia, and hypoparathyroidism. Thyroid storm may occur due to accidental removal of the parathyroid glands and may occur within 1 to 7 days after surgery. Check for Trousseau's sign (hand and fingers can go into spasm) or Chvostek's sign (touching facial nerve in front of the ear, which will produce twitching of the patient's upper lip).

> **KEY NOTE:** Convulsions, arrhythmias, tetany, spasms, and stridor are due to decreased calcium.

AUTOIMMUNE SKIN DISORDERS

Psoriasis vulgaris: Chronic, recurrent, and genetic systemic disease that is due to overstimulation of T-cells
  Signs and symptoms: Skin thickens; silvery white scales that have a symmetrical distribution arranged in lines, especially on the knees, back, and elbows; may cause arthritis
  Medical management: Suppress T-cell activation by using corticosteroids, ultraviolet therapy, and photochemotherapy
  Complications: Bone marrow depression, liver damage, and GI bleeding
Vitiligo: An immune system disorder that destroys the melanocytes (pigment cells) in the skin, which will cause well-defined irregular white patches and can be associated with other autoimmune disorders
  Signs and symptoms: Well-defined irregular white patches with white hair on different areas on the body
  Treatment: Phototherapy, immunosuppressant, and corticosteroid creams; psychological support is important because of the altered body image
Sjögren's syndrome: An autoimmune disorder in which the WBCs attack the exocrine glands that produce moisture; it can damage other organs as well
  Signs and symptoms: May be associated with lupus, patients 40 years old or older, joint pain, blurred vision, dental caries, and dryness of eyes and salivary glands
  Treatment: Consists of treating the symptoms

LIVER DISEASES

The liver is the largest internal organ in the body. The lobules of the liver contain rows of hepatic cells (hepatocytes). There are capillaries located between the rows of hepatic cells. The capillaries are lined with Kupffer cells, which remove bacteria and toxins from the blood. The blood arrives to the liver via the portal system. Bile is transported from the liver and stored in the gallbladder.
  Functions of the liver include:

- Carbohydrate is stored as glycogen and is converted to glucose
- Proteins are synthesized from amino acids and ammonia is converted to urea
- Fats are oxidized for energy
- Steroid hormones and drug metabolism
- Bile salt production, which is responsible for the digestion of fats and elimination of bilirubin
- Storage of glucose, minerals, and vitamins
- Filtration of blood and removal of bacteria and toxins

HEPATITIS

Hepatitis (inflammation of the liver) can be caused by viruses, bacteria, alcohol, toxins, infections, medications, and autoimmune processes. The symptoms of hepatitis are the same but the treatment may be different depending on the source of inflammation. Risk factors include sharing needles, having multiple sex partners, blood transfusions, being involved in the health care occupations, and working in sewer treatment plants.

Nonviral autoimmune hepatitis: Involves hardening of the liver and spider angiomas; begins in adulthood.

Symptoms: Pale-colored stools, abdominal pain, jaundice, and ascites. Ascites is excess fluid accumulated in the abdomen due to increased portal liver HTN that is caused by liver failure and a decreased albumin level. The bilirubin will present in the eyes first, and then the skin will show as a yellowish discoloration.

Tests: Antinuclear antibodies, anti-liver and kidney microsomes, smooth muscle antibodies, and liver biopsy. The liver plays a pivotal role in the clotting process because it synthesizes the clotting factors. When liver disease is present, there may be coagulopathy that has to be corrected before a liver biopsy with vitamin K or fresh frozen plasma. It is essential to evaluate prothrombin time prior to a liver biopsy.

Viral hepatitis:

Symptoms: Fatigue; nausea; joint aches; itching; jaundice; and elevated serum aminotransferase (AST) levels, elevated alanine aminotransferase (ALT), and elevated serum glutamic oxaloacetic transaminase (SGOT), which assess injury to liver cells; elevated serum bilirubin, elevated gamma-glutamyl transferase, and elevated alkaline phosphatase (measures hepatic excretory function), weakness, loss of appetite, ascites, light-colored stools, mental status changes, and encephalopathy.

Prevention: Hepatitis can be prevented by vaccines, immunoglobulins, or avoidance of exposure to viruses by not sharing needles or by not having multiple sex partners.

Treatment: Prednisone, cyclosporine, Imuran

Transmission:

Hepatitis A is spread by feces and contaminated food or water; it is spread via the fecal–oral route, and is seen with epidemics.

Hepatitis B spreads via infected blood and urine. It is transmitted from an infected mother to her baby at birth, through unprotected sex with an infected person, and by sharing equipment for injecting street drugs. Hepatitis B is not spread through food or water or by casual contact.

Hepatitis C spreads via contact with contaminated blood and needles shared during illegal drug use, posttransfusion from contaminated blood, and it is more prevalent with diseases that require frequent transfusions such as hemophiliacs or sickle cell crisis.

Stages of hepatitis:

Pre-icteric stage: 3 weeks; very contagious in this stage; arthralgia (joint pain); liver, spleen, and lymph nodes are enlarged

Icteric stage: 2 to 4 weeks; jaundice occurs because the body cannot metabolize bilirubin (clay-colored stools, dark urine, and liver tenderness)

Posticteric stage: begins with the disappearance of jaundice and lasts several months; vaccine for hepatitis B is Recombivax HB; three injections

The liver normally removes ammonia during urea synthesis, but blood ammonia elevates because the liver is damaged. The patient will require lactulose to treat this elevation or to prevent hepatic encephalopathy or coma. Asterixis is the jerking motion of the hands when flexed (associated with encephalopathy). Wernicke's encephalopathy is the acute phase of Wernicke–Korsakoff syndrome (acute mental confusion, ataxia [lack of coordination], and ophthalmoplegia [weakness or paralysis of the eye]).

WERNICKE–KORSAKOFF SYNDROME

Wernicke–Korsakoff syndrome, also called cerebral beriberi, is a severe memory disorder usually associated with chronic excessive alcohol consumption, although the direct cause is a deficiency in thiamin (vitamin B_1).

Signs and symptoms of alcohol withdrawal (within 4 to 6 hours): Nervousness, diaphoresis, tachypnea, HTN, and hyperthermia. At 48 hours since last drink:

Hallucinations, seizures, and delirium tremors. The baseline criteria for identifying delirium tremens include: a heart rate of 150 or greater, diastolic blood pressure higher than 100, a temperature in patients of 101°F or higher, and both agitation and active hallucinations.

Treatment: Treat with long-acting oral benzodiazepines such as diazepam (Valium), chlordiazepoxide (Librium, Librax), and lorazepam (Ativan); replacement of thiamine, multivitamins, and folate in IV fluids; and clonazepam (Klonopin).

CIRRHOSIS

Cirrhosis is the diffuse inflammation and fibrosis of the liver. There are different types of cirrhosis based on different causes:

- **Nutritional cirrhosis (portal cirrhosis):** Most prevalent type; due to a long history of alcoholism
- **Biliary cirrhosis:** Occurs because of liver bile-duct disease because the bile flow gets impeded
- **Postnecrotic cirrhosis:** Caused by chronic liver infections
- **Pigment cirrhosis:** This is also known as hemochromatosis, which is the inability to metabolize iron
  Signs and symptoms: Abdominal pain, enlarged liver and spleen, jaundice, elevated liver enzymes (bilirubin, ALT, AST, and SGOT), ascites (obstruction of the portal vein), and coagulation defects.
  Treatment: High-calorie, high-carbohydrate, low-fat, low-sodium, and low-protein diet; small meals. Vitamins, sodium intake restricted to 1 g/day, fluid restriction, Lasix, Aldactone (inhibits sodium and retains potassium), albumin IV, high Fowler's position to relieve respiratory distress, vitamin K (Aquamephyton), replacement of clotting factors (correct elevated PT with fresh frozen plasma), low-protein diet, and neomycin

HEPATIC COMA

Hepatic coma is the metabolic encephalopathy of the brain associated with liver failure.

Assess ammonia levels ($NHCO_3$), assess for airway obstruction due to decreased protective reflexes of the gag reflex, and assess for asterixis (an abnormal tremor of the hands when the patient is experiencing hepatic coma).

Symptoms: Slurred speech, restlessness, inability to write clearly

Treatment: Neomycin (antibiotic to decrease normal intestinal flora), lactulose (reduces ammonia levels), Flagyl (antibiotic used specifically for gastrointestinal infections), and liver transplant

INFLAMMATORY BOWEL DISEASES

Inflammatory bowel diseases are chronic inflammations of the digestive tract such as ulcerative colitis and Crohn's disease.

ULCERATIVE COLITIS

Ulcerative colitis is defined as inflammation of the large bowel. Potential causes include stress, autoimmunity, allergies, and infections (viral or bacterial).

Signs and symptoms: Abdominal tenderness and cramping, anorexia, bloody watery stools, tenesmus (constant feeling of need to defecate), and hyperactive bowel sounds

Diagnosis: Barium enema, biopsy by a sigmoidoscopy or colonoscopy, and lab work such as an erythrocyte sedimentation rate or C-reactive protein (CRP), which are signs of inflammation

Treatment: Depends on the advancement of the disease. Medications can consist of corticosteroids, aminosalicylates, immunosuppressants (cyclosporine), and biologics (TNP inhibitors); dietary changes should include consumption of fatty acids, probiotics, and vitamin supplements; surgery such as an ileostomy may be required

Ileostomy: Teach stoma assessment and care. If skin irritation is present apply the pouch 1/16th of an inch away from stoma and treat skin problems (candida–fungal). Reduce odor (avoid eggs, fish, onions, cabbage); enteric drugs may not be absorbed; and the patient needs a diet high in protein, carbohydrates, and calories; the patient is more prone to calculi (calcium oxalate)

CROHN'S DISEASE

Crohn's disease is an inflammation of the digestive tract. Crohn's disease often causes abdominal pain and diarrhea (malnutrition). Although it involves different areas of the digestive tract, the rectum is not involved. Crohn's disease involves edematous-heavy, reddish-purple areas called Peyer's patch. This disease may cause bleeding or necrosis. There is no cure. Intervention is geared toward reducing the symptoms of the disease.

Signs and symptoms: Abdominal pain, cramping, nausea, and diarrhea (often bloody); the intestinal tissue will have a cobblestone appearance

Diagnosis: Laboratory tests and an esophagogastroduodenoscopy

Treatment: Decrease diarrhea; administer steroids; replace electrolytes and water; administer total parenteral nutrition (TPN); antidiarrhea medications; assess nutritional intake by a calorie count; assess patient's stress and emotional status; patients with Crohn's disease may be unable to absorb vitamin B_{12} and may require a colectomy; the patient will then need ostomy teaching

RELATED NEUROLOGICAL SYSTEM DISORDERS

The central nervous system (CNS) is made up of the brain and the spinal cord, and the peripheral nervous system (PNS) is made up of the nerves. The brain collects, integrates, and interprets all stimuli and initiates and regulates voluntary and involuntary motor activity. Sensory nerves gather information from the environment, and the impulses are sent to the spinal cord, which transmits to the brain. The brain motor neurons deliver the instructions from the brain to the rest of the body via the spinal cord nerves.

The spinal cord extends from the upper border of the first cervical vertebra to the lower border of the first lumbar vertebra. The spinal cord is encased by the same membrane structure as the brain and is protected by the bony vertebrae of the spine. The spinal cord mediates the sensory-to-motor transmission path known as the REFLEX arc.

Neural horns are the H-shaped mass of neuron cell bodies in the spinal cord. This mass is divided into four horns, which consists mainly of two dorsal (posterior) horns in the spinal cord that relay sensation, and two ventral horns (anterior) that play a role in voluntary and reflex motor activity.

White matter surrounding the four horns consists of myelinated nerve fibers grouped in vertical columns or tracts. The dorsal horn white matter contains the ascending tracts (which carry impulses up the spinal cord to higher sensory areas). The ventral white matter contains the descending tracts (which carry impulses from the higher motor center down the spinal cord).

Motor impulse pathways:

- Travel from the brain to the muscles by way of the motor or descending pathway
- Begins in the frontal lobe and travel from the upper motor neurons to the lower motor neurons of the PNS
- Upper motor neurons originate in the brain and form two major systems: the pyramidal system and the extrapyramidal system.
  - **Pyramidal system** (corticospinal tract): Responsible for fine movements of skeletal muscle. At the medulla cortico-spinal fibers cross to the opposite side and continue down the spinal cord.
  - **Extrapyramidal system** (extracorticospinal tract): Controls gross motor movements.

Pain and temperature sensation enter the spinal cord through the dorsal horn. The ganglia are relay stations that allow sensations such as touch, pressure, and vibration to reach the spinal cord.

GUILLAIN–BARRÉ SYNDROME

Guillain–Barré syndrome is an immunological disorder that attacks the myelin sheath of the nerves. The cause is unknown, but it is preceded by an infectious illness such as a respiratory infection or the stomach flu.

Signs and symptoms: Begins with weakness, tingling, or loss of sensation, starting in the feet and legs and spreading to the upper body and arms, then paralysis. Other symptoms include difficulties with walking, eye movement, facial movement, speaking, chewing, breathing, and swallowing. The condition tends to progressively worsen for about 2 weeks. Symptoms reach a plateau and remain steady for 2 to 4 weeks; then recovery begins, usually lasting 6 to 12 months. It may take years to recover.

Diagnosis: Spinal tap (lumbar puncture) and electromyography (EMG), which interprets electrical activity in the muscle to determine whether the weakness is caused by muscle damage or nerve damage.

Treatment: Plasmapheresis, which consists of removing the plasma and separating it from the actual blood cells. The blood cells are then put back into the body, which manufactures more plasma to make up for what was removed. IV immunoglobulin contains healthy antibodies from blood donors.

AMYOTROPHIC LATERAL SCLEROSIS

Amyotrophic lateral sclerosis (ALS) attacks neurons in the brain and spinal cord, affecting voluntary control of the arms and legs. ALS attacks only motor neurons—the senses of sight, touch, hearing, taste, and smell are not affected.

Signs and symptoms: Abnormal fatigue of the arms and/or legs, slurred speech. Most people with ALS die from respiratory failure. ALS strikes between ages 40 and 60.

Diagnosis: EMG and nerve conduction velocity tests; blood and urine studies, including high-resolution serum protein electrophoresis; thyroid and PTH levels; 24-hour urine collection for heavy metals; spinal tap; x-rays; myelogram of cervical spine; and nerve biopsy.

Treatment: No treatment is available to cure or halt this disease. Symptoms can be treated with physical therapy, antidepressants, baclofen for stiff muscles, and nutritional supplements.

MULTIPLE SCLEROSIS

Multiple sclerosis is an autoimmune disorder that destroys and attacks the myelin sheath in the CNS and slows the conduction of nerve impulses. There are many remissions and exacerbations. Risk factors include being a Caucasian woman, between the ages of 20 and 40, and having the Epstein–Barr virus.

Signs and symptoms: Loss of control; blurred vision, usually in one eye; balance problems; heat sensitivity; incontinence of bowel and bladder; fatigue; dysphagia; pain; and ambulation and vision problems

Diagnosis: MRI, lumbar puncture

Treatment (depends on symptoms exhibited): Deep brain stimulators, which are implanted electrodes inserted in the brain to regulate brain impulses; and medications imitating interferon, which is a protein normally produced by the immune system that helps the body to be more resistant to viruses, bacteria, and other pathogens. There is a slow progression to this disease, and there is no cure.

MYASTHENIA GRAVIS

Myasthenia gravis (MG) is characterized by varying weakness of the body's skeletal muscles. It can be caused by infection, fever, and medications; it affects women younger than 40 and men older than 60. The large thymus may become malignant and the thymus may trigger antibodies that block acetylcholine. Nerve endings normally release acetylcholine, but the antibodies block and destroy receptors for acetylcholine at the neuromuscular junction. Hypothyroidism will worsen MG symptoms.

Signs and symptoms: Affects swallowing, speech, and eye muscles (diplopia, which usually occurs first); trouble swallowing (dysphagia); symptoms improve with rest

Diagnosis: Medical history, acetylcholine receptor antibodies, and EMG (measures electrical potential of muscle fibers)

Treatment: Treat with neostigmine, pyridostigmine, and prednisone; thymectomy may be needed. Administer medications to control symptoms and reduce muscle spasms, such as baclofen or a benzodiazepine. Cholinergic medications are used to reduce urinary problems and antidepressants are used for behavioral symptoms.

Emergency: Myasthenia crisis is a life-threatening situation due to severe weakness of the respiratory muscles. These patients will frequently require intubation, so respiratory evaluations to assess the diaphragm and the lungs are required. These tests would include vital capacity (amount of air exchanged after a maximum exhalation), tidal volume (amount of air exchanged with each breath), and inspiratory force (which will assess the chest muscle strength).

> **KEY NOTE:** Do not use beta-blockers, quinidine, quinine, or phenobarbital, because these drugs will worsen MG symptoms and increase muscular weakness.

SCLERODERMA

Progressive systemic sclerosis (scleroderma, meaning "hard skin"): A connective-tissue disease, it will affect many internal organs and causes muscle atrophy on the face and neck, with widespread vascular movement in the GI tract, lungs, and kidneys. Progressive systemic sclerosis is associated with certain environmental factors (plastics, coal, and silica dust).

Signs and symptoms: Calcium deposits in tissues, which causes hardening of the endothelial tissues; Raynaud's phenomenon, which causes intermittent vasospasm of the fingertips; esophageal sclerosis of the esophagus, causing reflex; sclerodactyly, which is tightening and edema of the digits; telangiectasias, which is capillary dilations that form vascular lesions on face, lips, and fingers

Treatment: Vasoactive: Calcium channel blockers (nifedipine); glucosteroids (prednisone); immunosuppressive agents (cyclosporine); for renal crisis and HTN: angiotensin-converting enzyme.

SYSTEMIC LUPUS

Systemic lupus is a chronic inflammatory disease, common in African American and Hispanic women who are usually between the ages of 20 and 45. It may come on suddenly or develop slowly, may be mild or severe, and may be temporary or permanent with exacerbations.

Signs and symptoms: "Butterfly" rash; photosensitivity; mucous membrane ulcers; arthritis; pericarditis (most common); abnormal amounts of urine protein; seizures; low counts of white or red blood cells, or PLTs; abnormal immune tests that include anti-DNA or anti-Smith antibodies; lupus anticoagulant; sedimentation rate and CRP; and fingers and toes that turn white or blue when exposed to cold or during stressful periods (Raynaud's phenomenon). Women with systemic lupus erythematosus can experience worsening of their symptoms prior to their menstrual periods. Some medications such as hydralazine, quinidine, Dilantin, salicylates, corticosteroids, isoniazid, and antimalarial medications can trigger lupus as a side effect.

Treatment: Nonsteroidal anti-inflammatory drugs, corticosteroids, hydroxychloroquine (Plaquenil) antimalarial, and immunosuppressive medications such as Cellcept.

Patients should avoid sunlight and use sunscreen, get an eye examination, and a get cardiac and lung work-up. Patients are at increased risk for developing cancers such as leukemia, lymphoma, and breast cancer.

RHEUMATOID ARTHRITIS

Rheumatoid arthritis is an autoimmune disease that causes chronic inflammation of the joints. Patients experience numerous remissions and exacerbations, and the disease is more common in women.

Signs and symptoms: Fatigue, loss of energy, lack of appetite, low-grade fever; it affects multiple joints in a symmetrical pattern that leads to a loss of cartilage and weakness of the bones as well as the muscles, resulting in joint deformity and loss of function

Diagnosis: Based on the joints involved, characteristic joint stiffness in the morning, the presence of blood rheumatoid factor, sedimentation rate, and CRP; diagnostic procedures would include arthrocentesis (needle aspiration), arthrogram (x-ray after injection), arthroscopy (surgical insertion of fiber-optic scope), electromyogram (EMG; a nerve conduction test using electrodes inserted into the pathway), indium scan (useful for detecting osteomyelitis [infection]), and bone scan for detecting osteoporosis

Treatment: The goals of treatment are to reduce joint inflammation, reduce pain and maximize joint function (do not massage joints), and prevent joint destruction and deformity. Aspirin, naproxen (Naprosyn), ibuprofen (Motrin), and cortisone are used to reduce pain and inflammation. Immunosuppressive drugs used to treat rheumatoid arthritis include methotrexate (very few side effects, but can cause liver cirrhosis); azathioprine (Imuran), cyclophosphamide (Cytoxan), and cyclosporine (Sandimmune). However these immunosuppressive medications will depress bone marrow function and cause anemia, a low white cell count, and low PLT counts. Cyclosporine can cause kidney damage and high blood pressure. Other treatments include regular exercise, such as swimming; physical and occupational therapy to maintain joint mobility and strengthen muscles; and splinting supports.

Intervention: Comprehensive treatment includes a combination of patient education, rest and exercise, joint protection, medications, and surgery

PHEOCHROMOCYTOMA

Pheochromocytoma is a rare, usually noncancerous (benign) tumor that develops in the core of an adrenal gland.

Signs and symptoms: Hypersecretion of epinephrine and norepinephrine, persistent HTN, increased HR, hyperglycemia, diaphoresis, tremor, and pounding headache.

Treatment: Avoid stress, take frequent rest breaks, avoid cold and stimulating foods, and have surgery to remove tumor.

CELIAC DISEASE

Celiac disease is an intolerance for gluten, a protein found in wheat, barley, rye, and oats. This intolerance creates an immune-mediated toxic reaction that causes damage to the small intestine and does not allow food to be properly absorbed.

Signs and symptoms: Growth failure, vomiting, bloated abdomen, steatorrhea (fatty foul stools), behavioral changes, and infections.

Treatment: Untreated celiac disease will cause vitamin D, K, and B_{12} as well as mineral deficiencies, central and PNS disorders, and pancreatic insufficiency.

Interventions: Lifelong diet compliance, reading all food labels, and supplemental vitamins.

CELIAC CRISIS

Celiac crisis is a deadly condition due to its side effects of malabsorption, severe dehydration, and diarrhea. Celiac crisis may occur in patients who have not yet been diagnosed with celiac disease.

Signs and symptoms: Patients suffer from severe diarrhea, dry mouth, lethargy, sunken eyes, shriveled and dry skin, low blood pressure, increased heart rate, fever, delirium, and unconsciousness. Babies with celiac crisis will have sunken fontanels. Celiac crisis will cause hypokalemia, hypomagnesemia, hypocalcemia, and hypoproteinemia.

Treatment: Replacement of K, Ca, Mg, and albumin; corticosteroids; and treat metabolic acidosis and dehydration

DIABETES MELLITUS

The pancreas produces necessary hormones to utilize carbohydrates, proteins, and fats. The cells that produce the hormones reside in the islets of Langerhans. Within the islets of Langerhans are three types of cells: alpha, beta, and delta. The alpha cells produce glucagon. Beta cells secret insulin. Insulin is used as a facilitator to move glucose across cell membranes and into the cell (it lowers serum glucose levels). Delta cells produce somatostatin, which inhibits the production of both glucagon and insulin.

The hormones involved in glucose metabolism include:

- **Glucagon**: Stimulates gluconeogenesis alpha cells in the pancreatic islets
- **Catecholamines** (epinephrine/norepinephrine): Produced from the adrenal medulla. Norepinephrine and epinephrine have opposing effects on insulin release (norepinephrine inhibits, epinephrine stimulates)
- **GH**: Increases blood glucose by inhibiting glucose uptake by cells; it also promotes glycogenolysis in muscle tissue
- **Corticosteroids**: Increase blood glucose by inducing glucose release from hepatocytes and inhibiting glucose uptake by cells

TYPE 1 DIABETES

Type 1 diabetes (insulin-dependent diabetes) is a chronic condition in which the pancreatic beta cells produce little or no insulin (patient must take insulin daily to live). It typically appears during adolescence, but can develop at any age. As glucose levels rise, glucose is spilled into the urine. Glucose is not available for energy so the body breaks down fat and protein from adipose tissue and muscles, resulting in ketone formation. This patient will be diagnosed with DKA.

Signs and symptoms: Blood sugar is higher than 240 mg/dL; diabetes mellitus is more common in Hispanics and African Americans; there is no cure and symptoms can develop suddenly

Risk factors: Family history, genetics, and autoimmune destruction of the islet cells caused by viral exposure such as the Epstein–Barr virus, mumps, or cytomegalovirus

Treatment: Prevention, with attention to meals, medicines, and alcohol intake; checking blood glucose before sports or exercise and having a snack if the level is below 100 mg/dL, and adjusting medication before physical activity; avoiding exercise if glucose levels are above 300 mg/dL or under 100 mg/dL; patient should inject insulin in sites away from the muscles that are used most during exercise

TYPE 2 DIABETES

Diabetes mellitus (type 2 diabetes) is a metabolic disease caused by a defect in the secretion of insulin or the inability to utilize insulin. The patient diagnosed with type 2 diabetes presents with these "classic" signs: polyuria, polyphagia, and polydipsia. The body is unable to utilize the available insulin. Research has shown that obesity results in insulin resistance.

Diagnosis: Fasting glucose (100–126 mg/dL); hemoglobin A1C (glycated hemoglobin, which measures glycemic levels over past 3 to 4 months, with recommended levels at 6%–7%); oral glucose tolerance test (2-hour postglucose load is positive if blood sugar 140–199 mg/dL); urinalysis (glucose, acetone, ketones); fasting glucose (100–126 mg/dL)

Risk factors: Obesity, HTN, elevated cholesterol, metabolic syndrome (truncal obesity); common among African Americans, Mexican Americans, and Native Americans; proper diet, exercise, and medication can help to maintain healthy serum glucose levels. However, there are many reasons for a type 2 diabetic to have uncontrolled glucose levels. When this occurs, the patient is at a risk for hyperglycemic hyperosmolar nonketotic syndrome, which is an emergency.

Complications: Common infections (bacterial and fungal), urinary tract infections, and carbuncles (abscesses larger than a boil) caused by *Staphylococcus aureus*; leg and foot ulcers; nephropathy; damage to capillaries that supply the glomerulus of kidneys that causes albuminuria and HTN; and accelerated coronary symptoms, including a increase in cholesterol and saturated fat that can accelerate atherosclerosis. Diabetes mellitus patients do not experience normal chest pain and may only exhibit pain in the shoulders, neck, or arms, and not in the chest. They present with a general malaise (vague feeling of illness) and diaphoresis; peripheral neuropathy with temporary episodes of pain and paresthesia; neurogenic bladder symptoms, including impotence, gastroparesis (delayed gastric emptying), vagus nerve damage (diagnosed by upper endoscopy and ultrasound), diabetic retinopathy (development of retinal microaneurysms that cause hemorrhages that will produce scar tissue); symptoms may only produce blurriness or can cause blindness (glaucoma). Hyperglycemia and hypoglycemia may not confirm the patient has diabetes mellitus. Each episode needs to be investigated.

Treatment and interventions: Administer metoclopramide (Reglan), which stimulates stomach muscle contractions to help empty the stomach, administer erythromycin, and the patient should eat six small meals a day. Dilated eye exams are required every 6 months with photocoagulation and vitrectomy, if required. Patients should inspect their feet daily, they should not go barefoot, and should not soak their feet. Patients should use only warm water to wash their feet and dry carefully between the toes (no hot water bottles or heating pads). Patients should wear comfortable shoes that fit well and protect the feet, they should not cross their legs for long periods, and they should not smoke. Monitor for signs of infection.

HYPOGLYCEMIA

Hypoglycemia means that a patient's blood sugar is less than 70 mg/dL.

Causes: May be caused by too much antidiabetic medicine; meals or snacks that are too small, delayed, or skipped; alcohol intake; use of beta-blockers (can mask symptoms); and exercising without supplementation

Signs and symptoms: Diaphoresis, tremors, tachycardia, and coldness; hypoglycemia can cause loss of consciousness

Immediate treatment required: Three or four glucose tablets (or 15 g of carbohydrate, 4 oz of any fruit juice, or 8 oz of milk); if unresponsive, give D50 IV or glucagon; recheck glucose level every 15 minutes until stabilized

Treatment: Prevention by addressing meals, medicines, alcohol intake, checking blood glucose before sports or exercise and having a snack if the level is below 100 mg/dL, and adjusting medication before physical activity

> **KEY NOTE:** With any change in a patient's mental status, the nurse should always check vital signs, O$_2$ saturation, and blood sugar first. This is an emergency situation, and an order is not required.

Causes of Hypoglycemia

- Medications such as insulin, oral hypoglycemics, alcohol, pentamidine, quinine, beta-blockers (can mask symptoms), and quinolones
- Adrenal insufficiency or failure (no cortisol)
- Pituitary insufficiency (no GH or cortisol)
- Liver failure or insufficiency (no glycogen stores)
- Autoimmune hypoglycemia
- Tumors such as insulinomas or retroperitoneal sarcoma

DIABETIC KETOACIDOSIS

When glucose is not available to a patient for energy because of the lack of insulin, the body breaks down fat and protein from adipose tissue and muscles, which results in ketones leading to acidosis. This patient will be diagnosed with DKA. This condition is more common among Hispanics and African Americans. This occurs when the blood sugar is higher than 240 mg/dL.

Signs and symptoms: Blood sugar that is higher than 240 mg/dL; rapid breathing (Kussmaul), dry skin and mouth, fruity breath odor, polydipsia, and dehydration. Excessive loss of fluids, severe nausea, and vomiting lead to hypovolemia and shock; as acidosis increases, H$^+$ ions move from extracellular fluid to intracellular fluid, and shift K into extracellular fluid. K levels may be normal or even elevated, but as the acidosis is corrected the K will decrease, causing severe hypokalemia if not treated.

Treatment: Rehydrate: fluids are the most important intervention; isotonic (20 mL/kg) followed by 200 to 8,000 mL over next 24 hours; reverse shock: administer albumin and dextran; hypokalemia: K re-enters cells along with glucose after insulin administration and is then excreted in urine with rehydration (monitor labs every 2 hours); replace potassium and magnesium; correct pH and administer insulin (note: Insulin enhances movement of phosphate into cells and can produce hypocalcemia); monitor anion gap and ketones, which will help determine resolution of pH balance; administer bicarbonate to patients with a pH of 7.1 or less; administer low-dosage regular insulin (5–10 units/hr); prevent reoccurrence; frequent blood glucose (every hour) and electrolytes (every 2 hours)

> **KEY NOTE:** While treating DKA, avoid precipitous drop in glucose. Bringing the glucose down rapidly can result in increased intracranial pressure due to water being pulled into the CSF. So D5NS will be administered if the blood sugar drops too fast until the anion gap is normal.

HYPERGLYCEMIC HYPEROSMOLAR NONKETOTIC SYNDROME

Hyperglycemic hyperosmolar nonketotic syndrome occurs because the beta cells of the pancreas do not produce enough insulin. Blood glucose levels may become very high—greater than 600 mg/dL—without the presence of ketones. Glucose is dumped in the urine, causing increased urination. Left untreated, diabetic hyperosmolar nonketotic syndrome can lead to coma and life-threatening dehydration. Osmolarity is elevated above 320 mOsm/kg. Hyperosmolarity is a condition in which the blood has a high concentration of salt (sodium), glucose, and other substances that normally cause water to move into the bloodstream.

Treatment: Fluids are the most important intervention; potassium is low due to diuresis and needs to be replaced; supplemental insulin may be required

DIABETES MEDICATIONS

Oral hypoglycemics are used for diabetes mellitus (type 2 diabetes) if interventions with dietary changes, exercise, and weight control do not control blood glucose levels. Oral hypoglycemics will decrease insulin resistance but a major side effect is hypoglycemia. The following medications are examples of oral hypoglycemics.

- Sulfonylureas will trigger insulin release by direct action on pancreatic beta cell. These drugs include tolbutamide (Orinase); chlorpropamide (Diabinese); glipizide (Glucotrol); glyburide (Diabeta, Micronase, Glynase); glimepiride (Amaryl)
- Meglitinides help the pancreas to produce insulin. This medication is taken shortly before meals to boost the insulin response to each meal. If a meal is skipped, the medication is also skipped. Includes drugs such as repaglinide (Prandin).
- Thiazolidinediones will help regulate glucose and fat metabolism, and includes drugs such as rosiglitazone (Avandia) and pioglitazone (Actos).
- Biguanide: Metformin is for the treatment of diabetes mellitus (type 2 diabetes). This drug can produce lactic acidosis. Medication needs to be stopped 48 hours before and after any contrast dye.
- Alpha-glucosidase inhibitors (Precose, Glyset) will prevent the digestion of carbohydrates in the small intestines.

DIABETES INTERVENTIONS

1. Prevent infection
2. Dietary intake plan individualized for the patient's lifestyle, economic status, and food preferences:
   - High-fiber carbohydrates should provide up to 60% of total daily calories (vegetables, fruits, beans, and whole grains). Use exchange list within each category
   - Fats should provide no more than 30% of daily calories. Best types of fats: monounsaturated (such as olive, peanut, and canola oils; avocados; and nuts) and omega-3 polyunsaturated (such as fish, flaxseed oil, and walnuts). Limit saturated and trans fats
   - Protein should provide 12% to 20% of daily calories. Patients with kidney disease should limit protein intake
   - Achieve and maintain ideal weight; lose weight if body mass index is 25 to 29 (overweight) or higher (obese)
3. Exercise: Prolonged exercise requires protein and complex carbohydrate snacks prior to exercise. Patients with sensitive feet should avoid running exercises; wear good, protective footwear.
4. When insulin is required for type 1 and type 2, the different types are discussed in the following table.

Drug	Onset	Peak	Duration	Side Effects
Humalog (lispro) NovoLog (aspart)	15 min	60–90 min	3–4 hr	Hypoglycemia
Regular (fast acting) (*Humulin R, Novolin R*)	30 min–1 hr	2–3 hr	4–6 hr	Hypoglycemia Regular insulin is the only insulin that can be given IV
Intermediate (cloudy) NPH	2 hr	6–8 hr	12–16 hr	Hypoglycemia
Long-acting Ultra Lente	2 hr	16–20 hr	24+ hr	Hypoglycemia
Long-acting insulin glargine (Lantus) (Apidra)	1–2 hr	None	24+ hr	Do not dilute or mix Lantus with any other insulin or solution Hypoglycemia

- When mixing a long-acting insulin and a short-acting insulin injection, remember to inject air into the cloudy, then the regular, and to withdraw the regular dose first and then the cloudy insulin.
- Insulin is given subcutaneously with rotation of sites. Do not massage or aspirate; insulin is best absorbed in abdomen.
- The *onset* is how soon the insulin starts to lower the glucose after administered.
- The *peak* is the time when the insulin is at its highest concentration in the body working to lower the blood glucose.
- The *duration* is how long the insulin lasts.
- Insulin side effects: Hypoglycemia, tissue hypertrophy

Somogyi effect: The tendency of the body to react to hypoglycemia by overcompensating, resulting in high blood sugar.
Treatment: Need to increase snacks or change intermediate-acting insulin dosing
Dawn phenomena: Abnormal increase in blood glucose level in the early morning between 2 a.m. and 6 a.m.
Treatment: Carbohydrates need to be avoided before bedtime; adjust the time, type of insulin, or the insulin dose

ENDOCRINE MATCHING EXERCISE

Match the appropriate gland or disease in the left column to the hormone or condition in the right column. Complete this exercise and return by preconference of next week's clinical.

Cushing's syndrome	Dwarfism
Adrenal cortex	Hyperthyroidism
Myxedema	Master gland
Gigantism	DM type I
Pituitary	Cortisol insufficiency
Parathyroid	Mineralocorticoid
Hyposecretion of growth hormone	DM type II
Graves' disease	Increased glucocorticoid
Addison's disease	Hypersecretion of GH
No insulin	Hypothyroidism
Hyperosmolar hyperglycemic nonketotic syndrome	Kidney stones

ANSWERS TO ENDOCRINE MATCHING EXERCISE

Match the appropriate gland or disease in the left column to the hormone or condition in the right column.

Cushing's syndrome	Increased glucocorticoid
Adrenal cortex	Mineralocorticoid
Myxedema	Hypothyroidism
Gigantism	Hypersecretion of GH
Pituitary	Master gland
Parathyroid	Kidney stones
Hyposecretion of growth hormone	Dwarfism
Graves' disease	Hyperthyroidism
Addison's disease	Cortisol insufficiency
No insulin	DM type I
Hyperosmolar hyperglycemic nonketotic syndrome	DM type II

CRITICAL THINKING EXERCISE #3

A 15-year-old female was admitted with DKA. She has been a type 1 diabetic for 12 years. She has not been feeling well for the past 3 days. She is admitted with Kussmaul breathing, lethargy, and nausea. She is an avid runner at school. She has been adjusting her insulin and diet because she was concerned about her weight. She has currently placed herself on a 1,200-calorie-a-day diet. She normally weighs 58.5 kg and is 165 cm tall. She currently weighs 53 kg.

		Lab Work	
Na 150	FBS 384	WBC 11	Osmolarity level 350
K 4.0	BUN 34	Hct 42	
Cl 110	Cr 1.2	ABG pH 7.30 PO_2 80	PCO_2 37 HCO_3 17
CO_2 16	Hb14	Hb A1C 10	

She is ordered a basic metabolic panel every 2 hours with blood sugar every hour, and ABGs every 8 hours. The patient has been placed on an insulin drip, and the nurse must mix the first bag of insulin administration. The patient was given 1,000 NSS bolus, and then NSS is given at 200/hr. On assessment, the patient had dry mucous membranes, delayed capillary refill, and has lost 10 pounds within the past 2 weeks.

Answer the following questions and return by preconference next week.

1. What is Kussmaul breathing?
2. Why is IV fluid given at such a fast rate?
3. How would the nurse first detect fluid overload?
4. Why are the lab work and ABGs checked so frequently?
5. What considerations would the nurse address with children with diabetes?
6. How would the nurse mix the first bag of insulin?

ANSWERS TO CRITICAL THINKING EXERCISE #3

1. Kussmaul breathing is a rapid deep breathing present in DKA due to the breakdown of ketones. The breath is characterized by a "fruity" odor.

2. The IV fluid is given at such a fast rate because the patient is severely dehydrated due to excessive fluid losses due to polyuria. The fluids needs to be replaced to maintain hemodynamic status.

3. The first sign of fluid overload is usually an increase in respiratory rate and crackles in the lungs, with a drop in oxygenation.

4. ABGs are done to see whether acidosis is resolving. When acidosis is being corrected, the potassium is moved by the sodium potassium pump from the serum extracellular to the intracellular, thereby decreasing the serum potassium level. Potassium will also be diluted by rehydration. It is essential to do repeat electrolytes to monitor changes.

5. Adolescent children need emotional and psychological support. Since the child is an adolescent, there may be a rebellion against guidance or the disease. Physical activity is important, but the patient needs to understanding dietary intake and the need for monitoring blood glucose levels before, during, and after activities.

6. Insulin is a high-alert drug, and when mixed it must be checked by another nurse. The nurse would mix 1 mL of regular insulin to 100 mL of normal saline to make a 1 to 1 concentration. The bag and tubing must be labeled properly with date, time, and initials.

WEEK 12 POSTCONFERENCE

Inquire whether students noticed an increase in WBCs in their assigned patients with infections due to medications such as steroids, or elevated temperature. Discuss with students how the body responds to pathogens and the role the blood cells have in protecting the body.

Discuss diabetes, whether diabetic patients understand this disease, and how compliant they are with diet and medication. Does the diabetic patient adhere to the diet in the home environment? Does the diabetic patient exercise? What patient teaching or guidance can be given to the patient? Inquire whether the students noticed a correlation in diabetes, obesity, and HTN.

Clinical instructors must attempt to use didactic instruction to aid the student in understanding theoretical knowledge. Students should understand "normal" health and the signs and symptoms of the disease processes. Offering weekly information with guidance tools should help the students develop an understanding of the various diseases and interventions for patient care.

Case scenarios are a great way to help the students understand the interventions that should be implemented in a variety of disease or health issues. Case scenarios also allow the clinical instructor to provide the students with a variety of information that may not available in the didactic setting.

Chapter 16

REPRODUCTIVE SYSTEM FUNCTIONS, ASSESSMENT, DISEASES, AND TREATMENTS

This chapter examines:

- Male and female reproductive systems
- Conception, contraception
- Hormones and age-related disorders
- Sexually transmitted diseases, and HIV/AIDS

Week 13 discusses the normal functioning of the reproductive system and some of the many diseases that affect the reproductive system.

WEEK 13 PRECONFERENCE

Hand out:
- Medication forms (Viagra and Provera)
- Body surface area calculation quiz
- Reproductive system quiz
- Reproductive survey exercise
- Critical thinking exercise

Collect:
- Medication forms (Prednisone and Benadryl)
- Endocrine matching exercise
- Hematology exercise
- Critical thinking exercises
- Concept maps
- Care plans
- Physical assessment form
- Journals
- Additional assignments (makeup assignments, shadow forms, etc.)

Students often find it difficult to discuss and conduct reproductive system assessments. Discussing sexuality, sexual activity, and reproduction is often difficult for the patient as well. This type of information is very personal, and the patient is often too embarrassed to discuss this topic. However, students should understand the importance of collecting this data. The patient's reproductive history, sexual partners, and sexually transmitted diseases must be addressed because they can affect the patient's health. Encourage students to maintain a professional demeanor whenever they are discussing reproductive system issues with patients.

THE MALE AND FEMALE REPRODUCTIVE SYSTEMS

The male reproductive system is designed to produce and transport sperm into the female reproductive system. Within the scrotum (a protective sac) are two testes that house seminiferous tubules in which the spermatozoa develop. The sperm (once formed) travel from the testes through the ducts (ductus deferens and ejaculatory) and then out through the urethra.

The ejaculatory gland passes through the prostate gland. This anatomical association is the reason why men who have had prostate surgery may have ejaculation problems or urinary problems status post prostate surgery. The seminal vesicles, prostate, and Cowper's (bulbourethral) glands produce semen and the fluid that surrounds the semen.

The penis consists of erectile tissue that becomes firm on arousal. The skin covering the penis is smooth. The tip of the penis (glans) is initially covered by folds of skin (foreskin, or prepuce) that are often removed (by circumcision) based on health or religious practices.

The female reproductive system is designed to accept male sperm in a jointly contributory effort to conceive. The function of the ovaries is to ovulate as well as to produce estrogen and progesterone (hormones). The ovaries house follicles that contain oocytes. It is estimated that there are millions of follicles present at birth. However, the oocytes are often absorbed into the body (atresia), thereby decreasing in number throughout a woman's reproductive life span.

Each month, a mature ovum is released from the ovary. The ovum travels down the Fallopian tube. The gonadotropic hormones (follicle-stimulating hormone [FSH] and luteinizing hormone [LH]) stimulate this occurrence. The sperm meets the ovum within the Fallopian tube. Fertilization occurs in the distal portion of the Fallopian tube.

Students should review the three layers of the uterus (the outer layer [perimetrium], the middle layer [myometrium], and the inner layer [endometrium]) and review as well the internal and external structures of the reproductive system.

The cervix (lower portion of the uterus) extends into the vagina. The cervical canal permits the expulsion of menses during menstruation. The cervical opening also allows sperm to enter. The cervix's epithelial cells stretch during labor to allow expulsion of the fetus. The vagina is lined with squamous epithelium. The vagina contains cervical mucus, which assists in protecting the vagina against infections.

The female breasts develop during puberty. The areola is the dark center of the breast. The nipple is centered within the areola. The alveoli (or acini) secrete milk when the woman's hormones stimulate milk production. Milk flows through the lactiferous duct to the sinuses. The nipple has multiple pores that allow milk to flow during lactation. Fatty tissue supports this glandular system. The shape and size of the female breast vary in each individual woman.

The bilateral breast lymphatic system drains into the axillary and infra- and supraclavicular channels. Due to this close proximity, breast cancer often will metastasize to other parts of the body using the lymphatic system as a transport modality.

The hypothalamus produces gonadotropin-releasing hormones (GnRH) that stimulate the anterior pituitary to secrete FSH and LH. The FSH stimulates ovum maturity. LH stimulates ovulation or rupture of the follicle. The follicle produces both estrogen (which suppresses FSH) and inhibin (a hormone that inhibits GnRH and FSH). Prolactin stimulates growth of the mammary glands (stimulating milk production during lactation). Progesterone assists in developing and maintaining female sexual characteristics. Progesterone also assists in the preparation of the endometrium for potential fertilization.

Infertility may occur when the male is diagnosed with no or low sperm count, or when the female is diagnosed with anatomical abnormalities (abnormal Fallopian tubes) or failure to ovulate. Mumps is one of the most significant childhood diseases that affect male fertility. Also, exposure to pesticides will influence male fertility. Women diagnosed with endometriosis may also have infertility. Fertilization interventions may assist a couple to conceive. In vitro fertilization is a process in which ova (eggs) are extracted from the woman by a physician, placed in a sterile dish, fertilized by sperm, and then inserted into the uterus.

The uterus performs a normal monthly menstrual cycle stimulated by the hypothalamus and anterior pituitary. If the ovum is not fertilized, menstruation occurs. Once the ovum is released, the ovarian follicle continues to secret estrogen and progesterone. During this time, the endometrium begins to change. The growth of blood vessels allows an increase in vascular blood supply. If fertilization occurs, the follicle continues to produce estrogen and progesterone. If fertilization does not occur, the blood-rich lining of the endometrium sloughs off (menses).

Sexual responses aid in the potential for fertilization. In the male, the excitement phase occurs, resulting in penile erection. The erection occurs when venous sinuses within the erectile tissue becomes engorged with blood. The penis skin tightens, allowing easier entry into the vagina. When orgasm occurs, there is a muscular contraction of the penile and urethra (ejaculation). Sperm is propelled out through the meatus during ejaculation.

In the female, the excitement phase occurs, resulting in increased vaginal lubrication, and the clitoris becomes engorged. When orgasm occurs, the cervical opening relaxes slightly, aiding in the probability of sperm entry.

CONTRACEPTION

For women who do not wish to become pregnant, contraception can be used as a preventative measure. When choosing a birth control or birth prevention method, a woman should determine whether there is a risk for sexual transmitted diseases (STDs). Many birth control methods do not offer protection from STDs.

Barrier methods of contraceptive are devices such as an intrauterine device (IUD), a sponge, or a diaphragm (not all inclusive). IUD contraceptives (which are inserted by a physician) may become dislodged or cause excessive bleeding. The sponge (non-prescription) is inserted by the woman into the vagina to prevent sperm from entering the cervix. The sponge must be left in place for 6 hours after intercourse. The sponge may increase the risk of toxic shock syndrome if left in place longer than directed. The diaphragm is fitted snuggly over the cervix (by the woman) to prevent sperm entry; however, the diaphragm may become dislodged during sexual intercourse. Women may also use a spermicide. This chemical is inserted into the vagina for killing sperm. Spermicides may cause vaginal irritation or an allergic reaction.

Birth control pills allow for continual birth control protection when taken as prescribed. However, there are increased health risks with taking birth control pills such as dizziness, nausea, blood clots, stroke, and others. Birth control pills use hormones to fool the body into believing that no fertilization has occurred; thus, a regular monthly menstrual flow occurs.

Men can choose to use condoms to aid in birth control or birth prevention. Condoms are made of latex, fit over the penis, and collect the sperm during ejaculation. The advantages of the condom are its protection against STDs. However, complaints of decreased sensitivity and occasional condom breakage have been noted. Men can have a surgical procedure, called a vasectomy, which allows for a permanent solution to birth prevention.

When a patient enters the hospital, data must be collected. The patient's history must include information relating the reproductive systems. Data on the female patient should include menstrual history (age initiated, regularity, and characteristics). Data on preventative health measures should also be collected (routine pap smears, mammograms, monthly breast self-examination, etc.).

FEMALE REPRODUCTIVE SYSTEM DISORDERS

A common disorder for women is premenstrual syndrome (PMS). Although the etiology is not clearly understood, the mood swings and emotional behaviors can tax interpersonal relationships. Presenting physiological symptoms may include breast pain, abdominal bloating, and cephalgia. Treatment is based on symptoms. Some antidepressants been prescribed with great success.

Endometriosis happens when the endometrial cells live outside the uterus. This causes masses of aberrant growths of endometrial tissue throughout pelvis. Endometrial cells that are normally shed during the menstrual period start living outside the uterus. These cells respond to hormonal changes. The signs and symptoms of endometriosis consist of chronic pelvic pain, irregular uterine bleeding, the uterus fixed and tender to movement, and the ovaries enlarged. Endometriosis causes infertility because of pelvic adhesions, tubal obstruction, and decreased ovarian function. The disease is diagnosed with ultrasound and laparoscopy. Laparoscopy is a procedure in which a tube (laparoscope) is placed into the abdomen to inspect the internal organs after the abdomen cavity is filled with carbon dioxide through a small incision made near the navel. Endometriosis is treated with nonsteroidal anti-inflammatory drugs (NSAIDs), oral contraceptives, progestins, and surgery.

Dysmenorrhea is severe pain felt hours before the menses actually occur. Therapy for treatment of dysmenorrhea includes birth control pills, heat, NSAIDs, and exercise. Acupuncture therapy and the use of a TENS (transcutaneous nerve stimulation) unit has also been reported to help.

As aging occurs, perimenopause (changes in the menstrual cycle) and postmenopause (cessation of menses) occur. Perimenopause symptoms may present with heavy menstrual bleeding, or decreased flow, or irregularity of menses. Women are still vulnerable to becoming pregnant during perimenopause.

Women can present with symptoms of postmenopause due to surgical intervention (total abdominal hysterectomy), due to the effects of certain pharmaceuticals, or due to aging. As women age, estrogen and progesterone levels decline. Vasomotor affects (hot flashes) occur in postmenopausal women. There is also an increased risk of osteoporosis. Vaginal dryness occurs, which can make sexual intercourse painful. Hormone replacement therapy (HRT) to treat menopause symptoms is controversial. Research has shown that HRT increases the risk of CVA, breast cancer, and deep vein thrombosis (DVT).

Uterine fibroids (leiomyomas) may present with abnormal uterine bleeding and pain. The etiology of uterine fibroids is unknown. However, uterine fibroids do appear to be dependent on hormonal levels. The surgical removal of large fibroids may be necessary if the fibroids result in excessive uterine bleeding that causes severe anemia.

Ovarian cysts occur but the etiology is unknown. Ovarian cysts may be benign or may develop into a neoplasm. A health risk that may occur with a benign ovarian cyst is that the cyst growth can become large and cause twisting of the ovary or occlusion of blood flow. Surgical intervention is the treatment of choice when an ovarian cyst is large and symptomatic.

Cervical cancer is a preventable health disorder. Mortality from cervical cancer is related to lack of health screening and intervention. The symptom of vaginal discharge may initially be clear, but then changes to dark and often becomes odorous. Menses flow progresses from spotting to heavy.

Ovarian cancer initially may present with vague symptoms, such as abdominal cramps, bloating, and a change in bowel habits. As the cancer continues to develop, abdominal girth increases, abdominal pain develops, and ascites occurs. There is currently no screening tool for ovarian cancer, although a transvaginal ultrasound can be ordered to determine whether an ovarian mass is present. Treatment for ovarian cancer is chemotherapy and surgery (salpingo-oophorectomy).

As women age, their musculature weakens, and their internal structures may lose support and result in a prolapsed uterus. The prolapsed uterus can be diagnosed in stages. Stage one occurs when the cervix has descended and occupies the vaginal canal. As the uterine prolapse reaches the second stage, the cervix is at the vaginal orifice. The cervix has dropped through the vaginal opening. The uterine prolapse can be accompanied by a cystocele (prolapsed of the bladder) or rectocele (prolapse of the rectum).

Treatment for the uterine prolapse can be surgery or insertion of a pessary (a device placed within the vagina to support the uterus).

Cystoceles and rectoceles result from weakened vaginal walls. With a cystocele, voiding may not completely empty the bladder (which now protrudes into the vagina), resulting in a higher risk for urinary tract infections (UTIs). A rectocele may cause difficulty with defecation. The pessary device may aid in preventing complications. Women are also encouraged to participate in Kegel exercises to strengthen the perineal muscles.

MALE REPRODUCTIVE SYSTEM DISORDERS

As men age, they experience reproductive system problems. When the prostate gland enlarges, it causes urinary problems. This condition is called benign prostatic hyperplasia (BPH; also known as benign prostatic hypertrophy). There is difficulty in bladder emptying due to obstruction by the enlarged prostate. Initial symptoms may present as resistance to voiding. Symptoms can also present as difficulty initiating the void, intermittent starting and stopping of urine flow, and urine dribbling after voiding is completed. Residual urine can cause frequent UTIs.

Treatment can be drug therapy (5-alpha-reductase inhibitors) to reduce the size of the prostate gland. A transurethral resection of the prostate (TURP) is a surgical procedure performed to remove enlarged prostate tissue. The procedure is performed by using a resectoscope. The resectoscope is inserted into the urethra. Prostate tissue is surgically removed. Bleeding can occlude the bladder, so a large three-way catheter is inserted into the bladder and continuous bladder irrigation is initiated. The continuous bladder irrigation may continue for 1 to several days (dependent on the amount of blood flow). Initially, there will be hematuria for 24 hours after surgery. After surgery, the catheter will be taped tightly to the leg (traction) to help decrease bleeding. Do not release that traction unless indicated by the physician. Also monitor hourly the bladder irrigation to ensure that the catheter does not become clogged by clots.

Prostate cancer is usually a slow-growing tumor of the prostate. Symptoms often mask those of BPH (urine hesitancy, dribbling, and retention). As with all cancers, early detection and treatment are necessary. Screening involves testing for prostate-specific antigen (PSA) and a digital rectal examination (DRE). In some cases, the cancer may grow more rapidly. The PSA can be a useful tool to diagnose the tumor. The larger the PSA number, the larger the tumor. Treatment includes monitoring, surgery, or radiation.

Hypospadia is an abnormal positioning of the urethral meatus. The meatus is on the ventral (underneath) surface of the penis. Epispadias is the positioning of the urethral meatus on the dorsal (above) surface of the penis. Both hypospadia and epispadias are abnormal urological birth defects. Treatment is surgical repair.

Orchitis is the inflammation of the testes. Causes include mumps, infections, or syphilis. Treatment consists of antibiotics, pain relievers, and bed rest.

Testicular torsion (twisting of the spermatic cord) is a medical emergency and can result in severe pain and swelling. Diagnosis can be determined via ultrasound. Treatment is surgical repair.

Testicular cancer presents with a small "lump" in the scrotum (usually painless). Diagnosis of testicular cancer can be determined via ultrasound. Treatment is an orchiectomy (surgical removal of the testis).

BODY SURFACE AREA

Body surface area (BSA) is a calculated measurement of the surface area of a body. BSA is frequently used when calculating dosages of medicines used both in chemotherapy and with children to prevent overdosing and underdosing.

BSA can be calculated two different ways, depending on whether the patient's weight and height are measured in pounds and inches or in kilograms and centimeters:

$$\sqrt{\frac{\text{Weight (lbs)} \times \text{inches}}{3,131}}$$

For example, if a patient weighs 100 pounds and is 5 feet tall (60 inches), $100 \times 60 = 6,000$

$6,000/3,131 = 1.9$, $\sqrt{1.9} = 1.4$ m²

The following version of the formula needs pounds converted to kilograms and inches converted to centimeters (remember, 2.54 cm = 1 inch).

$$\sqrt{\frac{\text{Weight (kg)} \times \text{cm}}{3,600 \text{ conversion factor}}}$$

SEXUALLY TRANSMITTED DISEASES

Data must be collected on any patient history of STDs. STDs are also known as venereal diseases. STD statistics are on the rise due to earlier ages of sexual behavior and increased population numbers due to greater longevity.

Acute salpingitis, or pelvic inflammatory disorder (PID), is acquired from a sexually transmitted disease exposure that is characterized by a sudden fever of 100.4°F, suprapubic pain and tenderness, a rigid lower abdominal musculature, purulent discharge, and adnexal masses. Complications include ectopic pregnancy, infertility, and reinfection caused by *Neisseria gonorrhea* and chlamydia.

Gonorrhea, chlamydia, syphilis, herpes, and genital warts are several STDs that may present in the genital regions but also may spread to other body areas. Gonorrhea is spread by the infected host via direct contact. Gonorrhea can occur in the vaginal area, orally, or anally. Men notice purulent drainage from the penis or swollen, painful testes and will seek treatment. Women may be unaware of the infection even though an inflammatory response occurs. Untreated, the infection can lead to tubal pregnancies, infertility, and pelvic pain from fibrous scarring and strictures. Babies born to mothers with gonorrhea are at high risk for blindness. For this reason, erythromycin ointment or silver nitrate solution is instilled in the eyes of newborn babies.

Rocephin is the drug of choice for adult treatment for gonorrhea. Ciprofloxacin and Levaquin have also been used. Both partners should be treated to prevent the "ping-pong" re-exposure problem that may occur. Patient education is important in the treatment of gonorrhea. The patient must refrain from both sexual activity and the consumption of alcohol during the treatment period. Gonorrhea must be reported to the public health department.

Syphilis can enter the body through small breaks in the skin (occurring during intercourse) or mucus membranes. Syphilis can also be spread by needle sharing (among IV drug users). Chancres present during the primary stage of syphilis. The chancres are lesions that may present on the penis, vagina, rectum, or orally. The second stage of syphilis presents with flulike symptoms. The bacteria are spread systemically and a generalized rash may appear. The third stage may not be noticeable. The immune system attempts to fight the infection. The final stage presents with a high risk of morbidity. The pathogen can affect the heart valves, cause aneurysms and heart failure, and damage bone and liver. The syphilis pathogen causes neurosyphilis, resulting in degeneration of the brain tissue and causing deterioration of cognitive function. Penicillin is the drug of choice for syphilis. Although this disease is treatable, the damage occurring in the final stages of syphilis prior to treatment is irreversible.

The most commonly reported STD is chlamydia. Women present with purulent drainage (cervicitis), frequent urination, pelvic inflammatory disease (PID), and pain during intercourse. Men present with epididymitis and urethral discharge. Treatment includes Zithromax or doxycycline and refraining from sexual activity for 7 days status post antibiotics.

OTHER STDs

- **Genital herpes** enters through breaks in the mucosa or through the mucus membranes. The virus travels to the nerve ganglion and remains inside the human host for the entire life span. Herpes type 1 (HSV type 1) results in infections above the umbilicus. Herpes type 2 (HSV type 2) results in genital infections (below the umbilicus), presenting with small, fluid-filled vesicles that appear on the penis, scrotum, vagina, cervix, or perineal areas. The fluid within the vesicles will spread the infected virus. The vesicles will rupture in 1 to 3 days and leave ulcers; the initial infection lasts 7 to 10 days. An infection can reoccur without warning; however, stress and the menstrual cycle may trigger an outbreak. Once the vesicles break, they leave an ulcer that can be painful. Antiviral medications such as Acyclovir and Valtrex are used to treat herpes.
- **Pediculosis pubis (crab lice)** symptoms include severe itching and little dark spots adjacent to pubic hair. Diagnosis is made by physical examination of the hair. Lice may be present in three different stages ranging from the eggs to a fully developed louse that resembles a crab. Lice are spread through physical contact. Medication to kill the lice must be carefully administered because the lotion or shampoo is toxic to the nervous system.
- Exposure to the **human papillomavirus** (HPV) can cause painless, cauliflower-like patches of genital warts. The HPV virus enters the body through small skin breaks during sexual intercourse. The epithelial cells infected by the HPV proliferate, resulting in abnormal cell growth. Warts may appear on the penis, scrotum, anal area, urethra, vulva, vagina, and cervix. HPV is common among sexually active females; risk factors include early age of menarche and multiple sexual partners. The HPV virus is linked to cervical cancer in women. Treatment involves chemical or laser ablation of the warts.
- **Trichomoniasis** symptoms include malodorous vaginal drainage (worse during menstruation), vulva erythematous, "strawberry appearance"; and yellow-green, foul-smelling drainage. Diagnosis would include a physical exam and lab test of the vaginal fluid or urethral fluid to look for the Trichomonas parasite. Treatment would consist of administering an antibiotic such as metronidazole.
- **Candidiasis** symptoms include intense itching, thick white drainage, and vulva erythematous. Predisposing causes include use of contraceptives or antibiotics and a more alkaline vaginal pH that will occur during pregnancy from increased glycogen and can also occur as a result of an immunosuppressive disease such as diabetes mellitus. Candidiasis can occur in the mouth, vagina, and urinary tract system. It is diagnosed by pelvic examination and examination of the vaginal drainage. Candidiasis is treated with antifungal medications.

HIV/AIDS

HIV is caused by a retrovirus and is characterized by progressive immune system impairment. T-helper cells are infected more readily than any other cells. T cells are white blood cells that initiate or suppress immunity. Once inside the host, HIV attaches to the target (T-helper) cell membrane by way of its receptor molecule, $CD4^+$. The T cells are destroyed, which makes the person more susceptible to infections and unusual cancers. There is no cure for HIV/AIDS. HIV is infectious even if the person is asymptomatic.

It is only transmitted through blood, semen, vaginal fluids, and breast milk. There is an aggressive treatment called HAART (highly active antiretroviral therapy) that will suppress HIV viral replication. However, the toxicity of the drugs used with this treatment is one of the problems with patient compliance. Seroconversion is the production of antibodies for HIV. Antibodies usually are detected in 4 to 12 weeks but can take from 6 months up to 10 years (2–5 years is average). However, the infected person can spread the disease before seroconversion. $CD4^+$ is the most significant laboratory study for a person infected with HIV.

AIDS is HIV accompanied by opportunistic infections that include:

- Pneumocystis carinii pneumonia (PCP), a fungal pneumonia caused by yeast
- Oropharyngeal or esophageal candidiasis, common yeast infections
- Cytomegalovirus (CMV), a virus that causes mononucleosis-like symptoms that can be toxic to a fetus; the virus stays alive and dormant in the patient's body
- Mycobacterium tuberculosis

Signs and symptoms of AIDS include wasting syndrome (weight loss), diarrhea, chronic weakness, and fever. Associated metabolic disorders such as lipodystrophy result in changes in body appearance (including increased abdominal girth, buffalo humps, wasting of fat from face, and breast enlargement); elevated serum cholesterol and triglycerides; and increased insulin resistance.

Other advanced-stage diseases of AIDS include:

- AIDS dementia complex, which is seen in advanced stages of AIDS
- Toxoplasmosis is a parasitic infectious disease that causes lesions of the central nervous system; it can be acquired from cleaning a cat litter box or consuming contaminated meat or water; patients with AIDS can be susceptible to this disease
- Leukoencephalopathy, which causes destruction of the white matter in the brain

Medication Forms

Listed in the vertical box is a medication. For each of the remaining boxes, list the following:

Box 1: List a laboratory result you would need to monitor. Explain the significance of the laboratory test to the medication.
Box 2: List one food that may interact with the medication. Explain the significance of the food item to the medication.
Box 3: List one patient educational instruction you would give to the patient regarding the medication. Explain the significance of the instruction to the medication.

List other educational information you could provide this patient. Are there websites you can refer? What about travel overseas and health issues? How should the medication be stored? Does the medication being administered interfere with other medications?

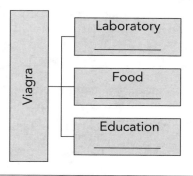

Listed in the vertical box is a medication. For each of the remaining boxes, list the following:

Box 1: List a laboratory result you would need to monitor. Explain the significance of the laboratory test to the medication.
Box 2: List one food that may interact with the medication. Explain the significance of the food item to the medication.
Box 3: List one patient educational instruction you would give to the patient regarding the medication. Explain the significance of the instruction to the medication.

List other educational information you could provide this patient. Are there websites you can refer? What about travel overseas and health issues? How should the medication be stored? Does the medication being administered interfere with other medications?

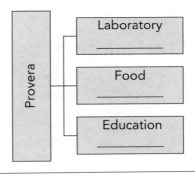

BODY SURFACE AREA CALCULATION QUIZ

Answer the following question and return by preconference next week.

1. The patient is receiving Cisplatin for ovarian cancer. The dose ordered is 80 mg/m². The patient's height is 165 cm (65 inches) and her weight is 100 kg (220 lbs). How many milligrams of Cisplatin would the patient receive?
2. For a child who weighs 30 pounds and is 30 inches tall. 35 mg/m² of medication A is ordered. How many milligrams should the child receive?

ANSWERS TO BODY SURFACE AREA CALCULATION QUIZ

1. There are many formulas to calculate BSA.
   The formula used here is the Mostellar formula for calculating BSA using centimeters to express height and kilograms to express weight:

$$\sqrt{\frac{165\,\text{cm} \times 100\,\text{kg}}{3,600}} = 2.139\,\text{m}^2$$

This height and weight would produce a BSA of 2.14 m².
80 mg/m² × 2.139 m² = 171.12 mg or 171 mg
The patient should receive 171 mg of Cisplatin.

2. For pediatric calculations, the Mostellar formula can also be used expressing height in inches and weight in pounds:

$$\sqrt{\frac{\text{Weight (lbs)} \times \text{inches}}{3,131}}$$

$$\sqrt{\frac{30\,lbs \times 30\,inches}{3,131}} = 0.537\,m^2$$

$0.537\ m^2 \times 35\ mg/m^2 = 18.795\ mg$

The child should receive 18.8 mg of medication A.

REPRODUCTIVE SURVEY EXERCISE

Instructions: Make copies of the following form and then complete the follow-ing survey by interviewing two women and two men in the reproductive age range (between ages 21 and 40). The reproductive survey exercise results are due by preconference next week.

1. Are you aware of the self-screening assessment that you should perform monthly? Yearly?
2. Do you perform those self-screening assessments? Why or why not?
3. Does your family have a history of reproductive diseases or cancer?
4. Do you participate in your annual health screening?
5. What tests does your primary physician perform?
6. If you found a symptom (such as a mass or discharge), where would you research for more information?
7. Do you find discussing the reproductive system difficult?
8. Where did you learn about health screening or self-assessment?
9. Do you have lifestyle habits that put you at greater risk?
10. Do you use birth control? What type do you use and what made you choose that type?

REPRODUCTIVE SYSTEM QUIZ

Complete the following questions and return by preconference next week.

1. What laboratory test is performed to test for prostate cancer?
2. What gland passes through the prostate gland?
3. What term is used to describe when the urethral meatus in the man is on the dorsal surface?
4. Where does sperm meet the ovum?
5. The female breasts develop during what stage of life?
6. Which hormone stimulates milk production?
7. Which hormone assists in maintaining female sexual characteristics?
8. What is the infectious childhood disease that will affect male fertility?
9. If the ovum is not fertilized, what is the discharge of blood called?
10. What medical conditions of the bowel and bladder result from weakened vaginal walls?
11. What medications are used to prevent unwanted pregnancies?
12. What is the male surgical form of birth control?
13. Where do ectopic pregnancies occur?
14. What term is used to describe the cessation of menses in the aging female?
15. A TURP is performed for what medical condition?

ANSWERS TO REPRODUCTIVE SYSTEM QUIZ

1. PSA
2. Ejaculatory gland
3. Epispadias
4. In the fallopian tube

5. Puberty
6. Prolactin
7. Progesterone
8. Mumps
9. Menses
10. Cystocele and rectocele
11. Contraceptives
12. Vasectomy
13. Fallopian tube
14. Menopause
15. Enlarged prostate

CRITICAL THINKING EXERCISE

A 40-year-old African American male is admitted for surgical radical prostatectomy for prostate cancer. His past medical history involves atrial fibrillation and hyperlipidemia, and he continues to smoke two packs of cigarettes a day. He is a full-time radiology technician. His initial PSA was 6ng/mL. His lab work shows calcium 14mg/dL, potassium 4 mEq/L, sodium 135, and phosphorous 2 mg/dL. He is having some periods of confusion. Initial CAT scan of brain is negative. Pupils are equal and reactive.

Answer the following questions and return by preconference next week.

1. What is PSA and what does it indicate?
2. Does a positive PSA indicate cancer?
3. What are this patient's risk factors?
4. What is a radical prostatectomy?
5. What are the side effects of a prostatectomy?
6. What is the normal level of calcium?
7. What are the effects of high calcium levels?
8. What are the primary causes of hypercalcemia and what other diseases can cause it?
9. What is the normal phosphorous level?
10. How are high calcium levels resolved?

ANSWERS TO CRITICAL THINKING EXERCISE

1. PSA is a protein that is produced by the prostate gland. PSA levels of 4.0 ng/mL or lower are normal.
2. There can false positive PSA tests. An elevated PSA could be due to an inflammation or due to drug use and does not necessarily indicate cancer.
   A urine culture should be performed to rule out infection, and a biopsy should be performed to confirm cancer.
3. The risk factors are his age, race, smoking history, and his exposure to radiation.
4. It is an operation that removes the prostate and surrounding tissues.
5. Side effects may include urinary and bowel incontinence and erectile dysfunction.
6. The normal level of calcium is 8 to 10 mg/dL. High levels of calcium are caused by different types of cancer, immobility, dehydration, nausea, and vomiting.
7. Elevated calcium levels can cause muscle twitching, confusion, and coma.
8. High levels of calcium are caused by different types of cancer, immobility, dehydration, nausea, and vomiting. Other diseases that can cause hypercalcemia are: bone cancer, hyperparathyroidism, vitamin D toxicity, granulomatous diseases, Cushings disease, and Addison's disease.
9. The normal phosphorous level is 3 to 4.5 mg/dL. Calcium and phosphorous have an inverse relationship—so when calcium is high, the phosphorous will be low.
10. Address the underlying cause, rehydration, exercise, bisphosphonates, and calcitonin.

WEEK 13 POSTCONFERENCE

Discuss the reproductive system with the students. Did their assigned patients have any reproductive system abnormalities? Were there any specific treatments or interventions? Did the patients have a past medical history of reproductive system treatments or interventions? Inquire why it is important to know the patient's current and past reproductive history.

Inform students that final evaluations will be discussed individually next week. Students should have been given positive and directive feedback throughout the entire clinical course. Students must understand that final grades will be tallied based on clinical observations, assignments, the midterm evaluation, and attendance.

Inquire whether students have any questions regarding clinical materials, resources, or didactic skills.

Inform students that next week the students will give the clinical unit a gift to reflect their gratitude for promoting a learning environment for the group.

Request that students e-mail to you questions on any topic that may need further clarification. Additional resources can be supplied at the next clinical to assist with explaining these topics.

PART IV

THE POSTCONFERENCE AND TRANSITION INTO NURSING PRACTICE

CAREER GOALS AND PLANNING: PROFESSIONAL IDENTITY, JOB SEARCH, AND LICENSING EXAM

This chapter examines:

- Transitioning from school into the health care profession
- Career goals and professional identity
- Guides for students for the job application process
- Midterm and final evaluation tool and criteria

WEEK 14 PRECONFERENCE

Hand out:
- Final evaluations
- Sample cover letter
- Sample résumé

Collect:
- Medication forms
- Reproductive system quiz
- Reproductive survey exercise
- Body surface area calculation quiz
- Critical thinking exercise
- Concept maps
- Care plans
- Physical assessment forms
- Journals

Instruct the students that their final evaluations will be viewed and discussed individually. Students are expected to sign, date, and return their evaluations to the clinical instructor by the beginning of postconference. A copy of the evaluation can be made available, if the student so desires. Student grades will be posted at the completion of the clinical course. Assignments submitted late will be graded according to the syllabus guidelines. Any assignment not completed and submitted by the end of the last clinical day will be given a zero.

Evaluations are based on observation, participation, and attendance. Final grades are based on assignments and on the ability to meet the requirements of the clinical class, as stated in the course syllabus.

The final clinical class will also be a time of celebration. Students and the instructor will deliver a gratuity gift to the clinical unit as a token of their appreciation for allowing the students the learning experience. Students are requested to donate time, funds, and ideas for the clinical gift.

GRADUATION

Although there are many topics in nursing that must be taught and learned in classes, students have often voiced their concern that they have received little guidance on how to plan for future nursing positions. Once school is complete, students find themselves frustrated due to the lack of available positions for graduate nurses. For this reason, inform the students that today's class and materials will attempt to provide them with guidance on planning their future nursing careers and on ways to become more marketable.

Students must understand that the process of becoming marketable requires time and energy. Students should seek additional learning experiences that can enhance their résumés. Instructors can guide the students by offering the following suggestions:

- Join a nursing organization (National Student Nurses Association [NSNA]).
- Complete a certification course (Advanced Cardiovascular Life Support [ACLS]).
- Contact local health care facilities for volunteer opportunities. Although the student may not be able to perform in the "nurse" capacity, participation can offer networking connections.
- Apply for a patient care technician position. The health care facility can then determine whether the student's work ethic matches the facility's expectations. This process can benefit both the health care facility and the student. The facility has already invested in the student. The student is familiar with the facility and may be offered a nursing position before it is offered to an outside applicant.
- Participate in school organizations.
- Join online nursing networks (e.g., LinkedIn).

REFERENCE LETTERS

Whether the student is in the final courses of the nursing program, early in the program, or somewhere in between, guidance on preparation for job seeking, reference letters, and well-written résumés can assist the students to prepare for their future professions.

Students should consider three sources (faculty, employers, or personal contacts) when requesting letters of recommendation. It is never too early to begin planning for who may be one of three resources for a reference letter. The student should give the person writing the reference letter all the accurate information necessary to portray the capabilities and current experience of the student. Busy schedules and responsibilities may require time for each chosen referrer to complete a reference letter; therefore, planning ahead will offer both the student and the referrers less frustration and stress.

Students should offer the following information: the student's name, program, courses the student may have taken with the faculty member (if applicable), experiences (work, school, and personal) that may apply, credentials, organizations, participation in volunteer opportunities, work–study program, and leadership roles in study groups.

Instructors should learn the proper format for writing a reference letter. There are several ways to write a professional reference, but it is always important to include your contact information in the event the receiver wishes to request further information or clarify a matter included in the letter. A sample reference letter is included below to offer new instructors a format to follow.

REFERENCE LETTER FORMAT

KEY NOTE: Most employers want to see the letter printed on the school's letterhead.

123 Main Street (this should be the referrer's address)
Your town, state, zip code

The current date

Future employer
Company name (if applicable)
Employer address
Employer city, state, zip code

Salutation (more details on salutations to follow)

The first paragraph should be an introduction explaining who is writing the letter and why.

The second paragraph should discuss the student, what position the student is applying for, and informational facts regarding the student.

The third paragraph should include examples confirming the student's ability and skills.

The last paragraph should be the conclusion of the letter (always end in a positive way).

Choosing how to close the letter may prove difficult. The writer may not want to appear overly familiar by writing, "Yours Sincerely." By using "Respectfully yours," instead the letter can end in a professional manner.

Remember to leave enough space to allow a signature between the ending and your typed name.

Salutations can be worrisome if the writer does not know the name of the intended receiver. If the intended receiver is known, the salutation should be "Dear (receiver's name)." If the intended receiver's name is unknown, it is perfectly acceptable to write, "Dear Sir," "Dear Madam," or "To whom it may concern." It is important to maintain a professional manner when writing a reference letter.

Certain confidential personal information should not be included in a reference letter. Confidential personal information can be the student's age, religious preference, marital status, sexual preference, and so on. Do not mention any student weaknesses such as a chronic health issues. Remember, the reference letter should focus on the positive and guide the receiver toward the student's strengths.

In the event that you as the instructor believe that you cannot successful recommend the student, it is perfectly all right to explain to the student your regrets about not being able to write a letter. Be honest. Explaining that you do not remember a student, or have a busy schedule, or feel as though you would not have information to contribute that would benefit the student is much better than writing a letter that is vague or generic.

With much of the world going paperless and students becoming so technology savvy, reference follow-up requests may come to you in the form of an e-mail. The potential employer may ask the referrer to complete a generic survey based on knowledge of the student. Many companies prefer to speak to the referrer on the telephone. Let the student know if you have limitations on your ability to respond. Many instructors do not wish to offer a home telephone number. Some instructors do not open e-mails from individuals whom the instructor may not recognize.

Sample Letter of Recommendation

123 Main Street
City, state, zip code

December 17, 2013

Ms. Mary Miller
Health Care Facility
Get Well Street
New York, New York 10036-8002

Dear Ms. Miller,

Our university has a very structured and intense nursing program. As an instructor in the BSN program, I have the opportunity to instruct as well as observe nursing students throughout the 4-year program. It is therefore my pleasure to write a reference letter for Nancy Nurse.

Nancy has informed me she is applying for a staff nurse position in your adult medical–surgical unit. Nancy scored well in both her medical–surgical classes. She volunteered this summer in her local community to assist in the annual wellness fair. Nancy has worked part-time as a patient care technician (PCT) at the geriatric center. Nancy often went the extra mile by offering to spend her free hours assisting the elderly women of the geriatric center with their craft bazaar items. The proceeds go to help provide socks and slippers for those less fortunate.

Nancy attended my theoretical course as well as my didactic course in the fall of 2013. As a student in my didactic course, Nancy often requested additional learning experiences. Nancy demonstrated exceptional skills in performing assessments and interventions. Nancy has been a leader to her study group and frequently guided her fellow students to complete their practicum projects. Nancy has been a member of the university's student association and has held the position of secretary on the student counsel.

It is for all the above reasons that I do not hesitate to recommend Nancy Nurse for her applied position. If you have any further questions, please feel free to contact me.

Respectfully,
Deborah Wirwicz, RN, MSN

RÉSUMÉS

There was a time when an applicant needed only to complete an application form. In today's market, it is usually necessary to provide a résumé and references. What is a résumé and what should a résumé contain? A résumé is a document that offers the employer a summary of work experiences, positions held, duration of employment, and the applicant's educational level.

A cover letter is often included with the résumé. With today's technology, applicants apply for most employment positions online. It is therefore suggested that any résumé developed should be saved on the computer or on a thumb drive for easy uploading to online job application sites. Examples of a résumé and cover letter are included in this chapter.

There are professional sites that will offer to produce excellent résumés (at a cost); however, it is wise to remember that employers do conduct thorough background searches. Keep the résumé true. Do not embellish job skills or education. Discrepancies may not be apparent immediately, but can surface at a later date and cause not only embarrassment but also a potential job loss.

Most résumés contain limited work histories (10 years); however, if the applicant has skills from a job 15 years ago that would qualify the applicant for the position, it is appropriate to add that employer to the résumé. It is also helpful to flag that job (see example). Before summiting your résumé, it may be helpful to have a mentor or family member read your résumé and view the résumé as if they were an employer seeking an applicant. Always use action verbs in your résumé.

Sample Cover Letter

Name
Address
City, state, zip code
Telephone number
E-mail address/fax

Date

Name (of employer contact)
Title (within the corporation)
Name of corporation
Address
City, state, zip code

Dear Mr./Mrs./Ms. (last name)

I would appreciate an opportunity to interview for one of the available positions in the new graduate nurse program. Please accept the attached résumé as an application for one of the new graduate nurse positions that were recently advertised. I have graduated from the School of Nursing baccalaureate program with honors. In addition to my 14-week practicum experience on a pediatric medical–surgical unit, I have worked as a nursing assistant for 3 years at a children's hospital.

Your hospital has been rated number one in multidisciplinary pediatric procedures. Your organization provides a comprehensive orientation program that provides opportunities for new skills and experiences prior to taking on responsibilities as an independent registered nurse.

I feel that I would be a suitable applicant for your organization because of my previous skills and experience. During clinicals, I was able to analyze patient information based on a detailed assessment of the physiological and psychological aspects of each patient. I identified problems that would affect the patient's outcome and initiated interventions with the help of other staff members. I participated in interdisciplinary teams to improve my patients' outcomes. I administered medication in all forms using the five rights of medication administration. I was prompt with my attendance and thorough with my documentation.

I am experienced with computer charting, proficient in Spanish and French, and was class president of the Student Nurses Association. I am currently Basic Life Support–trained and am pursuing a Pediatric Advanced Life Support certification.

I look forward to hearing back from you to set up an appointment for an interview with you and your staff. If you have any questions prior to that time, please do not hesitate to contact me.

Thank you for your time and consideration.

Sincerely,
John Doe

Sample Résumé

Nancy Nurse
123 Main Street
City, state, zip code
Telephone number
E-mail address

Objectives (optional): This is a short summary explaining what the applicant wants. Often this space can be used for accomplishments.

Education
Best University
December 2013
BSN
(May add GPA, Honor Society, etc.)
High school (Do not add if graduated more than 5 years ago.)

Work Experiences
Most recent employer
Job title held
Duration of employment
List job duties

Additional Information

Include organization memberships, volunteer opportunities, hobbies, and any other leadership roles, educational experiences, or skill development opportunities.

References on Request (optional)

Employers may require your reference contacts' names and information on the application.

INTERVIEW DAY

Once you have received notice of a job interview, you must prepare for it. Note the time and place. Go to the site ahead of time and acquaint yourself with where the interview is going to be held. This will help you to avoid being late and confused. Also, you can ask other individuals at the facility how they like their jobs at this organization. Do the employees look happy? Do they take the time to assist you if you ask for directions? You can obtain a lot of information about the organization just by observing its employees' attitudes and responses. This may give you an insight into the organization's "climate" before your interview.

The employer will ask questions of you, but you must also be prepared to ask questions of your own. Lists of questions to expect and proposed question to ask are set forth below. Investigate the organization: What are its mission and goals, who founded it, when was it founded? This information is on its website. Practice in advance your answers to the questions you may be asked. This will show the employer that you have taken an interest in their organization. Show up ahead of time and in proper attire (professional business suit) with your credentials such as photo identification (state ID card or driver's license), Social Security card or other government-required ID, nursing license, BLS, ACLS, letters of recommendation, and so on. Be aware of your body language—sit upright, relax and lean slightly forward, and keep your hands folded comfortably in your lap. Make appropriate eye contact but avoid staring. When leaving, thank the interviewer for giving you this opportunity to be interviewed.

QUESTIONS YOU MAY BE ASKED

1. Why did you choose nursing as a career?
2. Why do you think that you are a qualified applicant for this job?

3. How did you deal with a challenging and difficult situation? Give me an example.
4. When you experienced a difficult coworker, how did you handle the situation?
5. You have come across a patient who is experiencing a decreased level of consciousness. What should your nursing actions be? (Note: Do not get complicated with this answer—respond with taking vital signs, pulse oximetry, and blood sugar, calling a rapid response.)
6. Who is your nursing theorist?

QUESTIONS TO ASK

1. What shifts are offered here, 8- or 12-hour shifts?
2. What is the nurse–patient ratio and how is it calculated?
3. What is the longevity of the nurse manager and the nurses?
4. How long is the preceptorship for new nurses?
5. What are the expectations for this job?
6. What are the major long-term goals for this organization?

PROFESSIONAL IDENTITY

Novice nurses must learn to form a professional identity. What is a professional identity? Professional identity is the nurse's own self-concept. The nurse must learn how to perform in the role of the nurse, be knowledgeable, hone didactic skills, and demonstrate professional standards while meeting the professional code of ethics and conduct. Nurses must learn to perform in the role of advocate for their patients.

As a member of a growing profession, the nurse must learn to incorporate evidence-based practice into his or her professional practice. The nurse must continue to seek knowledge and develop new skills in order to one day achieve professional confidence and competence. Having a strong professional identity allows nurses to incorporate autonomy into their practice while honesty and trust reflect their integrity.

The public is becoming more aware of the role in today's society of the professional nurse. The nurse lobbies in Congress for better patient care. The nurse performs in various roles and holds various positions. The nurse may be at the patient's bedside or may visit the patient via telecommunications.

New nurses are oriented to their new role of caregiver by a preceptor. The new nurse should welcome any new learning experiences. Ask questions and request positive feedback. Constructive criticism is offered to improve a person's performance. Constructive criticism should not be taken as a personal assault. Learn from the information given to you. Gather information from various health team members.

If the particular health care organization does not meet your needs, always give 2 weeks' notice as a professional courtesy, and leave with a positive attitude. Many health care organizations are owned by one holding company, and if the nurse leaves one site on unpleasant terms, he or she will then be "banned" from rehire not only from that particular site but also from every other health care site within that organization. This may prove to be a challenge to obtaining another job.

The new nurse has a long professional career ahead. Learning ways to develop a professional identity can also help the nurse to become more proficient.

CAREER GOALS

People chose their career goals for various reasons. Some chose their career goal based on a personal passion, while others may chose a career they like so much that it doesn't feel like work. Some prefer careers that offer challenges and excitement, and yet others may want careers with less stress. Career goals can vary tremendously. Careers can be chosen based on the probability of promotions, financial rewards, short-term employment versus long-term employment (job security), better benefits, effective management versus self-direction, creativity, collaboration, bonuses, available training—the list goes on.

Each student must perform a self-analysis. Each student should determine what career goal he or she is interested in. Is the career goal achievable? Does the student have the knowledge and skills to perform the chosen career goal? If the student does not currently possess the knowledge and skills to attain the career goal, will the employer provide a mentor? Does the student have the ability to master the necessary skills?

Students have the opportunity while in college to engage academic counselors. Encourage the students to utilize these resources. Once the students recognize what may be their career goals, instruct them to contact the various organizations in which members of their desired career participate. Shadowing someone in a career of choice can allow a brief but accurate insight into that career. The student can ask questions as well as personally visualize the career in a nutshell. Employers are more likely to express interest in the student if the student demonstrates initiative.

MIDTERM AND FINAL EVALUATIONS

The clinical instructor should use the following form to evaluate students for midterm and final evaluations. The evaluation is user-friendly and therefore requires little instruction.

Clinical Evaluation

Check the appropriate box to reflect the student's level of knowledge or skill.

Student _____   Date _____   Course _____

Core Learning Outcome	Satisfactory Behavior	Needs Improvement	Unsatisfactory Behavior
1. Practices within an established framework for the adult system			
2. Assesses patient physiological, cultural, spiritual, and developmental variables			
3. Assesses patients' internal/external environment lines of defense			
4. Selects appropriate nursing diagnoses in priority order			
5. Identifies disease process, signs, and symptoms for nursing diagnosis			
6. Able to identify specific, measurable goals and short-term outcomes for patient system			
7. Able to choose nursing prevention and intervention, appropriate diagnosis, and outcomes			
8. Able to prioritize needs based on physiological necessity			
9. Implements nursing prevention/interventions safely			
10. Maintains a safe environment for the patient			

(continued)

11. Administers medications safely (if applicable)			
12. Follows guidelines for infection control			
13. Provides care in an organized and timely manner			
14. Maintains professional behavior; adheres to dress protocol			
15. Complies with attendance protocols			
16. Communicates appropriate information to other health team members			
17. Documents assessment findings according to protocol			
18. Demonstrates legal and ethical behavior			
19. Seeks out new learning opportunities			

Clinical Evaluation Criteria

Core Learning Outcome	Satisfactory Behavior	Needs Improvement	Unsatisfactory Behavior
1. Practices within an established framework for the adult system; demonstrates knowledge of the physiological systems of the adult	Frequently demonstrates system-based knowledge of the physiological systems of the adult, with minimal instructor assistance	Requires constant instructor assistance with knowledge of the physiological systems of the adult	Unable to assess knowledge of the physiological systems of the adult
2. Assesses patient physiological, cultural, spiritual, and developmental variables	Frequently able to assess patient system variables, with minimal instructor assistance	Requires constant one-on-one guidance to assess patient system variables	Unable to assess patient system variables, even with instructor's assistance
3. Assesses patients' internal/external environment lines of defense	Frequently able to assess patients' internal/external environment lines of defense, with minimal instructor assistance	Requires constant one-on-one guidance to assess patients' internal/external environment lines of defense	Unable to assess patients' internal/external environment lines of defense, even with instructor assistance
4. Selects appropriate nursing diagnoses in priority order with instructor assistance	Frequently selects 85% of nursing diagnoses appropriate to patient's assessment, with minimal instructor assistance	Requires constant instructor assistance to select nursing diagnosis appropriate to patient's diagnosis	Unable to select any appropriate nursing diagnosis, even with instructor assistance

(continued)

Core Learning Outcome	Satisfactory Behavior	Needs Improvement	Unsatisfactory Behavior
5. Identifies disease process, signs, and symptoms for nursing diagnosis	Frequently able to identify disease process, signs, and symptoms for nursing diagnosis, with minimal instructor assistance	Requires constant instructor assistance to identify disease process, signs, and symptoms for nursing diagnosis	Unable to identify disease process, signs, and symptoms for nursing diagnosis, even with instructor assistance
6. Able to identify specific, measurable goals and short-term outcomes for patient system	Requires minimal instructor assistance to identify specific, measurable goals and short-term outcomes for patient system	Requires constant instructor assistance to identify specific, measurable goals and short-term outcomes for patient system	Unable to identify specific, measurable goals and short-term outcomes for patient system, even with instructor assistance
7. Able to choose nursing prevention and intervention, appropriate diagnosis, and outcomes	Frequently able to choose nursing prevention and intervention, appropriate diagnosis, and outcomes, with minimal instructor assistance	Requires constant instructor assistance to choose nursing prevention and intervention, appropriate diagnosis, and outcomes	Unable to identify and choose nursing prevention and intervention, appropriate diagnosis, and outcomes, even with instructor assistance
8. Able to prioritize needs based on physiological necessity	Frequently able to prioritize needs based on physiological necessity, with minimal instructor assistance	Requires constant instructor assistance to prioritize needs based on physiological necessity	Unable to prioritize needs based on physiological necessity, even with instructor's assistance
9. Implements nursing prevention/ interventions safely	Implements nursing prevention/ interventions safely, with minimal instructor assistance	Requires constant instructor assistance to implement nursing prevention/ interventions safely	Demonstrates unsafe behavior to patient system when implementing nursing prevention/ interventions
10. Maintains a safe environment for the patient	Corrects environmental hazards that could result in patient system injury	Requires constant instructor assistance to correct environmental hazards that could result in patient system injury	Does not correct hazards that could result in patient injury and/or does not seek instructor assistance
11. Administers medications safely (if applicable)	Administers medications correctly using six rights of medication administration and is able to discuss all prescribed medications, actions, side effects, and nursing implications	Makes frequent errors in dosage calculations, dose administered route, time, the right patient, and documentation, even with the instructor's assistance; not prepared to discuss medications	Unable to administer medications without instructor's assistance and not aware of all prescribed medications, actions, side effects, and nursing implications
12. Follows guidelines for infection control	Follows guidelines for infection control, with minimal instructor assistance	Requires constant instructor assistance to follow guidelines for infection control	Violates guidelines for infection control despite instructor assistance

(continued)

Core Learning Outcome	Satisfactory Behavior	Needs Improvement	Unsatisfactory Behavior
13. Provides care in an organized and timely manner	Uses time management skills to complete nursing care within allotted clinical time	Requires constant instructor assistance to complete nursing care within allotted clinical time	Does not demonstrate time management skills or disregards time constraints
14. Maintains professional behavior; adheres to dress protocol	Demonstrates positive attitude toward the patient, health team members, and institution; complies with dress protocol	Disregards program rules concerning behavior in clinical area; does not argue but does not change behavior after criticism; and requires reminders to comply with dress protocol	Displays consistently negative attitude toward the patient or members of the health care team; argumentative; and does not comply with dress protocol
15. Complies with attendance protocols	Attends 100% of scheduled clinical	Attends 80% or more of scheduled clinical	Consistently late and missing at least two clinical classes; does not notify the instructor of absences or lateness
16. Communicates appropriate information to other health team members	Communicates essential patient information to other health team members with minimal prompting from instructor	Requires constant prompting from instructor to communicate essential patient information to other health team members	No attempt is made to communicate essential patient information to other health team members
17. Documents assessment findings according to protocol	Frequently able to document assessment findings with minimal instructor assistance	Requires constant guidance from instructor to accurately document assessment findings	Unable to document assessment findings, even with guidance from instructor
18. Demonstrates legal and ethical behavior	Demonstrates respect for patient's culture, dignity, and confidentiality. Follows nursing legal guidelines	Requires constant guidance from instructor to not disclose personal information; needs instruction on legal matters	Breaches confidentiality; falsifies records; treats the patient with disrespect; demonstrates behaviors such as stealing, assault, and violation of the Nurse Practice Act
19. Seeks out new learning opportunities	Discloses new learning with others	Has to be encouraged to either participate in or to discuss new learning experiences	Unmotivated to learn or does not seek new learning experiences

Instructors should use the evaluation tool to inform each student of his or her strengths and weaknesses. Note, however, that a student who frequently is graded with "needs improvement" or "unsatisfactory behavior" does not successfully meet the goals necessary to pass the clinical class. The instructor must make arrangements for the student to meet with the dean of nursing to discuss what type of remediation can be undertaken.

Instructors can grade each box with the following values: Each box checked with "satisfactory behavior" has a value of 3 points. Each box checked with "needs improvement" has a value of 2 points. Each box checked with "unsatisfactory behavior" has a value of 1 point. Students must tally a total of 78 points, in total, to pass the clinical class.

HOW TO PREPARE FOR STATE BOARDS AND LICENSING

1. Decide where you want to be licensed. It may be an advantage to be licensed in a compact state that will allow the nurse to work in several states. (A compact state allows a nurse to work under multistate jurisdictions with his or her current licensure without having to apply for licensure in other compact states.)
2. Review the procedures and requirements for taking the nursing boards.
3. Go to the National Board of Nursing website to review the categories that will be on the test.
4. Review what items you are allowed to take to the test, how long the test going to last (expect approximately 6 hours), how many test questions there will be, and how many breaks you are allowed to take. You may need to get up and stretch.
5. Be organized with your study routine and commit a certain amount of time and effort to study. Ascertain what your weaknesses are and what topics need more work. Make flash cards and CDs of standard information (BP parameters, drug brand and generic names, etc.). The student can also make CDs that can be listened to while performing other tasks in order to reinforce information. Memorize the mnemonics that are provided in this book. Set up a study group. Try to answer a question a minute. Go with your "glimmer" thought (first thought) and do not change the answer.
6. Learn how to pick up the key words when reviewing questions. Determine what is important to the question, that is, what are they asking for. Never pick an answer that has "always, never, or must" in it—these are called "absolutes."
7. Get plenty of rest and relaxation.
8. An assessment answer should be picked as the first task to be done unless there is an emergency. Assessment can also be described as collection, auscultation, or palpation. Assessment should always be done before an intervention to prevent performing the wrong intervention.
9. Answer the questions that address the patient's body, not the machine or equipment.
10. Know what licensed practical nurses (LPNs) and unlicensed personnel are allowed to do and what is within their scope of practice. Any teaching, evaluation, medications, or unstable patients are the responsibility of only the registered nurse. LPNs can monitor blood transfusions but cannot check or hang the blood. LPNs not allowed to intravenously push medications.
11. Never pick an answer that delays care or treatment (such as calling the doctor first when the patient's oxygen saturation is extremely low). Apply oxygen first and then call the doctor.
12. There are questions in which the nurse needs to identify the doctor first.
13. Practice your math skills. Be able to do math conversions of micrograms to grams; to calculate an IV solution to mcg/kg/min, mcg/min, and mcg/hr; and to calculate the drip factor. Be sure to answer the math question that is actually being asked, especially in regards to rounding off to the nearest whole number, tenth, hundredth, or thousandth.
14. Pick the most important intervention. There may be two or more answers that are completely similar or alike, so the correct answer would be the one that is left. Be sure to read the question very carefully. What exactly are they asking for?
15. Questions that are phrased to imply patient understanding or misunderstanding of instructions or comprehension of disease process have to be carefully read to pick the appropriate answer. For example: "What answer would indicate that the client *understands* the instructions?" or the question would state "What indicates that the client *needs* additional instructions?" Look for these key words.
16. When asking patients questions, eliminate the "why" questions.
17. If you have never heard of it. . . please don't pick it!
18. If one nurse discovers another nurse's mistake, it is always appropriate to speak to that nurse before going to management. If the situation persists, then address it with management.

19. Deal with actual problems before potential problems and select the answer that is most important to the patient's well-being.
20. Assess the question for clues that may direct you to the correct answer.
21. Make certain that you know your normal values for laboratory tests such as electrolytes, arterial blood gases (ABGs), vital signs, and therapeutic drug levels.
22. Know your drug classifications.
23. The day before the test, stop studying early, do something relaxing, and get rest. It is wise to have someone else drive you to the test—but don't study on the way to the test, it will only create more anxiety. Walk in confidently and reassure yourself that you will pass the state boards.

WEEK 14 POSTCONFERENCE

Collect final evaluations (make certain each student's signature is on his or her evaluation). Initiate a discussion on how the students feel about their learning experiences in this clinical. Remind students to review the material to keep it fresh in their minds. Any topics they are weak in should be reread. It is helpful to the students to suggest they complete the questions at the end of each chapter in their medical–surgical textbooks. This will help them to identify their strengths and weaknesses.

Instruct students to research their areas of interest. Remind students that applying for a nursing position requires careful planning. Referrers should be considered. Résumés should be tweaked to ensure they display current and appropriate information. Remind students to dress appropriately for their scheduled interviews, and to use proper language. They should never answer questions with "yeah" or "nope." They should always thank the interviewers for their time. They should question the interviewer as to the date on which they should expect to know that the position was filled. This can relieve a lot of stressful waiting.

Remind the students to network. Students should ask family, friends, and coworkers if they know of a position that may be in their desired fields. Most importantly, they must never stop learning and must keep informed of the changes occurring in the nursing profession. Advise the students to subscribe to a nursing magazine or journal, join a nursing association, or research nursing materials. Nursing is a lifelong learning profession.

Chapter 18

MAKEUP ASSIGNMENTS

This chapter examines:

- Meeting required didactic hours
- Makeup exercises for missed and cancelled clinical classes

MAKEUP ASSIGNMENTS

Nursing programs require a specific amount of didactic hours. Students who miss a clinical class must make up the missed hours. This chapter presents a set of detailed assignments that can be used by students to make up missed class hours. A student who misses a class can be instructed to develop a well-researched 45-minute presentation on the assigned topic to give to the clinical group in postconference. The presentation can be submitted via e-mail if the student is absent on the last clinical day.

Any assignment must require the number of hours of effort that would have been spent in a clinical setting. If clinical hours have been missed because of bad weather, the required assignment can be supplemented. It is suggested that students should not be penalized for missing a clinical class because of bad weather if the supplemental assignment is completed appropriately and submitted. So the assignments must be detailed and must require research into a particular subject using evidence-based, peer-reviewed articles and books as sources of information. A clinical 8-hour makeup day is arranged at the end of clinical to ensure that students have the hours needed. The school will arrange a makeup day at a predetermined site before classes end for the semester. All students who have lost a clinical day due to a preapproved excuse are required to attend.

LABORATORY ASSIGNMENT

Provide detailed answers to the following questions:

1. What is the purpose of drawing peak and trough levels of a medication, and why is it important to gather this information?
2. What is the purpose of a random medication level, and why is this data important?
3. In what ways can the phlebotomy department make laboratory specimen errors? Include patient identification errors in your discussion.
4. How does the creatinine level play a role in both medication dosing and drug levels?
5. What are the normal levels of the following medications?
   a. Lithium
   b. Digoxin
   c. Vancomycin
   d. Valproic acid
   e. Potassium
   f. Gentamycin
   g. Coumadin
   h. Heparin

PHARMACOLOGY ASSIGNMENT

List the side effects for the following medications that are a major concern for nurses:

1. Antianxiety medications
2. Herbal supplements
3. Antiarrhythmic medications
4. Antibiotic medications
5. Anticholinergic medications
6. Antidepressant medications
7. Antidiabetic medications
8. Antihistamine medications

VULNERABLE POPULATION ASSIGNMENT

List two problems and their corresponding nursing solutions for the following situations:

1. Elderly woman who lives alone but falls frequently.
2. HIV patient unemployed due to frequent illnesses.
3. Single mother with two children (ages 4 and 6) living in a one-bedroom home. Youngest child has asthma.
4. Elderly widowed man who no longer socializes and has lost weight.
5. Female 87 years old who lives alone and has 15 cats.

CANCER ASSIGNMENT

List two symptoms for each of the following types of cancer. Also discuss one diagnostic test and treatment for each:

1. Non-Hodgkin's lymphoma
2. Glioblastoma
3. Small cell carcinoma
4. Prostate cancer
5. Breast cancer
6. Uterine cancer
7. Skin cancer

HOLISTIC ASSIGNMENT

1. Why is it important to know whether a patient has a drug, food, or environmental allergy?
2. What is the significance of knowing the allergic response?
3. What is the importance of asking whether the patient uses over-the-counter (OTC) medications or herbal supplements?
4. Explain how the following items can interact with medications. (List those medication(s) with which they can interact.)
   a. Smoking
   b. Diet
   c. OTC medications
   d. Herbal supplements
   e. Street drugs
   f. Activities

STANDARD OF CARE ASSIGNMENT

Research the qualifications and rules for the provision of medication that are required by the State Board of Nursing. Write a two-page report on your findings in American Psychological Association (APA) format with references to at least five peer-reviewed journal articles.

PROFESSIONAL CHARACTERISTICS ASSIGNMENT

1. Explain how ethics guide a nurse's behavior when providing patient care.
2. Explain the importance of beneficence, nonmaleficence, veracity, autonomy, justice, and fidelity in nursing.

3. Briefly describe the following:
   a. Code of conduct
   b. Standards of practice
   c. Nurse Practice Act
   d. Scope of practice

NURSING DOCUMENTATION STYLES ASSIGNMENT

Research the different types of nursing documentation styles.

1. Include an example of each style in your report.
2. Provide a short list of the pros and cons of each style.

PATIENT SLEEP PROBLEMS ASSIGNMENT

Sleep (or the lack of sleep) is a common complaint of hospitalized patients. Provide brief, research-based answers to the following questions:

1. What is insomnia?
2. How does lack of sleep affect the patient?
3. How does sleep affect the body?
4. What steps can the nurse take to improve the sleep process for the patient?
5. What is a hospital-induced psychosis? What can be done to prevent it?

CONCLUSION

It is with great hope that the writers, editors, and publisher have provided a thorough and complete program that will assist in your teaching experience. Please feel free to submit your feedback regarding this book to the publisher.

DRUG NAMES, MECHANISMS, DESCRIPTIONS, AND CONTRAINDICATIONS

Nurses must possess a wide range of knowledge about the vast number of drugs currently available, including their classification, actions and indications, routes of administration, appropriate dosages, side effects and adverse reactions, and antidotes (if available). To facilitate comprehension and retention of this essential information, the drug classification is often aligned for teaching purposes with the procedure, body system, or disease process in which it is used. In this way, the learner is better able to connect the use of a particular drug with a patient's clinical situation. By recognizing the disease process affecting a particular client, the nurse can confirm what drugs should be administered to that client. The discussion that follows includes relevant information about common drugs although it is not all-inclusive. Drug dosage has been deliberately omitted and should always be cross-checked against reliable sources. Also highlighted are notes that represent the content and concepts frequently tested in nursing.

ANALGESICS AND ANTI-INFLAMMATORY DRUGS

Analgesics are drugs used to provide relief from pain. Included in this category are non-narcotic, nonsteroidal anti-inflammatory drugs (NSAIDs) and narcotic drugs. Some analgesics also have anti-inflammatory effects. Corticosteroids are drugs used to treat a variety of conditions by acting to suppress inflammation and the immune system.

Category/Drug	Actions/ Indications	Adverse Effects	Nursing Considerations
Nonnarcotic Analgesics			
NSAIDs Suffix: -profen (fenoprofen, ibuprofen, ketoprofen) Suffix: -fenac (bromfenac, diclofenac, nepafenac) Examples: Acetic acids: indomethacin (Indocin), sulindac (Clinoril); Fenamates (Ponstel); celecoxib (Celebrex);	NSAIDs block cyclooxygenase-2 (COX-2), an enzyme that causes pain and inflammation COX-2 inhibitors selectively block the COX-2 enzyme and therefore have a lower risk of causing stomach or intestine ulcers than other NSAIDs These drugs inhibit the production of prostaglandins	▪ Nausea ▪ Vomiting ▪ Diarrhea ▪ Constipation ▪ Rash ▪ Dizziness	NOTE: NSAIDs carry the risk of myocardial infarction and stroke. ▪ Fenamates (e.g., Ponstel) are used to treat rheumatoid arthritis ▪ Ketorolac (Toradol) is the only NSAID that is available for administration orally, intramuscularly (IM), intravenously (IV), or topically

(*continued*)

Category/Drug	Actions/ Indications	Adverse Effects	Nursing Considerations
oxicams (Feldene); Propionic acids: naproxen (Naprosyn); ketorolac tromethamine (Toradol)	Ketorolac tromethamine (Toradol) is similar to morphine and is used for short-term management of moderately severe acute pain		■ Ketorolac is contraindicated in patients with a patent ductus arteriosus, renal or hepatic impairment, anemia, myocardial infarction, or stroke

Narcotics

NOTE: The antidote for narcotics is naloxone (Narcan), which is used to reverse respiratory depression.

Category/Drug	Actions/ Indications	Adverse Effects	Nursing Considerations
Demerol (meperidine)	Acts as an agonist at specific opioid receptors in the central nervous system (CNS) to produce analgesia, euphoria, and sedation	■ Mood changes (e.g., euphoria, dysphoria) ■ Weakness ■ Headache ■ Agitation ■ Tremor and involuntary muscle movements	■ Give the smallest effective dose for the shortest period of time
Fentanyl	Buccal form is used to treat "breakthrough" cancer pain that is not controlled by other medications; also used as a pain reliever and anesthetic in pre-procedures	■ Drowsiness ■ Lightheadedness ■ Weakness and fatigue	■ Fentanyl is 100 times stronger than morphine
Morphine	Indicated for the relief of pain in patients who require opioid analgesics for more than a few days; interacts predominantly with the opioid mu-receptor; also produces respiratory depression by direct action on the brainstem respiratory centers.	■ Respiratory depression ■ Bradycardia ■ Seizure (convulsions) ■ May also cause itching of the face, mouth, and eyes, which can be treated with promethazine	■ Contraindicated in patients with pancreatitis as morphine induces "spasm" in the sphincter of Oddi
Oxycodone (OxyContin)	Decreases pain by binding to the opiate receptors in the CNS	■ Respiratory depression ■ Flushing ■ Physical and psychological dependence	■ Monitor the patient's response closely, especially when giving sustained-release preparations

Corticosteroids

Category/Drug	Actions/ Indications	Adverse Effects	Nursing Considerations
Examples: Betamethasone, prednisone, Solu-Cortef IV, Solu-Medrol IV	Steroids have a wide range of uses reflecting their anti-inflammatory and immunosuppressive properties Individual agents may be	■ Dizziness ■ Mood swings ■ Hyperglycemia ■ Weight gain ■ Electrolyte imbalance ■ Extreme fatigue	■ Administer with meals NOTE: When discontinuing these drugs, gradually decrease the dosage to prevent adrenal crisis.

Category/Drug	Actions/ Indications	Adverse Effects	Nursing Considerations
(methylpredni-solone), dexa-methasone	available in several different prepara-tions (i.e., oral, IV, topical) Betamethasone accelerates fetal lung maturity and reduces intracranial hemorrhage in premature infants Prednisone sup-presses the normal immune response Dexamethasone is used primarily in the treatment of brain edema	■ Unusual bleeding ■ Black stools ■ Swelling ■ Leukocytosis ■ immune suppression increases the risk of infections (especially fungal) ■ Prednisone toxicity results in Cushing's syndrome (buffalo hump, moon face, high glucose levels, and hypertension)	

ANESTHETICS AND OTHER DRUGS GIVEN DURING SURGERY

Anesthetics are drugs that cause a reversible loss of sensation. Most anesthetics can cause respiratory depression, hypotension, and arrhythmias. A less common, but important and potentially fatal adverse reaction is malignant hyperthermia. As the result of an inherited condition, susceptible individuals develop hyperthermia, rhabdomyolysis, and muscle rigidity following administration of certain anesthetics. Without prompt treatment with dantrolene, death often occurs.

Keep in mind that, when an anesthetic is administered to induce paralysis, a seda-tive should always be administered first

Category/Drug	Actions/ Indications	Adverse Effects	Nursing Considerations
Anesthetics			
Etomidate	Short-acting IV anesthetic used for short-term procedures or to induce general anesthesia	■ Injection site pain ■ Eye movements ■ Skeletal movements	■ Unlike many other anesthetics, this drug does not cause hypotension
Ketamine	Used to induce and maintain general anesthesia in children	■ Hallucinations ■ Respiratory depression ■ Cardiovascular side effects	■ Closely monitor of vital signs during administration
Pancuronium bromide (Pavulon)	Competitive acetylcholine antagonist used as a muscle relaxant for intubation or for quick-onset surgery	■ Skeletal muscle weakness ■ Respiratory insufficiency ■ Apnea	■ This drug does not induce sleep; when administered with other anesthetic drugs, an additive effect occurs ■ Use caution when administering to patients with myasthenia gravis

(continued)

Category/Drug	Actions/ Indications	Adverse Effects	Nursing Considerations
			■ *Antidote*: The effects of this drug can be partially reversed by administration of an anticholinesterase drug, such as neostigmine and pyridostigmine
Propofol	Used for sedation and hypnosis	■ Metabolic acidosis ■ Hyperlipidemia	■ Use aseptic technique when administering this drug ■ Change the IV tubing used to administer the drug every 12 hours
Succinylcholine (Anectine)	Binds to the nicotinic M receptors for acetylcholine; used for relaxing muscles during surgery or when on a ventilator; also used during anesthesia for tube insertion	■ Hypotension ■ Bradycardia ■ Respiratory paralysis ■ Dystonia ■ Akathisia ■ Malignant hyperthermia ■ Increased intraocular pressure	■ Because this drug increases intraocular pressure, it should not be used in patients with penetrating eye injuries ■ Other contraindications include glaucoma, blood electrolyte abnormalities, malignant hyperthermia, or kidney or liver disease
Thiopental sodium (pentothal sodium)	Acts on the gamma aminobutyric acid (GABA) receptor in the brain and spinal cord; a rapid-onset, short-acting barbiturate general anesthetic	■ Cardiovascular depression ■ Respiratory depression	■ Contraindications include liver disease, Addison's disease, myxedema, and heart disease
Antimuscarinic agents			
Glycopyrrolate [Robinul])	Given preoperatively to reduce respiratory and gastric secretions	■ Dry mouth (xerostomia) ■ Urinary retention ■ Blurred vision and photophobia (due to dilation of pupils [mydriasis]) ■ Increased ocular tension ■ Tachycardia	■ Contraindications include glaucoma, asthma, and prostatic hypertrophy

ANTICOAGULANTS

Anticoagulants are drugs that prevent the clotting of blood.

KEY NOTE: Always monitor the patient's coagulant level and obtain a complete blood count (CBC) before administering these drugs. Monitor for any type of bleeding.

Category/Drug	Actions/ Indications	Adverse Effects	Nursing Considerations
Aspirin	Platelet inhibitor, anti-inflammatory, analgesic, antipyretic	■ Gastrointestinal (GI) bleeding ■ Heartburn ■ Nausea ■ Tinnitus	■ Contraindications include hemophilia and bleeding ulcers
Fibrinolytic agents Examples: alteplase, reteplase, urokinase, streptokinase, tissue plasminogen activator (tPA)	Converts plasminogen to plasmin, which in turn leaves fibrin, thereby causing clot dissolution and restoration of blood flow to ischemic tissues	■ Severe internal bleeding ■ Allergic reaction	NOTE: Before administering a fibrinolytic agent, all appropriate blood levels (e.g., coagulation levels, fibrinogen, hemoglobin [Hgb]/hematocrit [HCT] levels) should be obtained and all appropriate tubes (e.g., Foley, nasogastric), should be inserted. Avoid removing any tube or IV line for 48 hours post-infusion
Enoxaparin sodium (Lovenox)	Low-molecular-weight heparin	■ Bleeding	■ Given subcutaneously in the lower abdomen ■ Avoid administering within 1 inch of the umbilicus ■ When giving enoxaparin, there is no need to monitor coagulation levels
Heparin	Inhibits coagulation by forming an antithrombin that prevents the conversion of prothrombin to thrombin and by preventing liberation of thromboplastin from platelets Used in the treatment of deep vein thrombosis (DVT), atrial fibrillation, and disseminated intravascular coagulation	■ Heparin-induced thrombocytopenia (HITT), characterized by low platelet count	■ If HITT occurs, immediately stop heparin and administer argatroban instead ■ Has a short half-life (time required for the drug to fall to half its value as measured at the beginning of the time period) ■ Activated partial thromboplastin time (APTT) is 1.5–2 times the normal laboratory value NOTE: Heparin does not prevent formed clots.
Warfarin (Coumadin)	Inhibits the synthesis of vitamin K clotting factors	■ Increased risk of serious bleeding	■ Prothrombin time [PT] should be 1.5–2 times the normal laboratory value ■ Monitor closely when patients are also taking drugs that increase the international normalized ratio (INR) (e.g., steroids, metronidazole [Flagyl], salicylates, quinidine) NOTE: Teach the patient to avoid a diet rich in vitamin K (e.g., green leafy vegetables such as kale, brussel sprouts, mustard greens) and liquids such as green tea, cranberry juice, and alcohol.

(continued)

ANTIMICROBIALS

Antimicrobials are drugs that destroy or inhibit the growth of micro-organisms. This classification includes antibiotic, antifungal, antiparasitic, and antiviral drugs. There are various methods by which antimicrobials can destroy or inhibit micro-organisms:

- Inhibition of bacterial cell wall synthesis, which weakens the cell wall
  Agents used: cephalosporins, daptomycin, penicillins
- Inhibition of protein synthesis, which disrupts protein synthesis of microbes but does not disrupt normal cells
  Agents used: aminoglycosides, clindamycin, erythromycin, tetracycline
- Inhibition of metabolic pathways for nucleic acid synthesis, which requires folate
  Agents used: fluoroquinolones, rifampin
- Disruption of cell wall permeability, which causes cells to leak components that are vital to survival

> **KEY NOTE:** Always check for allergies before administering antibiotics (especially penicillin [PCN]). Make sure culture and sensitivity has been done before administration of the first dose of an antibiotic.

Category	Drug	Actions/ Indications	Adverse Effects	Nursing Considerations
Antibiotic Agents				
Aminoglycosides Suffix: -mycin	Amikacin	Used to treat infections with *Acinetobacter* and *Enterobacter* species	■ Kidney damage ■ Hearing loss	■ Closely monitor renal function and vestibulocochlear nerve function
	Gentamicin	Used to treat gram-negative organisms, *Staphylococcus*, *Proteus*, and *Pseudomonas*	■ Kidney damage	■ Blood level should usually be 5–10 mcg/mL for peak concentration and less than 2 mcg/mL for trough concentration; dosage is also adjusted based on creatinine level
	Neomycin	Kills bacteria in the intestinal tract, keeps ammonia levels low, and prevents hepatic encephalopathy Used prophylactically, especially prior to GI surgery	■ Nausea and vomiting ■ Diarrhea ■ Allergic reaction	■ Has the highest risk of toxicity of all aminoglycosides
	Strepto mycin	Used to treat infective endocarditis and tuberculosis	■ Nausea and vomiting ■ Loss of appetite	■ Be alert to symptoms of ototoxicity

Category	Drug	Actions/Indications	Adverse Effects	Nursing Considerations
	Tobramycin	Used in various severe or life-threatening gram-negative infections (e.g., meningitis in neonates; brucellosis)	■ Allergic reaction ■ Changes in hearing ■ Dizziness	■ Ineffective orally, so for systemic use it can only be given IV or IM, or administered and inhaled via nebulizer for *Pseudomonas* infection
	Erythromycin (EES, E-Mycin)	Used to treat respiratory, skin, and lung conditions	■ Nephrotoxic and ototoxic effects, including impaired balance and ringing in the ears ■ GI disturbances ■ Arrhythmia with prolonged QT intervals (start of Q wave to end of T wave measurement)	■ Monitor liver function in patients receiving prolonged therapy
Antiseptics	Nitrofurantoin (Macrodantin)	Used to treat urinary tract infections Interferes with bacterial enzyme systems	■ Peripheral neuropathy ■ Acute and chronic pulmonary reactions	■ Be alert to signs of urinary tract superinfections ■ Assess for nausea
Beta-lactam antibiotics	*Cephalosporins* Prefixes: cef-, ceph- Examples: cefaclor (Ceclor), cefixime, cephalexin	Broad-spectrum antibiotic used to treat urinary tract infections (UTIs)	■ Candidiasis, pseudomembranous colitis (*Clostridium difficile*) ■ Maculopapular rash ■ Nephrotoxicity ■ CNS symptoms	■ Contraindications include PCN allergies, liver disease, and jaundice
	Monobactams Example: aztreonam	Inhibits cell wall synthesis Used in the management of infections caused by gram-negative aerobic bacteria such as *Pseudomonas*	■ Rash ■ Diarrhea ■ Nausea and vomiting	■ Patients with kidney and liver disease are more likely to experience side effects

(continued)

Category	Drug	Actions/ Indications	Adverse Effects	Nursing Considerations
	Carbapenems Example: imipenem	High resistance to bacterial enzymes Used to treat *Escherichia coli* and *Klebsiella* pneumonia and other infections not readily treated by other antibiotics	■ High risk of seizures	■ Ensure close monitoring of patients who are highly vulnerable to CNS effects
Broad-spectrum antibacterial agents	*Fluoroquinolones* Suffix: -floxacin Examples: levofloxacin (Levaquin), azithromycin (Zithromax), ciprofloxacin (Cipro)	Used for community-acquired pneumonia and urinary tract infections	■ Peripheral neuropathy ■ Prolonged QT interval ■ Hepatotoxicity ■ CNS effects ■ *Clostridium difficile–* associated diarrhea	■ Do not administer with antacids
	Tetracycline Suffix: -cycline: Examples: demeclocycline, doxycycline, minocycline, tetracycline	Used for upper and lower respiratory tract infections, skin and soft tissue infections	■ Photosensitivity ■ Tooth discoloration ■ Hypoglycemia ■ Increased digoxin levels	■ Advise the patients to avoid dairy products and antacids
Gram-positive antibacterial penicillin antibiotics	Amoxicillin (Amoxil), penicillin, Augmentin, and ampicillin	Binds to bacterial cell wall; used to treat gram-positive infections such as streptococcus, staphylococcus, listeria, and clostridium	■ Anaphylaxis ■ Seizures ■ Superinfection ■ Hypersensitivity	■ Contraindications include PCN allergies and liver disease
Macrolide antibiotics	Erythromycin, azithromycin (Zithromax), and clarithromycin (Biaxin)	Used to treat chlamydial infection, acute bacterial exacerbation of chronic bronchitis, cirrhosis, and kidney problems	■ GI side effects ■ Prolonged QT interval ■ Ototoxicity ■ Bradycardia	■ Advise the patient to avoid grapefruit juice

Category	Drug	Actions/ Indications	Adverse Effects	Nursing Considerations
Oxazolidinones	Linezolid (Zyvox)	Used for gram-negative infections (e.g., pneumonia, meningitis)	■ GI disturbances (most common)	■ Should not be used by patients taking medications that inhibit monoamine oxidases A or B (MAO-A or MAO-B inhibitors)
PCP antimicrobial	Pentami-dine	Antimicrobial used to prevent and treat *Pneumocystis pneumonia* (PCP) in HIV patients	■ Prolonged QT interval ■ Nephrotoxicity ■ Stevens–Johnson syndrome ■ Leukopenia	■ Can cause allergic and toxic side effects, especially to pancreas
Quinolone antibiotics (broad spectrum) Suffix: -floxacin	Cipro-floxacin, levofloxa-cin, moxi-floxacin, ofloxacin	Inhibits bacteria by inhibiting DNA gyrase. Used to treat a wide range of infections.	■ Tendon rupture ■ Prolonged QT interval ■ Torsades de pointes	■ Give 1 hour before or 2 hours after antacids or milk products
Sulfa antibiotics	Sulfameth-oxa-zole–tri-methoprim (Bactrim), sulfadia-zine, sul-famethoxa-zole	Anti-infective and anti-inflammatory drugs used to treat PCP pneumonia and other infections	■ Slow heart rate, weak pulse ■ Severe tingling, numbness, and muscle weakness ■ Steven–Johnson syndrome ■ Blood dyscrasias (anemia) ■ Crystalluria (crystallization in renal tubules) and severe renal damage	■ Contraindicated in patients with a sulfa allergy ■ Advise the patient to avoid foods and fluids that are acidic, avoid alcohol, drink and 1.5 L of water per day ■ Patients must have a urine pH less than 5.5
Vancomycin	Tricyclic glyco-peptide antibiotic that is the only drug in its class	Used to treat serious infec-tions caused by gram-positive bacteria known or suspected to be resistant to other antibiotics	■ Ototoxicity and nephrotoxicity	■ Can cause histamine release, resulting in an anaphylactic response known as "red man syndrome"

(continued)

Category	Drug	Actions/ Indications	Adverse Effects	Nursing Considerations
Antifungal Agents				
Azoles Suffix: -nazole	Clotri- mazole (Mycelex), fluconazole (Diflucan), keto- conazole (Nizoral)	Stops the growth of the yeast (*Candida*) that causes thrush	■ Nausea ■ Stomach pain ■ Itchy skin ■ Possible allergic reaction	■ Monitor for an allergic response: patients allergic to other azole antifungals may be allergic to fluconazole
	Mycostatin (Nystatin)	Used to treat fungal skin infections	■ Redness, itching, or hy- persensitivity	■ Generally well- tolerated even with prolonged therapy
Antiparasitic Agents				
Antihelmintics Suffix: -dazole	Meben dazole	Used to treat- ment pinworm, whipworm, roundworm, and hookworm	■ Diarrhea	■ Warn patients that the drug may turn stools red or cause urine to have an asparagus-like smell
Antiviral Agents				
Suffixes: -tadine, -vir	Cidofovir, ganciclovir	Anticytomeg- alovirus (anti- CMV)	■ Kidney damage	■ Monitor patient for hypersensitivity reactions, ■ white blood cell count (neutropenia), ■ stomatitis, ■ blood pressure, ■ Monitor HIV RNA assay, CD4 counts, liver function, kidney function, CBC, ■ blood glucose, and serum amylase and triglyceride levels (these will ■ determine the effectiveness and toxicity of the drug)
	Amanta- dine, rim- antadine, zanamivir	Antiflu	■ Agitation ■ Headache ■ Nausea	

Category	Drug	Actions/ Indications	Adverse Effects	Nursing Considerations
	Adefovir, entecavir, ribavirin	Anti-hepatitis	■ Weakness ■ Headache ■ Abdominal pain	
	Acyclovir; famciclovir (for herpes zoster, genital herpes, and chickenpox [varicella])	Anti-herpes	■ Nausea and vomiting ■ Abdominal pain	
	Abacavir, ritonavir, tenofovir	Anti-HIV	■ Nausea ■ Headache ■ Fatigue ■ Vomiting	
	Nucleoside analogs— lamivudine, stavudine, telbivu-dine, zido-vudine	Used to treat hepatitis B and C, herpes simplex, and HIV infections	■ Stomach upset ■ Possible peripheral neuropathy	

ANTIPYRETICS

Antipyretics are fever-reducing drugs.

Drug	Actions	Indications	Adverse Effects	Nursing Considerations
Aspirin (acetylsalicylic acid [ASA])	Inhibits prostaglandin (necessary for normal cell function)	Used as an analgesic, antipyretic, anti-inflammatory, and an antiplatelet, and enhances anticoagulants	■ GI ulcers, stomach bleeding, and tinnitus	■ *Antidote*: Salicylate poisoning can be rapidly fatal; administer charcoal to reduce absorption of the drug NOTE: Young children with fever or flu-like symptoms should not be given aspirin because of the risk of developing Reye's syndrome (characterized by rash and detrimental effects to many organs, especially the brain (encephalitis) and liver)

(*continued*)

Drug	Actions	Indications	Adverse Effects	Nursing Considerations
Para-aminophenol derivatives: acetaminophen (Tylenol, other trade names)	Produces analgesia by elevation of the pain threshold	Has antipyretic and analgesic effects	■ Can cause liver insufficiency and blood dyscrasias	■ Phenylketonuria patients should avoid Tylenol with aspartame (NutraSweet) and children's Tylenol) *Antidote:* N-acetylcysteine (Mucomyst) or charcoal NOTE: Do not take more than 1 g (1000 mg) of Tylenol per dose or 4 g (4000 mg) per day. Do not use alcohol with Tylenol

CARDIAC DRUGS

Cardiac drugs encompass a wide range of drugs used alone or in combination to treat diseases of the heart (arrhythmias, defects) and vasculature (coronary artery disease).

Category	Drug	Actions/ Indications	Adverse Effects	Nursing Considerations
Antihypertensives				
Alpha-adrenergic inhibitors Example: doxazosin mesylate (Cardura)	Relaxes smooth muscle surrounding blood vessels	Benign prostatic hypertro-phy (BPH), gestational hyperten-sion	■ Syncope ■ Significant hypotension ■ Bradycardia ■ Paresthesia ■ Thrombocy topenia ■ Decreased or absent reflexes	■ Can negatively affect cataract surgery
Alpha agonists Examples: clonidine (Catapres), methyldopa (Aldomet, Aldoril)	Stimulates alpha-receptors in the brain, enhancing blood flow in peripheral arteries, decreasing resistance, and decreasing blood pressure	Hyper-tension, gestational hyperten-sion	■ May cause renal failure ■ Hemolytic anemia ■ Black tongue ■ Aggravation of angina pectoris ■ Congestive heart failure (CHF) ■ Bone marrow suppression ■ Toxic epidermal necrolysis	■ Must obtain baseline CBC before initiating medication

Category	Drug	Actions/ Indications	Adverse Effects	Nursing Considerations
Alpha blockers, anti-adrenergic Suffix: -pril Examples: captopril (Capoten), enalapril (Vasotec)	Blocks conversion of angiotensin I to angiotensin	Hypertension, heart failure, diabetic neuropathy	■ Renal problems ■ Hypotension ■ Angioedema of extremities, face, lips, mucous membranes, and tongue	■ Be sure that patient is not pregnant before beginning treatment
Angiotensin II receptor antagonists Suffix: -sartan Examples: irbesartan (Avapro), losartan, valsartan	Blocks the action of angiotensin, resulting in dilation of blood vessels and decrease in blood pressure	Used in diabetic patients with kidney problems to treat hypertension and heart failure	■ Hypotension ■ Arrhythmias ■ Conduction disorder	■ Caution is indicated when these drugs are used in combination with potassium-sparing diuretics or NSAIDs
Beta-1–selective (cardioselective) adrenoceptor blocking agents Suffix: -olol Examples: atenolol (Tenormin), metoprolol, nadolol (Corgard), pindolol, propranolol, timolol	Reduces the force of contraction of heart muscle and lowers blood pressure	Used to treat hypertension, angina pectoris, and migraines	■ Side effects are generally mild and transient	NOTE: If beta-blocker eye drops such as timolol are used, pressure must be applied to the lacrimal duct for 5 seconds to minimize the occurrence of systemic bradycardia or hypotension. Patients with bronchospastic disease should not receive beta blockers. Beta blockers can also mask the symptoms of hypoglycemia
Calcium channel blockers Suffix: -dipine Examples: benzothiazides—diltiazem hydrochloride (Cardizem); dihydropyridines—nifedipine, nicardipine, felodipine, amlodipine; verapamil	Negative inotropic agents that inhibit calcium transport into myocardial and smooth muscle cells, inhibit atrioventricular conduction, and decrease sinoatrial (SA) node automaticity	Used to treat migraines, hypertension, supraventricular tachyarrhythmias (e.g., atrial fibrillation, atrial flutter, and paroxysmal supraventricular tachycardia), and exertional angina pectoris	■ Heart block ■ Liver insufficiency ■ Angioedema ■ Stevens–Johnson syndrome ■ Constipation ■ Headache ■ Nausea ■ Rash ■ Edema ■ Sexual dysfunction	■ Advise the patient to avoid grapefruit juice

(continued)

Category	Drug	Actions/ Indications	Adverse Effects	Nursing Considerations
Hydralazine (Apresoline)	Vasodilator	Used to treat hypertension	■ Shortness of breath, skin rash, edema	■ Use with caution in patients with suspected coronary artery disease
Nipride	Vasodilator	Administered to reduce afterload, and as an antidote for ergot alkaloid poisoning	■ Anemia ■ Bradycardia ■ Hypotension ■ Encephalopathy, or other conditions in which intracranial pressure is increased, causes confusion, tremors, and arrhythmias	■ Drug is sensitive to light ■ Byproduct is cyanide; monitor thiocyanate serum toxicity
Antiarrhythmic drugs				
Adenosine	Slows conduction time through the A-V node	Used for paroxysmal supraventricular tachycardia (PSVT)	■ Breathing problems ■ Chest pain	■ Contraindicated in patients with second- or third-degree A-V block, sick sinus syndrome, or symptomatic bradycardia
Atropine	Blunts the increased vagal tones and increases heart rate	May be used in the operating room to reduces secretions Also used as an antidote for inadvertent overdose of cholinergic drugs	■ Dry mouth ■ Blurred vision ■ photophobia ■ Tachycardia	■ Contraindicated in patients with glaucoma, pyloric stenosis, or BPH
Calcium channel blockers (see above, under Antihypertensives)				

Category	Drug	Actions/ Indications	Adverse Effects	Nursing Considerations
Glycosides Example: digoxin (Lanoxin)	Increases the strength and vigor of heart contractions	Used to treat mild to moderate heart failure and atrial fibrillation	■ Heart block ■ Nausea and vomiting ■ Visual disturbances (blurred or yellow vision) ■ Digitalis increases ventricular irritability and could convert a rhythm to ventricular fibrillation following cardioversion	■ Check apical pulse; if less than 60 bpm, hold medication. ■ Check digoxin and potassium levels prior to administration; digoxin blood levels should be 0.8–2.0 mg/mL ■ Potassium-depleting diuretics are the major contributing factor to digitalis toxicity ■ *Antidote:* digoxin immune Fab (Digibind)

Drugs Used to Treat Congestive Heart Failure (CHF)

Category	Drug	Actions/ Indications	Adverse Effects	Nursing Considerations
Nesiritide (Natrecor)	Human B-type natriuretic peptide that relaxes and dilates blood vessels	Improves breathing in patients with CHF failure	■ Headache ■ Dizziness ■ Nausea and vomiting ■ Back pain	■ Do not administer for more than 48 hours in patients with acutely decompensated CHF ■ Monitor blood pressure
Phosphodiesterase (PDE) 3 inhibitors	Vasodilation; increases contractility and heart rate	Used to treat acute decompensated heart failure, and reduce preload and afterload	■ Hypotension ■ Arrhythmias ■ Cutaneous flushing	■ Mothers who are breast feeding should be instructed to discontinue this practice for the duration of drug treatment

Drugs Used to Treat High Serum Cholesterol Levels

Category	Drug	Actions/ Indications	Adverse Effects	Nursing Considerations
Atorvastatin (Lipitor)	Lipid-lowering HMG-CoA reductase inhibitor	Used to manage hypercholesterolemia, prevent stroke, and lower total low-density lipoprotein (LDL) cholesterol and triglyceride levels	■ Muscle pain ■ Fever ■ Dark-colored urine ■ Fatigue	■ Evaluate fat consumption ■ Monitor liver function tests ■ Advise the patient to avoid grapefruit juice and follow dietary restrictions

(continued)

Category	Drug	Actions/ Indications	Adverse Effects	Nursing Considerations
Drug Used to Treat Pulmonary Hypertension				
Phosphodiesterase (PDE) 5 inhibitors Suffix: -afil (e.g., vardenafil, tadalafil) Examples: milrinone	Vasodilation; these agents relax muscles around blood vessels, promoting dilation	Used to treat pulmonary hypertension, anti-inflammatory agent for COPD, asthma, and impotence.	■ Headache ■ Tremors ■ Easy bruising	NOTE: Patients cannot take nitrates with (PDE) 5 inhibitors
Drugs Used to Treat Ventricular Arrhythmias				
Amiodarone (Cordarone)	Multiple and complex effects on the electrical activity of the heart, normalizing heart rhythm	Can be used for atrial and ventricular arrhythmias	■ Pulmonary toxicity (most serious reaction)	■ Concurrent administration with numerous drugs (e.g., antibiotics, other cardiac drugs) can increase toxicity ■ Advise the patient to avoid grapefruit juice and St. John's wort
Bretylium	Adrenergic neuron blocking	Used to treat life-threatening ventricular arrhythmias when other drugs are ineffective	■ Dizziness, lightheaded-ness, faintness	■ This drug has been discontinued; however, generic formulations may be available
Disopyramide (Norpace), procainamide (Pronestyl), and quinidine	Prolongs repolarization	Used to treat abnormal heart rhythms	■ Dizziness	■ Advise the patient to avoid taking with alcohol
Lidocaine HCI (Xylocaine)	Accelerates repolarization	Used to prevent and treat ventricular tachycardia	■ CNS symptoms (lidocaine toxicity) include slurred speech, tonic–clonic seizures	■ May cause cardiac toxicity, hypotension, and bradycardia
Vasoconstrictors				
NOTE: All vasoconstrictor medications should be administered via a central line.				
Dopamine	Positive inotrope that increases peripheral vascular resistance and arterial blood pressure	Used to treat low blood pressure due to shock and other serious medical conditions	■ Ectopic heart-beats ■ Tachycardia ■ Angina ■ Palpitations ■ Vasoconstric-tion ■ Hypotension ■ Dyspnea ■ Nausea and vomiting ■ Headache	■ Contraindicated in patients with pheochromocy-toma, uncor-rected tach-yarrhythmias, or ventricular fibrillation

Category	Drug	Actions/ Indications	Adverse Effects	Nursing Considerations
Epinephrine (Adrenalin)	Positive inotrope that increases peripheral vascular resistance and arterial blood pressure	Relieves respiratory distress due to bronchospasm, allergic reactions, cardiac arrest	■ Anxiety ■ Headache ■ Fear ■ Palpitations	■ Contraindicated in patients with narrow-angle glaucoma ■ Use caution with elderly patients who have cardiovascular disease, hypertension, diabetes mellitus, or hyperthyroidism
Norepinephrine	Positive inotrope that increases peripheral vascular resistance and arterial blood pressure	Used to treat life-threatening hypotension that occurs with some medical conditions	■ Headache ■ Severe hypertension ■ Reflex bradycardia	■ Contraindicated in patients with mesenteric or peripheral vascular thrombosis because it may increase ischemia
Phenylephrine (Neo-Synephrine)	Positive inotrope that increases peripheral vascular resistance and arterial blood pressure	Used to treat nasal or sinus congestion or congestion of the eustachian tubes	■ Restlessness ■ Anxiety ■ Nervousness ■ Dizziness	■ Contains sulfites that may cause allergic reactions in certain individuals (e.g., asthma patients)
Vasopressin antidiuretic hormone (ADH) (Pitressin)	Increases urine osmolality and decreases water excretion	Used in prevention and treatment of diabetes insipidus, to control bleeding, and for management in septic shock patients not responding to high doses of inotropes	■ Local gangrene ■ Coronary thrombosis (chest pain) ■ Mesenteric infarction ■ Venous thrombosis ■ Infarction and necrosis of the small bowel ■ Peripheral emboli	■ *Antidote:* phentolamine (Regitine) for extravasation ■ Carefully monitor ST segment for ischemia

(continued)

Vasodilators

Nitrates Examples: nitroglycerin, isosorbide mononitrate (Imdur); available in sublingual (Nitrospan oral), transdermal, IV, or spray formulations	Decreases preload and afterload	Used to treat heart conditions such as angina, coronary heart disease, and chronic heart failure Dilates healthy vessels, reduces cardiac oxygen demand, and causes increased flow through collateral coronary vessels	■ Flushing ■ Syncope ■ Hypotension ■ Headache	■ Systolic blood pressure should be maintained at greater than or equal to 100 ■ If pain persists, the patient's condition is considered unstable and further diagnostic tests are required
Beta-adrenergic agonists Examples: dobutamine, isoproterenol, and epinephrine	Acts on the beta- receptors to increase myocardial contractility and stroke volume and open calcium channels Dobutamine stimulates beta receptors	Used to treat cardiogenic shock and acute heart failure	■ Hypertension ■ Angina ■ Arrhythmia ■ Tachycardia	■ Contraindicated in patients with a history of heart valve problems, adrenal gland tumor, in- creased irregular heartbeat, or an enlarged left ventricle caused by narrowing of the aortic blood vessel

CHEMOTHERAPEUTIC DRUGS

Chemotherapeutic (antineoplastic) drugs are used for palliative or curative effects in the treatment of patients with cancer. These agents inhibit different phases of the cell cycle, inhibiting DNA replication, cell division, or growth.

KEY NOTE: Chemotherapy causes bone marrow depression, resulting in leucopenia and anemia. Loss of hair and damage to the oral mucosa are common side effects. Fertility may also be affected. Patients should be instructed to use a soft toothbrush; because there is increased risk of infection, they should also avoid crowds and practice good hand washing.

Alkylating Agents

Nitrogen mustard (Mustine, other trade names) Suffix: -mustine	Prevents mitosis, thus interfering with cell replication	Used to treat certain types of brain tumors and multiple myeloma	■ Missed menstrual periods ■ Painful rash ■ Dizziness ■ Joint pain	■ Administer only under the supervision of a physician experienced in anticancer medications

Anthracycline Antibiotics

Suffix: -bicin Examples: doxorubicin (Adriamycin, other trade names), epirubicin, idarubicin, valrubicin	Targets DNA	Used to treat leukemias (doxorubicin, idarubicin), lymphomas (doxorubicin, epirubicin), breast, uterine, and ovarian cancers (epirubicin), bladder cancer (valrubicin), and lung cancer (epirubicin)	■ Labeled as a vesicant (a chemical that causes extensive tissue damage and blistering if it escapes from the veins) ■ Bone marrow depression, leukopenia, and thrombocytopenia ■ Major side effect is heart failure	■ Must be administered by a carefully trained nurse under the supervision of a physician experienced in anticancer medications
Daunomycin	Attacks cancer cells during cell division	Treats cancer of the bladder, breast, head, neck, liver, and lung; leukemia; lymphoma; mesothelioma; and multiple myeloma	■ Anemia ■ Leucopenia ■ Stomatitis	■ Patients with CHF who are immuno-suppressed cannot take this drug
Mitomycin (Mutamycin)	Potent DNA cross-linker	Used to treat cancer of the stomach and pancreas	■ Severe anemia ■ Thrombocytopenia, and ■ Irreversible renal failure (hemolytic uremic syndrome)	■ Do not administer to patients with shingles or chickenpox

Antimetabolites

5-fluorouracil (5-FU), methotrexate, mustargen	Interferes with synthesis of nucleic acid; causes direct damage to DNA, preventing cancer cells from reproducing	Used to treat numerous cancers	■ Nausea and vomiting ■ Mouth sores	■ Monitor the patient for symptoms of dehydration

Hormones

Tamoxifen, flutamide	Interferes with steroid hormones that bind to steroid receptors	Used to treat female and male breast cancer, endometrial cancer, and prostate cancer	■ Edema ■ Hypertension ■ Diabetes mellitus ■ Cushing's syndrome	■ Advise the patient of the importance of having estrogen receptors tested

(continued)

Kinase Inhibitors				
Suffix: -nib Examples: dasatinib, erlotinib, imatinib, sorafenib	Interferes with repair of DNA	Used to treat various cancers and polycystic kidney disease	■ QT prolongation	■ May decrease fertility in men and women
Miscellaneous				
383.8 pt	Blocks amino acids	Used to treat chronic myelogenous leukemia, ovarian cancer, and melanoma	■ Hepatotoxicity	■ Be alert for signs of serious infection or bleeding
Plant Alkaloids				
Vincristine (Oncovin)	Disrupts mitosis	Leukemias, lymphomas, and childhood cancers	■ Extravasation ■ Neurotoxicity ■ Hair loss ■ Bone marrow suppression	■ Advise the patient to avoid grapefruit or grapefruit juice, which can change the blood level of the drug

DIABETIC MEDICATIONS

All patients who take diabetic medications are at risk for hypoglycemia. Control of blood glucose requires a thorough knowledge of the onset, peak, and duration of action of each drug being taken by the patient. In addition, there are numerous drugs that may cause either hypoglycemia (e.g., beta blockers) or hyperglycemia (e.g., steroids).

Category	Drug	Actions/Indications	Adverse Effects	Nursing Considerations
Oral antidiabetic drugs	*Alpha-glucosidase inhibitors*	Prevents digestion of carbohydrates	■ Flatulence ■ Diarrhea	■ Initiate therapy with a low dose and increase to desired amount
	Metformin (Glucophage)	Increases the sensitivity of the liver, muscle, fat, and other tissues to the uptake and effects of insulin	■ Abdominal discomfort ■ Cough or hoarseness ■ Decreased appetite	■ Can cause lactic acidosis ■ The drug must be stopped 2 days before an IV contrast test and should not be restarted until 2 days after the test
	Sulfonylureas: glipizide, glyburide, glibenclamide, glimepiride	Reduces blood glucose by stimulating the pancreas to produce more insulin	■ Nausea ■ Diarrhea ■ Constipation ■ Dizziness	■ Because many drugs can interact with sulfonylureas, it is important that patients report all drugs that they are taking

Category	Drug	Actions/Indications	Adverse Effects	Nursing Considerations
	Thiazolidinediones: rosiglitazone (Avandia), pioglitazone (Actos)	Attaches to insulin receptors; makes cells more sensitive to insulin and facilitates removing glucose from blood	Upper respiratory tract infection, headache, back pain	Concurrent use of rifampin may decrease effectiveness
Insulin		Allows body to process glucose and avoid complications from hyperglycemia		NOTE: When mixing a long-acting insulin and a short-acting insulin, care must be taken to avoid contaminating the bottle containing the long-acting insulin. Patients taking steroid medications (e.g., prednisone) may require extra insulin
	Short-acting analogs: Humulin Regular, Novolin	Onset: within 30 minutes Peak: within 2 hours Duration: 6 hours	■ Hypo-glycemia (headache, hunger, weakness, sweating)	Because of its rapid onset, a short-acting insulin analog should not be administered to the patient until a meal is provided NOTE: Regular insulin is the only insulin that can be given by the IV route
	Rapid-acting analogs: Insulin NovaLog aspart, insulin lispro (Humalog), insulin glulisine (Aprida)	Onset: within minutes Peak: within 2 hours Duration: 4 hours	■ Site reactions (pain, redness, irritation)	■ Administered by subcutaneous injection in the abdominal wall, thigh, or upper arm
	Immediate-acting: Lente, NPH	Onset: within 2 hours Peak: within 4 hours Duration: 16 hours	■ Hypoglyce-mia ■ Hyperglyce-mia	■ Administered by subcutaneous injection
	Long-acting: Ultralente, Lantus, Levemir	Onset: within 1 hour Duration: 24 hours	■ Hypoglyce-mia	■ Do not mix or dilute Lantus with any other solution or insulin
	Long-acting analogs: insulin glargine, insulin detemir	Onset: within 2 hours Duration: 24 hours	■ Hypoglyce-mia	■ Administered by subcutaneous injection

DIURETICS

Diuretics are used to treat fluid overload.

> **KEY NOTE:** Before administration of a diuretic, it is essential to obtain both a current blood pressure reading and serum electrolyte levels. Do not administer the drug if the systolic pressure is 100 mmHg or lower or the patient has hypocalcemia, hypercalcemia, or hypomagnesemia.

Drug	Actions	Indications	Adverse Effects	Nursing Considerations
Bumetanide (Bumex)	Works on the ascending limb of the loop of Henle	Used to treat edema associated with CHF, hepatic disease, and renal disease, including nephrotic syndrome	■ Dizziness ■ Dehydration	■ Administer before furosemide (Lasix) when the patient is taking both diuretics
Carbonic anhydrase inhibitors Example: acetazolamide (Diamox)	Suppresses carbonic anhydrase, which converts carbon dioxide and water to carbonic acid	Used to treat glaucoma, acute mountain sickness, CHF, and seizure disorders	■ Numbness and tingling in fingers and toes ■ Increased risk of developing calcium oxalate and calcium phosphate kidney stones	■ Contraindicated in patients with sickle cell anemia, allergy to sulfa medications, liver or kidney disease, adrenal gland failure (Addison's disease), or women who are pregnant
Chlorothiazide sodium (Diuril)	Helps kidneys remove excess fluid from the body	Used to treat CHF, hypertension, or renal insufficiency	■ Nausea and vomiting ■ Excessive urine production ■ Dehydration ■ Hypokalemia ■ Hypomagnesia	■ Contraindications: sulfa allergy

Drug	Actions	Indica-tions	Adverse Effects	Nursing Considerations
Furosemide (Lasix)	Hinders the absorption of sodium and chloride in the proximal and distal tubules and in the loop of Henle	Used to treat edema associated with CHF	■ Can damage the structures of the inner ear, causing tinnitus, dizziness, and disequilibrium	■ Contraindicated in patients with allergies to sulfa drugs ■ Teach the patient to avoid corticosteroids, adrenocorticotropic hormone (ACTH), licorice in large amounts (will deplete potassium), and prolonged use of laxatives ■ Digitalis therapy may exaggerate the metabolic effects of hypokalemia, especially myocardial effects ■ Ototoxicity is associated with rapid injection, dehydration, and electrolyte depletion
Osmotic diuretics Example: mannitol	Induces osmotic stress	Used to prevent and treat acute renal failure, reduce intracranial pressure in cerebral edema, reduce intraocular pressure, and promote excretion of toxic substances in urine	■ Chest discomfort ■ Cough ■ Difficulty breathing	■ Contraindicated in patients with a history of heart failure
Potassium-sparing diuretics Examples: triamterene, Dyazide, spironol-actone (Aldactone)	Blocks sodium and water reabsorp-tion in the kidneys	Used in the manage-ment of hyperten-sion, CHF, cirrhosis of the liver, nephrotic syndrome, and edema	■ Abdominal pain ■ Nausea and vomiting ■ Rash	■ Do not promote the excretion of potassium in patients taking these drugs ■ Monitor for hyperkalemia ■ Advise the patient to avoid the use of salt substitutes (which contain potassium); instead, patients should follow a low-sodium diet

(*continued*)

Drug	Actions	Indications	Adverse Effects	Nursing Considerations
Thiazide diuretics Example: hydrochlorothiazide (Hydrodiuril)	Acts in the distal tubule and diluting segment of Henle	Used in the management of hypertension, to treat edema, and as an antidiuretic in patients with diabetes insipidus	■ Weakness ■ Low blood pressure ■ Light sensitivity	■ May worsen kidney dysfunction
Thiazide-like diuretic: metolazone (Zaroxolyn)	Causes the kidneys to eliminate certain chemicals that allow large amounts of water to be eliminated	Used to treat edema resulting from CHF and nephrotic syndrome	■ Hyponatremia or hypokalemia ■ Sensitivity reactions (angioedema, bronchospasms) ■ Hyperglycemia ■ Increase in serum uric acid ■ Orthostatic hypotension ■ Hyperparathyroidism ■ Systemic lupus erythematosus	■ Administer 30 minutes before furosemide (Lasix) when the patient is taking both diuretics

GASTROINTESTINAL MEDICATIONS

Drugs used to treat gastrointestinal conditions.

Drug	Actions/ Indications	Adverse Effects	Nursing Considerations
Antacids			
Aluminum hydroxide (Amphojel), magnesium hydroxide (Milk of Magnesia; MOM).	Used for relief of GI discomfort or to reduce phosphate levels in	■ Aluminum-containing antacids can cause osteoporosis	■ Products such as Ascriptin contain significant amounts of aluminum hydroxide combined with buffered aspirin
	patients with kidney conditions	and should be avoided by women after menopause and by patients with renal disease	■ Antacids containing aluminum, calcium, or magnesium may bind phosphate in the gut, leading to hypophosphatemia (low phosphate levels) when used chronically.
H$_2$ antagonists Examples: ranitidine (Zantac, Tritec), famotidine (Pepcid), nizatidine (Axid), cimetidine (Tagamet)	Reduces the amount of stomach acid secreted by glands in the lining of the stomach	■ Can deplete calcium, folic acid, iron, vitamin B$_{12}$, vitamin D, and zinc	■ Most common side effect is headache but famotidine (Pepcid) can affect the platelet count

Drug	Actions/ Indications	Adverse Effects	Nursing Considerations
Proton pump inhibitors Examples: clopidogrel (Plavix), pantoprazole (Protonix), esomeprazole (Nexium)	Reduces stomach acid levels	■ Risk of fracture Inhibits active transport of magnesium in the intestine and can cause hypomagnesemia, hyponatremia, liver and kidney failure, and Stevens–Johnson syndrome.	■ Patients taking clopidogrel (Plavix) should avoid taking esomeprazole (Nexium) because it will reduce clopidogrel's effectiveness by half
Antidiarrheals			
Imodium	Used to control acute diarrhea and chronic diarrhea associated with inflammatory bowel disease Contains a narcotic-like drug that slows the action of the intestines and the passage of stool	■ Dizziness ■ Drowsiness ■ Constipation ■ Skin rash	■ Chronic diarrhea usually responds within 10 days ■ If improvement does not occur within this time, it is unlikely that symptoms will be controlled by further admin- istration
Paregoric (anhydrous morphine)	Used to treat diarrhea	■ Lightheaded- ness ■ Dizziness ■ Sedation ■ Nausea and vomiting	■ Can produce drug dependence
Subsalicylate (Kaopectate), bismuth subsalicylate (Pepto-Bismol)	Slows expulsion of fluids into the digestive system by irritated tissues by "coating" them.	■ Dark tongue ■ Dark stools ■ Anxiety ■ Loss of hearing	■ Contraindicated in clients who are allergic to aspirin ■ Patients with glaucoma, prostate symptoms, or liver or kidney disease should not use antidiarrheal preparations ■ Do not administer to children who may have the flu or chickenpox as salicylates increase the risk of Reye's syndrome
Sucralfate	Coats the stomach and treats ulcers of the upper gastrointesti- nal tract	■ Constipation	■ Be aware of drug interactions; schedule other medications accordingly

(continued)

Drug	Actions/ Indications	Adverse Effects	Nursing Considerations
Antiemetics			
Benzamides Example: metoclopramide (Reglan)	Used to treat nausea or vomiting due to diabetic gastroparesis	■ Most serious complication is irreversible tardive dyskinesis	NOTE: Teach the patient to report tremors or other involuntary movements
Chlorpromazine (Thorazine)	Used to treat certain mental and behavioral disorders Controls nausea and vomiting, nervousness before surgery, and hiccups	■ Coma ■ CNS or bone marrow depression ■ Reye's syndrome	■ Establish baseline blood pressure (in standing and recumbent positions), and pulse, before initiating treatment
Haloperidol (Haldol)	Has antiemetic and neuroleptic actions Used to treat schizophrenia Relieves pain, nausea, and vomiting	■ Cardiovascular symptoms (hypotension, arrhythmias, and QT prolongation) ■ Dystonia ■ Tardive dyskinesia	■ Monitor patient's mental status daily
Ondansetron (Zofran)	Treats nausea resulting from chemotherapy and surgery	■ Temporary vision loss ■ Bradycardia ■ Anxiety ■ Agitation	■ Adjust dosage in patients with impaired renal function ■ Contraindicated in with liver disease, CHF, and electrolyte imbalance
Phenothiazine, promethazine (Phenergan)	Antihistamine; causes sedation (sleep) to assist in controlling postoperative pain, nausea, vomiting, and motion sickness	■ Dizziness ■ Drowsiness ■ Blurred vision ■ Tinnitus	■ May suppress cough reflex and cause thickening of bronchial secretions
Prochlorperazine (Compazine)	Antiemetic, antipsychotic, tranquilizer	■ Extrapyramidal effects such as involuntary muscle movements, hypotension, fatigue, anxiety, and agitation	■ Position nauseated patients who have received this drug carefully to prevent aspiration of vomitus

Drug	Actions/ Indications	Adverse Effects	Nursing Considerations
Trimethobenza-mide (Tigan)	Used to treat postoperative nausea and vomiting, and gastroenteritis	■ Drowsiness ■ Dizziness ■ Blurred vision ■ Headache	■ Contraindications: narrow-angle glaucoma, prostate conditions, severe hypotension, or cardiac arrhythmia ■ Adjust dosage in patients withimpaired renal function
Pancreatic Enzyme Supplements			
Pancrelipase (Creon, Ultrase), Pancrease	Used as replacement therapy in pancreatic insufficiency and cystic fibrosis	■ Stomach ache ■ Bowel obstruction or bloating	■ Administer prior to food ingestion
Laxatives			
Docusate (Colace, Peri-Colace)	Stool softener and laxative	■ Mild diarrhea or nausea	■ Assess bowel movements, diarrhea
Lactulose	Osmotic laxative; binds with urea to remove ammonia Used to treat chronic con-stipation, and to prevent or treat hepatic encephalopa-thy	■ Diarrhea ■ Nausea ■ Bloating ■ Stomach pain	NOTE: If the patient is confused because of alcohol abuse, obtain an ammonia level
Magnesium citrate	Used to empty bowels prior to surgery or colonoscopy	■ Mild abdomi-nal discomfort or nausea	■ Overuse may cause persistent diarrhea, dehydration, and mineral imbalances (e.g., hypomagnesemia) NOTE: do not use in patients with kidney disease
Senokot	Stimulant laxative	■ Stomach cramps ■ Bloating ■ Mild diarrhea	■ May alter the color or urine and feces

IMMUNOSUPPRESSANTS

Immunosuppressant drugs suppress or reduce the strength of the body's immune system.

Drug	Actions/ Indications	Adverse Effects	Nursing Considerations
Antirejection Drugs			
Mycophenolate mofetil (CellCept)	Prevents kidney rejection by suppressing T- and B-lymphocyte formation	■ Electrolyte imbalance ■ Leucopenia	■ Teach patients to avoid taking simultaneously with antacids ■ Assess for signs for organ rejection ■ Monitor hepatic function

(continued)

Drug	Actions/ Indications	Adverse Effects	Nursing Considerations
Tacrolimus (Prograf)	Prevents kidney rejection by inactivating T lymphocytes	■ Ascites ■ Hyperglycemia ■ Electrolyte imbalance ■ Thrombocytopenia ■ Hypertension	NOTE: Advise the patient to avoid grapefruit and shellfish
Drugs Used to Treat HIV			
Fusion inhibitors (T-20)	Helps prevent HIV from entering and infecting human cells	■ Kidney problems ■ Hypotension ■ Paralysis ■ Severe rash ■ Difficulty breathing	■ Give at ordered times around the clock ■ Assess for bone marrow suppression, anemia, leukopenia, and granulocytopenia
Non-nucleoside reverse transcriptase inhibitors (NNRTIs)	Blocks viral replication of HIV by binding to the enzyme reverse transcriptase		■ Resistance to single-medicine NNRTI treatment develops quickly; for this reason, these drugs should be used only in combination with other antiretroviral agents to treat HIV infection or to prevent or delay the development of resistance
Protease inhibitors	Used to treat or prevent infection by viruses, including HIV and Hepatitis C.		■ Assess for stomach upset, nausea, and diarrhea

IV FLUIDS

IV fluids are used to maintain water balance or as replacement or restorative therapy.

IV Fluid	Actions	Indications	Nursing Considerations
Crystalloids			
0.45% sodium chloride solution	_Hypotonic:_ Causes a sudden fluid shift out of the blood vessels and into cells that can cause cardiovascular collapse Expands the intracellular compartment	Used for dehydration, gastric fluid loss, and cellular dehydration from excessive diuresis.	■ Do not give hypotonic solutions to patients at risk for third space fluid shifts, especially with cerebral edema; these fluids make the patient retain more water and salt, increase tendency for edema, and the patient may become hypokalemic.

IV Fluid	Actions	Indications	Nursing Considerations
0.9% sodium chloride solution and lactated Ringer's solution	*Isotonic*: Correlates with the osmolality of plasma, temporarily expands the extracellular compartment during times of circulatory insufficiency Replenishes sodium and chloride losses so that fluid stays in the intravascular space	Used to treat diabetic ketoacidosis, in the early treatment of burns, and in adrenal insufficiency Ringer's lactate is frequently used during surgical procedures	■ Lactated Ringer's solution contains potassium, sodium, chloride, and calcium ■ Ringer's lactate is contraindicated in patients with liver disease because they cannot metabolize it ■ Also classified as crystalloids are normal saline and lactated Ringer's solution
5% dextrose in 0.9% sodium chloride solution, 3% normal saline solution, and dextrose 10% in water	*Hypertonic*: Pulls water from the intracellular space into the extracellular space, causing the cells to shrink and allowing fluid volume and intracranial pressure (ICP) to increase	Used to treat severe hyponatremia and to provide calories for energy	■ Will cause fluid overload in patients with a history of heart failure or hypertension ■ Can cause hyperglycemia, leading to osmotic diuresis and hyperosmolar coma
Colloids			
Albumin, hetastarch (Hespan)	Stays in the circulation, enabling much smaller amounts to be used for the same volume expansion	Increases plasma volume during shock caused by burns, bleeding, surgery, or other forms of trauma	■ Administration of 250 mL of albumin is equal to 4 L of normal saline ■ Can cause edema and can also trigger anaphylaxis

NEUROLOGICAL AND PSYCHOACTIVE DRUGS

These drugs are used to treat various neurological, cognitive, and psychological disorders.

Drug	Actions/ Indications	Adverse Effects	Nursing Considerations
Anticonvulsant/Anti-Seizure Medications			
Barbiturates Suffix: -bital Examples: secobarbital, phenobarbital, allobarbital	Sedative, hypnotic, anticonvulsant, and CNS depressant effects	■ Lethargy ■ Respiratory depression	■ Therapeutic blood level of phenobarbital is 10–25 mcg/mL

(*continued*)

Drug	Actions/ Indications	Adverse Effects	Nursing Considerations
Carbamazepine (Tegretol)	Used for bipolar disorder and seizure disorder if the patient cannot take valproate (Depakote)	■ Dizziness ■ Nausea ■ Headache	■ Does not cause significant side effects
Divalproex sodium (Depakote)	Blocks sodium or calcium channels; for treatment of epilepsy or bipolar mania	■ Nausea and vomiting ■ Gastrointestinal distress ■ May cause fatal hepatitis and pancreatitis	■ Therapeutic blood level of valproate is 50–100 mcg/mL ■ Rapid onset of action
Fosphenytoin	Treats certain types of seizures (e.g., status epilepticus)	■ Dizziness ■ Drowsiness ■ Headache ■ Dry mouth	■ Discontinue infusion and notify physician if rash appears ■ Be prepared to substitute an alternative therapy rapidly to prevent withdrawal-precipitated seizures; substitute when unable to use phenytoin (Dilantin)
Levetiracetam (Keppra)	Inhibits spread of seizure activity in the brain	■ Suicidal ideation ■ Hypertension ■ Drowsiness	■ Drug levels may be obtained to monitor compliance
Oxcarbazepine (Trileptal)	Alternative to valproate (Depakote) for patients with milder symptoms	■ Acute infection of nose, throat, and sinuses ■ Vertigo ■ Double vision	■ Low long-term risk
Phenytoin (Dilantin)	Anticonvulsant; inhibits seizure activity	■ Mild skin rash ■ Dizziness ■ Sleep problems ■ Headache ■ Joint pain	■ Must be given slowly ■ Therapeutic drug level of phenytoin is 10–20 mcg/mL ■ Toxicity symptoms include poor gait and coordination, slurred speech, nausea, lethargy, and diplopia Contraindicated in pregnancy as it may cause fetal Dilantin syndrome (craniofacial anomalies, mental retardation), drug-induced lupus, life-threatening skin reactions (Stevens–Johnson syndrome), toxic epidermal necrolysis, life- threatening liver failure, and pancreatitis NOTE: This drug is only compatible in normal saline. An increased risk of adverse cardiovascular reactions is associated with rapid administration

Drug	Actions/ Indications	Adverse Effects	Nursing Considerations
Verapamil (Calan)	Used for drug-resistant epilepsy	■ Constipation ■ Headache	■ Possible alternative antiseizure medication for pregnant women ■ Low incidence of side effects

Drugs Used to Treat Other Neurological Diseases and Psychological Disorders

Attention Deficit Disorder

Dextroampheta-mines: methylpheni-date (Ritalin)	Used for attention deficit disorder	■ Severe nervousness ■ Chest pain ■ SVTs ■ Hypertension ■ Uncontrollable head, mouth, neck, arm, or leg movements	NOTE: Supervise drug withdrawal carefully following prolonged use. Abrupt withdrawal may result in severe depression and psychotic behavior

Migraines

Serotonin 5-HT$_1$ receptor agonists Suffix: -triptan Examples: naratriptan (Amerge), almotriptan	Stimulation of receptors results in vasoconstriction	■ Dizziness ■ Drowsiness ■ Tiredness	■ Contraindicated in patients with history, symptoms, or signs of ischemic cardiac, cerebrovascular, or peripheral vascular syndromes

Myasthenia Gravis

Acetylcholinesterase inhibitors Examples: neostigmine, pyridostigmine	Inhibits the cholinesterase enzyme from breaking down acetylcholine Used to treat myasthenia gravis, glaucoma, and Alzheimer's disease	■ Muscle twitching ■ Blurred vision	NOTE: Neostigmine and pyridostigmine are the antidote to anticholinergic poisoning

Parkinson's Disease

Benztropine mesylate (Cogentin)	Antidyskinetic; used as an adjunct in the treatment of all forms of parkinsonism and in control of extrapyramidal disorders	■ Abdominal cramps ■ Bloating ■ Dizziness ■ Dry mouth	■ Can produce anhidrosis (absence of sweating), resulting in heat stroke ■ Contraindicated in patients with angle-closure glaucoma
Levodopa	Metabolized to dopamine in the body Used to treat symptoms of stiffness, tremors, spasms, and poor muscle control in Parkinson's disease	■ Uncontrolled movements of body parts ■ Irregular heartbeat	■ May cause a drug-induced extrapyramidal disorder ■ Contraindicated in patients taking monoamine oxidase inhibitors (MAOIs) and in those with narrow-angle glaucoma or malignant melanoma

(continued)

Drug	Actions/Indications	Adverse Effects	Nursing Considerations
Sinemet	Used to treat Parkinson's disease	<ul><li>Mild nausea</li><li>Dry mouth</li><li>Loss of appetite</li><li>Headache</li><li>May cause drowsiness</li></ul>	<ul><li>May turn sweat, saliva, and urine reddish brown</li></ul>
Trihexyphenidyl (Artane)	Antidyskinetic; used to treat the symptoms of Parkinson's disease and tremors caused by other medical problems or drugs	<ul><li>Dry mouth</li><li>Blurred vision</li><li>Drowsiness or dizziness</li></ul>	<ul><li>Adverse effects are usually dose related and may be minimized by dosage reduction</li><li>Older adults appear to be more sensitive to the drug effects and adjustment of standard adult dosages may be needed</li></ul>
Anxiety			
Azapirones Example: buspirone (BuSpar)	Used as anxiolytics, for generalized anxiety disorder; added to antidepressants such as selective serotonin reuptake inhibitors (SSRIs)	<ul><li>Dizziness</li><li>Nausea</li><li>Headaches</li><li>Nervousness</li></ul>	<ul><li>Monitor for therapeutic effectiveness</li><li>The desired response may begin within 7–10 days; however, optimal results generally take 3–4 weeks</li><li>Reinforce with the patient the importance of continuing treatment while drug response is being evaluated</li></ul>
Benzodiazepines Suffixes: -zolam, -zepam Examples: lorazepam (Ativan), alprazolam, midazolam, diazepam	Used for anxiety disorders; has sedative, hypnotic, anticonvulsant, muscle relaxant, and amnesic effects	<ul><li>CNS effects and respiratory depression</li><li>Ataxia</li><li>Renal and hepatic failure</li></ul>	<ul><li>Side effects are dose dependent</li><li>*Antidote for benzodiazepine overdosage:* flumazenil</li></ul>
Diphenhydramine (Benadryl)	Used as an anxiolytic and antihistamine; has potent anticholinergic effects	<ul><li>Motor impairment (ataxia)</li><li>Flushed skin</li><li>Photophobia</li></ul>	<ul><li>Monitor patients for drowsiness, dizziness, and fatigue</li></ul>

Drug	Actions/ Indications	Adverse Effects	Nursing Considerations
Antipsychotics			
Lithium	Used to treat bipolar disorder and syndrome of inappropriate antidiuretic hormone (SIADH) secretion	■ Hypothyroidism ■ Decreased renal function ■ Hyperparathy-roidism ■ Decreased sodium levels	■ Caution the patient to avoid NSAIDs, thiazide diuretics, and muscle relaxants ■ Monitor for signs and symptoms of lithium toxicity (persistent nausea, vomiting, diarrhea, ataxia, blurred vision, and ringing in the ears) ■ Lithium levels should be obtained 12 hours after the last dose NOTE: Fluid intake up to 3000 mL/daily is recommended, but patients should be instructed to avoid caffeine
Quetiapine (Seroquel)	Atypical (second-generation) antipsychotic; used for sleep problems and agitation, and in the treatment of bipolar disorder	■ Drowsiness ■ Dry mouth ■ Constipation ■ Weight gain	■ Monitor the patient for weight gain
Risperidone	Atypical (second-generation) antipsychotic; used in elderly patients at low dosage	■ Drowsiness ■ Dizziness ■ Dry mouth ■ Weight gain	■ Reassess the patient periodically and maintain on the lowest effective drug dose
Ziprasidone (Geodon)	Atypical (second-generation) antipsychotic; used to treat schizophrenia	■ Skin rash ■ Anxiety ■ Depressed mood ■ Headache	■ Causes less weight gain than olanzapine (Zyprexa)

(continued)

Drug	Actions/ Indications	Adverse Effects	Nursing Considerations
Other antipsychotic drugs Examples: chlorpromazine (Thorazine), thioridazine (Mellaril-S), loxapine (Loxitane), molindone (Moban), perphenazine (Trilafon), thiothixene (Navane), trifluoperazine (Stelazine), haloperidol (Haldol, Serenace), fluphenazine (Prolixin), droperidol, prochlorperazine	Used to treat schizophrenia	◾ Dry mouth ◾ Blurred vision ◾ Hypotension ◾ Irreversible degenerative pigmentary retinopathy ◾ Photosensitivity ◾ Blue-gray discoloration ◾ Orthostatic hypotension ◾ Lowered seizure threshold ◾ Ventricular arrhythmias ◾ Acute dystonia (spasms of tongue, neck, and back—mimics seizures), may occur 1–5 days after initial treatment; manage with antiparkinson drugs ◾ Parkinsonism (rigidity, tremors, masked expression, shuffling gait) may occur 5–30 days after initial treatment ◾ Akathisia (motor restlessness—not anxiety) may occur within 5–60 days; reduction in dosage is required or benzodiazepine must be administered	◾ May take up to 4 weeks to achieve a therapeutic effect NOTE: The combination of the following symptoms is considered a *crisis*: hyperthermia, dyspnea, seizures, and unstable blood pressure

Drug	Actions/ Indications	Adverse Effects	Nursing Considerations
		■ Akinesia (fatigue related) ■ Tardive dyskinesia (continuous movement of the mouth, jaw, hands, or legs) may occur after months to years of treatment ■ Rabbit syndrome (periorbital tremor) may occur after months to years of treatment; manage with antiparkinson drugs	
5-HT₂ antagonists Examples: fluphenazine (Prolixin), haloperidol (Haldol), olanzapine (Zyprexa), risperidone (Risperdal)	Used to treat schizophrenia and bipolar disorder, acute psychotic states, and delirium	■ Induces weight gain ■ High frequency of extrapyramidal motor side effects (dystonias, akathisia, pseudoparkinsonism) ■ Agranulocytosis ■ QT prolongation	■ Patients should not use alcohol and other CNS depressants because of the possible additive CNS depressant effects with concurrent use ■ Patients may develop hyperglycemia and diabetes
Depression			
Bupropion (Wellbutrin XL, Zyban)	Atypical antidepressant; assists in smoking cessation	■ Extrapyramidal symptoms ■ Grand mal seizures ■ Cardiac disease ■ Suicide risk	■ Patients should not take this medication with other medications that contain bupropion such as MAOIs
Monoamine oxidase inhibitors (MAOIs) Examples: isocarboxazid (Marplan), phenelzine (Nardil), tranylcypromine (Parnate)	Acts by inhibiting the activity of monoamine oxidase Used to treat panic disorders, social phobia, atypical depression, bulimia, post-traumatic stress disorder, and borderline personality disorder	■ Metallic, bitter taste ■ Akathisia ("inner" restlessness that manifests with an inability to sit still or remain motionless)	■ Considered the last-line treatment because of numerous lethal dietary and drug interactions ■ Should not be administered in patients who take other psychoactive substances; common examples include SSRIs, tricyclic antidepressants, and meperidine

(continued)

Drug	Actions/ Indications	Adverse Effects	Nursing Considerations
		■ Ataxia (gross lack of coordination of muscle movements) ■ May cause weight gain	■ Reduces the breakdown of serotonin, epinephrine, and norepinephrine, resulting in a higher risk of serotonin syndrome or hypertensive crisis, lowering of the seizure threshold, hepatotoxicity, and suicide ■ May take up to 4–6 weeks for side effects to decrease NOTE: Patients must follow a tyramine-restricted diet (no aged cheeses, alcohol, nuts, canned meats, figs, bananas, soy sauce, or bouillon cubes)
Selective serotonin reuptake inhibitors (SSRIs) Examples: citalopram (Celexa), escitalopram (Lexapro) , fluoxetine (Prozac), paroxetine (Paxil), sertraline (Zoloft)	Used to treat depression and anxiety disorders by increasing serotonin levels	■ Persistent pulmonary hypertension ■ Orthostatic hypotension ■ Akathisia ■ Suicidal ideation ■ Syndrome of inappropriate antidiuretic hormone hypersecretion (SIADH)	NOTE: Treatment for approximately 3 weeks is required to evaluate desired response
Serotonin modulators Example: trazodone hydrochloride (Desyrel)	Used to treat major depressive episodes; inhibits reuptake of serotonin and directly increases the action of serotonin	■ Increased risk of suicide ■ Priapism (sustained and painful erection)	■ Monitor pulse rate and regularity before administration if the patient has preexisting cardiac disease
Serotonin– norepinephrine reuptake inhibitors (SNRIs) Examples: duloxetine (Cymbalta), venlafaxine (Effexor, Effexor XR)	Blocks the absorption of serotonin and norepinephrine in the brain	■ Nausea ■ Dry mouth ■ Sleepiness ■ Fatigue	NOTE: SNRIs can cause dangerously high levels of serotonin. This is known as serotonin syndrome (confusion, rapid or irregular heart rate, dilated pupils, fever, and unconsciousness)
Thioxanthene derivatives Examples: clomipramine (Anafranil), thiothixene (Navane)	Used for depression or schizophrenia	■ Motor impairment (ataxia) ■ Flushed skin ■ Photophobia	NOTE: These drugs may cause neuroleptic malignant syndrome (hyperpyrexia, muscle rigidity, altered mental status, and evidence of autonomic instability)

Drug	Actions/ Indications	Adverse Effects	Nursing Considerations
Tricyclic antidepressants (TCAs) Suffix: -tyline Examples: amitriptyline, nortriptyline, protriptyline	Used primarily for depression	■ Hypotension ■ Weight gain ■ Urinary retention ■ Photosensitivity ■ May cause blurred vision, change in urination, and drowsiness	■ Monitor for signs and symptoms of drowsiness and dizziness (initial stages of therapy), and institute measures to prevent falling ■ Monitor for overdose or suicidal ideation in patients who abuse alcohol

REPRODUCTIVE DRUGS: HORMONES

Reproductive drugs act upon the reproductive system and are important for the regulation of ovulation and menstruation.

Drug	Actions/ Indications	Adverse Effects	Nursing Considerations
Estrogen (Premarin) Suffix: -trel Examples: female hormones (progestin)— desogestrel, etonogestrel, norgestrel	A mixture of conjugated estrogens derived from natural sources used to treat postmenopausal symptoms	■ Increased risk of myocardial infarction, cerebrovascular accident (CVA), invasive breast cancer, endometrial cancer pulmonary emboli (PE), and DVT	■ Arrange for pretreatment and periodic (at least annual) history and physical exam, which should include assessment of blood pressure, breasts, abdomen, pelvic organs, and a Pap smear
Progesterone (Provera)	Used to induce bleeding in women who have amenorrhea	■ Increased risk of blood clots, stroke, heart attack, and breast cancer	■ Monitor for signs and symptoms of thrombophlebitis

RESPIRATORY DRUGS

Respiratory drugs are used to treat diseases of the pulmonary system (respiratory tract and lungs), including inflammatory and obstructive diseases, such as reactive airway and chronic obstructive pulmonary diseases.

Drug	Actions/ Indications	Adverse Effects	Nursing Considerations
Bronchodilators			
Anticholinergic drugs Examples: ipratropium bromide (Atrovent)	Used for chronic obstructive pulmonary disease	■ Headache ■ Dizziness ■ Dry mouth ■ Cough	■ Contraindicated in patients with renal and hepatic insufficiency

(continued)

Drug	Actions/ Indications	Adverse Effects	Nursing Considerations
	Blocks acetylcholine in the central and peripheral nervous system, inhibiting the parasympathetic response		■ *Antidote for anticholinergic poisoning:* physostigmine
Beta-2 adrenergic agonists Examples: albuterol (Ventolin), levosalbutamol (Xopenex), metaproterenol (Alupent)	Short acting; used for reversible obstructive airway disease	■ Arrhythmias ■ Seizure disorder ■ Hyperthyroidism ■ Nervousness ■ Tremors	■ Monitor respiratory and cardiac status
Beta-adrenergic bronchodilators Suffix: -terol Examples: arformoterol, formoterol, levalbuterol, salmeterol	Relaxes airway smooth muscle with subsequent bronchodilation	■ Tremors ■ Tachycardia ■ Hypokalemia	■ Can be used for acute and chronic conditions ■ Administer with caution to patients being treated with MAOIs and TCAs, or patients with ischemic heart disease, hypertension, or cardiac arrhythmias
Leukotriene receptor antagonists Examples: zafirlukast (Accolate), montelukast (Singulair)	Used for asthma and to reduce bronchospasm	■ Hepatic and renal insufficiency ■ Montelukast (Singulair) can cause severe behavior and mood-related changes	■ Monitor effectiveness carefully when used in combination with phenobarbital or other potent cytochrome P450 enzyme inducers
Steroid inhalers Examples: fluticasone/ salmeterol (Advair), flunisolide (AeroBid), triamcinolone acetonide (Azmacort), fluticasone propionate (Flovent), budesonide (Pulmicort), budesonide/ formoterol (Symbicort), beclomethasone (Beclovent)	Opens airways in the lungs to make breathing easier	■ Nausea ■ Diarrhea ■ Upset stomach ■ Dry mouth or throat	■ Instruct patient to rinse and gargle after each use of a steroid inhaler to prevent thrush (candidiasis)
Allergy and Asthma			
Acetylcysteine (Mucomyst)	Used for dissolving mucus, to treat Tylenol overdoses, and as a nephron-protective agent when IV contrast agents must be administered	■ Unusual or unpleasant smell while using the medication ■ White patches or sores inside the mouth or lips	■ Concurrent use with a beta blocker can cause dangerous reductions in heart rate

Drug	Actions/ Indications	Adverse Effects	Nursing Considerations
Dornase alfa (Pulmozyme)	Used for cystic fibrosis treatment and allergic reactions.	■ Sore/dry throat or hoarseness ■ Eye irritation and redness	■ Monitor for changes in blood glucose levels or unusual bleeding
Fexofenadine hydrochloride (Allegra)	Histamine H$_1$-receptor antagonist Used to treat seasonal allergic rhinitis and chronic idiopathic urticaria in adults and children 2 years of age and older	■ Headache ■ Diarrhea ■ Nausea and vomiting ■ Weakness	■ Do not administer with aluminum- and magnesium-containing antacids
Methylxanthine drugs Example: theophylline	Used in the treatment of chronic obstructive pulmonary disease (COPD) and asthma Positive inotropic that relaxes smooth muscles and increases heart muscle contractility and efficiency	■ Headache ■ Irritability ■ Sleeplessness	■ Normal blood level less than 20 mg/L ■ Caution the patient to avoid consuming large amounts of caffeine-containing beverages or supplements ■ Monitor for signs and symptoms of toxicity (nausea, diarrhea, increased heart rate, arrhythmias, and CNS excitation)
Terbutaline (Brethine)	Beta-adrenergic agonist used for asthma Tocolytic; can be used for preterm labor	■ Cardiac arrhythmia ■ Poorly controlled thyroid disease ■ Diabetes mellitus ■ Migraines ■ Cardiopulmonary arrhythmias or ischemia ■ Hypotension ■ Tachycardia ■ Hypokalemia	■ Assess baseline pulse and blood pressure before each dose

TUBERCULOSIS COMBINATION DRUGS

Tuberculosis (TB) combination drugs represent a variety of drugs used to treat tuberculosis.

KEY NOTE: The most difficult problem is compliance with the drug regimen due to the side effects.

Drug	Action	Adverse Effects	Nursing Considerations
Ethambutol	Bacteriostatic against actively growing TB bacilli; obstructs the formation of the cell wall	■ Optic neuritis	■ Assess the patient for infection at beginning of and during therapy
Isoniazid (INH)	Used in treating TB; bactericidal to rapidly dividing mycobacteria but bacteriostatic if the mycobacteria are slow-growing	■ Neuritis ■ Hepatitis	■ Can cause peripheral neuropathy, which is manifested by a tingling sensation of the extremities; this can be prevented through use of supplemental vitamin B_6 (pyridoxine)
Para-aminosalicylic acid (PAS)	Chemotherapeutic agent (the precise mechanism of action is unknown)	■ GI and liver toxicity	■ Be alert for adverse effects of medications
Pyrazinamide	A prodrug that stops the growth of *Mycobacterium tuberculosis*	■ Kidney or liver toxicity	■ Examine patients at regular intervals to look for signs of toxicity
Rifampin	Inhibits bacterial DNA-dependent RNA synthesis by inhibiting bacterial DNA-dependent RNA polymerase Used to treat TB	■ Hepatitis ■ Purpura (red or purple discolorations on the skin that do not blanch on applying pressure)	■ Colors body fluids reddish-orange
Streptomycin	Aminoglycoside that kills sensitive bacteria by stopping the production of essential proteins needed by the bacteria to survive	■ Cranial nerve VIII damage (auditory or acoustic nerve) ■ Kidney toxicity	■ Be alert for symptoms of ototoxicity

VITAMIN AND MINERAL SUPPLEMENTS

Vitamin and mineral supplements are used to treat various conditions caused by nutritional deficiencies.

Supplement	Action	Adverse Effects	Nursing Considerations
Iron (FE) Examples: ferrous sulfate (Feosol),	Ferrous sulfate is involved in oxygen transport and is essential for the regulation of cell growth and differentiation	■ Constipation ■ Black, tarry stools	■ Can be taken orally (give with vitamin C or on empty stomach), IM (Imferon via Z-track injection), or IV but must first give a test dose and observe for any reaction

Supplement	Action	Adverse Effects	Nursing Considerations
deferoxamine	Used to treat iron deficiency, anemia, and related conditions; signs and symptoms include difficulty maintaining body temperature, decreased immune function, and fatigue; patients may demonstrate signs of pica (eating nonnutritive substances such as dirt or clay when iron levels low)	■ Metallic taste ■ Overdosage may cause bluish-colored lips, fingernails, and palms of hands; and seizures	■ Instruct the patient that meat proteins and vitamin C will improve the absorption of nonheme iron ■ Do not administer concurrently with antacids, antibiotics, or calcium supplements or within 2 hours prior to or after taking ferrous sulfate NOTE: excessive milk consumption reduces the intake of other essential nutrients, especially iron
Sodium bicarbonate	Increases plasma bicarbonate levels, buffers excess hydrogen ion concentration, raises blood pH; leads to alkalinization of the urine, diminishing nephrotoxicity; used to treat acidosis and hyperkalemia	■ Nausea ■ Bloating and gas	■ Normal plasma levels are 24–31 mEq/L ■ Contraindications: hypochloremic alkalosis (from vomiting) and hypocalcemia
Vitamins A, D, E, K	Fat-soluble vitamins used to treat related vitamin deficiencies	■ Nausea and vomiting	■ Use with caution; can cause toxicity

OTHER DRUGS USED TO TREAT SPECIFIC MEDICAL DISORDERS

Prostatic Hypertrophy

Dutasteride (Avodart)	Androgen inhibitor; inhibits the enzyme responsible for converting testosterone into a metabolite that causes prostatic hyperplasia	■ Decreased libido ■ Impotence ■ Breast tenderness	■ Assess for incomplete bladder emptying

(continued)

Thyroid Disorders			
Potassium iodide (SSKI)	Prevents uptake of radioactive iodine by the thyroid Used to treat hyperthyroidism (goiter)	■ Diarrhea ■ Nausea and vomiting ■ Stomach pain	■ May cause a metallic taste in the mouth, fever, swelling of the front of the neck/throat (goiter), and signs of decreased thyroid gland function ■ Administer in juice, instructing the patient to sip through a straw
Thyroid hormone inhibitors Examples: propylthiouracil, methimazole (Tapazole)	Anti-thyroids treat hyperthyroidism	■ Headache ■ Drowsiness ■ Dizziness ■ Skin rash	■ Drug dosage must be tapered to discontinue
Urinary Disorders			
Phenazopyridine (Pyridium)	Urinary analgesic	■ Headache ■ Dizziness ■ Stomach upset	■ Causes orange or red discoloration of urine

MEDICAL ABBREVIATIONS

AAA	abdominal aortic aneurysm
ABG	arterial blood gas
ac	before meals
ad lib	as desired
AFB	acid-fast bacilli
AFib	atrial fibrillation
AI	aortic insufficiency
AICD	automatic implanted cardiac defibrillator
A&O	alert & oriented
AMA	against medical advice
amp	one ampule
ARDS	adult respiratory distress syndrome
ARF	acute renal failure
AROM	active range of motion
AS	aortic stenosis
ASA	aspirin
AVM	arterial venous malformation
BBB	bundle branch block
BE	barium enema
bid	twice a day
BKA	below the knee amputation
BLE	bilateral lower extremities
BM	bowel movement
BP	blood pressure
BPH	benign prostatic hypertrophy
BRP	bathroom privileges
BSO	bilateral salpingo-oophorectomy
BUE	bilateral upper extremities
BUN	blood urea nitrogen
BX	biopsy

CABG	coronary artery bypass graft
CAD	coronary artery disease
CATH	catheter
CBC	complete blood count
CBI	continuous bladder irrigation
CDI	clean, dry, & intact
CHEM	chemistry
CHF	congestive heart failure
CHI	closed head injury
CI	cardiac index
CNS	central nervous system
C/O	complaint of
CO	cardiac output
CO_2	carbon dioxide
COMP	comprehensive metabolic profile
COPD	chronic obstructive pulmonary disease
cp	chest pain
CPAP	continuous positive airway pressure
CPK	creatine phosphokinase
CPP	cerebral perfusion pressure
CPR	cardiopulmonary resuscitation
CPT	chest pulmonary therapy
Cr	creatinine
CRF	chronic renal failure
CRRT	continuous renal replacement therapy
C&S	culture & sensitivity
CSF	cerebral spinal fluid
CV	cardiovascular
CVA	cerebrovascular accident
CVP	central venous pressure
CXR	chest x-ray
Cysto	cystoscopy
D&C	dilation and curettage
D/C	discontinue
D5NS	dextrose 5% in normal saline
D5W	5% dextrose in water
DJD	degenerative joint disease
DM	diabetes mellitus
DNR	do not resuscitate
DOA	dead on arrival
DOE	dyspnea on exertion
DPT	diphtheria, pertussis, tetanus
Dsg	dressing
DTs	delirium tremens
DVT	deep vein thrombosis
Dx	diagnosis
EBL	estimated blood loss
Echo	echocardiogram
EEG	electroencephalogram
EENT	eyes, ears, nose, & throat
EF	ejection fraction
ELR	electrolyte and renal profile
ENDO	endoscopy
ERCP	endoscopic retrograde cholangiopancreatography
ESRD	end-stage renal disease
ET	endotracheal
ETOH	ethanol (alcohol)

ETT	endotracheal tube
F/U	follow-up
FBS	fasting blood sugar
FiO$_2$	fraction of inspired oxygen
FM	face mask
FSH	follicle-stimulating hormone
FX	fracture
GERD	gastroesophageal reflux disease
GI	gastrointestinal
GLU	glucose
GSW	gunshot wound
GU	genitourinary
HCTZ	hydrochlorothiazide
Hgb	hemoglobin
HgbA1C	glycated hemoglobin
HH	hematocrit & hemoglobin
HHFM	high-humidity face mask
HL	hep-lock
HOB	head of bed
HOH	hard of hearing
H&P	history & physical
HR	heart rate
HS	hour of sleep
ht	height
HTN	hypertension
Hx	history
IABP	intra-aortic balloon pump
ICP	intracranial pressure
I&D	incision & drainage
IM	intramuscular
INR	international normalized ratio
I&O	intake &output
IS	incentive spirometer
ITP	idiopathic thrombocytopenic purpura
IV	intravenous
IVPB	intravenous piggyback
JVD	jugular venous distention
KCL	potassium chloride
KUB	kidneys, ureters, bladder
KVO	keep vein open
LAP	laparotomy
LE	lower extremities
LLL	left lower lobe
LLQ	left lower quadrant
LMP	last menstrual period
LOC	level of consciousness
LOS	length of stay
LP	lumbar puncture
LR	Lactated Ringers
LVF	left ventricular function
MAE	moves all extremities
MAOI	monoamine oxidase inhibitors
MAP	mean arterial pressure
MAR	medication administration record
MI	myocardial infarction
Mmol	millimole
MOM	milk of magnesia

MVC	motor vehicle crash
MVI	multivitamin
NAD	no acute distress
NC	nasal cannula
neb	nebulizer
NGT	nasogastric tube
NH	nursing home
NKA	no known allergies
NKDA	no known drug allergies
NPO	nothing by mouth (nothing per os)
NRB	nonrebreather
NS	normal saline
NSAIDS	nonsteroidal anti-inflammatory drugs
NSR	normal sinus rhythm
NT	nasotracheal
NTG	nitroglycerin
N/V	nausea and vomiting
NWB	nonweight bearing
O_2	oxygen
OA	osteoarthritis
OB	occult blood
OOB	out of bed
OR	operating room
ORIF	open reduction with internal fixation
OT	occupational therapy
OTC	over the counter
PAC	premature atrial contraction
PACU	postanesthesia care unit
pc	after meals
PCA	patient-controlled analgesia
PCEA	percutaneous carotid endarterectomy
PCN	penicillin
PCWP	pulmonary capillary wedge pressure
PEA	pulseless electrical activity
PEG	percutaneous endoscopic gastrostomy
PERRLA	pupils equal, round, react to light and accommodation
PFS	patient/family services
PFT	pulmonary function test
PICC	peripherally inserted central catheter
PID	pelvic inflammatory disease
PMD	private medical doctor
PMH	past medical history
PMI	point of maximal impulse
PMP	postmenopausal
po	by mouth (per os)
POD	postoperative day
PRBC	packed red blood cells
prn	whenever necessary
PROM	passive range of motion
PSA	prostate specific antigen
Pt	patient
PT	physical therapy
PTCA	percutaneous transluminal coronary angioplasty
PTSD	posttraumatic stress disorder
PTT	partial thromboplastin time
PTX	pneumothorax
PUD	peptic ulcer disease

PVC	premature ventricular contraction
PVD	peripheral vascular disease
q	every
QA	quality assurance
R/O	rule out
SBO	small bowel obstruction
SDP	single-donor platelets
SI	suicidal ideation
SIADH	syndrome of inappropriate antidiuretic hormone secretion
SL	sublingual
SLE	systemic lupus erythematosus
SNF	skilled nursing facility
S/O	significant other
SOAP	subjective/objective assessment & plan
SOB	short of breath
S/P	status post
SPA	salt poor albumin
SQ/SC	subcutaneous
S/S	signs and symptoms
SVT	supraventricular tachycardia
SUPP	suppository
SX	symptoms
sz	seizures
TAH	total abdominal hysterectomy
TB	tuberculosis
T&C	type & cross
TCDB	turn, cough, deep breath
TEDS	thromboembolic stockings
TEE	transesophageal echocardiography
TENS	transcutaneous electrical nerve stimulation
TF	tube feeding
TIA	transient ischemic attack
TIBC	total iron binding capacity
tid	three times a day
TKA	total knee arthroplasty
TMJ	temporomandibular joint
TO	telephone order
TPN	total parenteral nutrition
TPR	temperature, pulse, respirations
T&S	type & screen
TURP	transurethral resection of prostate
UA	urinalysis
UC	urine culture
UD	unit dose
UGI	upper gastrointestinal series
UO	urine output
US	ultrasound
UTI	urinary tract infection
VM	venti-mask
VO	verbal order
VS	vital signs
VSS	vital signs stable
WC	wheelchair
WBAT	weight-bearing as tolerated
WDI	warm, dry, & intact
WNL	within normal limits
WPW	Wolff-Parkinson-White syndrome

ADDITIONAL READING

Adams, C. (2014). *How to evaluate student-performance measures in nursing classroom education*. Retrieved from http://www.ehow.com/how_7438049_evaluate-measures-nursing-classroom-education.html

Advanogy. (2014). *Overview of learning styles*. Retrieved from http://www.learning-styles-online.com/overview

American Association of Critical-Care Nurses. (2014). *Critical care*. Retrieved from http://www.aacn.org

American Cancer Society. (2014). *Types of cancer*. Retrieved from http://www.cancer.org

American Chronic Pain Association. (2014). *Medications and treatments*. Retrieved from http://theacpa.org

American Diabetic Association. (2014). *Diabetes mellitus*. Retrieved from http://www.diabetes.org

Atherton, J. S.(2013). *Learning and teaching; learning contracts*. Retrieved from http://www.learningandteaching.info/teaching/learning_contracts.htm

Bates, B. (1979). *A guide to physical examination*. Philadelphia, PA: J. B.Lippincott Company.

Centers for Disease Control and Prevention. (2014). *Common eye disorders*. Retrieved from http://www.cdc.gov/visionhealth/basic_information/eye_disorders.htm

Distance Learning Centers. (2012). *How to evaluate nursing students*. Retrieved from http://dlsii.com/blog/online-classroom/how-to-evaluate-nursing-students

Emergency Nurses Association. (2014). *Emergency nursing*. Retrieved from www.ena.org

Encyclopedia of Surgery. (2014). *Patient controlled analgesia*. Retrieved from http://www.surgeryencyclopedia.com/La-Pa/Patient-Controlled-Analgesia.html

Federal Emergency Management Agency. (2014). *Emergency medical care and triage*. Retrieved from training.fema.gov

Gooder, V. (2011). *Nurses' perceptions of a (BCMA) Bar-coded Medication Administration System*. Retrieved from http://ojni.org/issues

Hanson, J. (2014). *How to prioritize nursing care plans for multiple patients*. Retrieved from http://www.ehow.com/how_7508427_prioritize-care-plans-multiple-patients

Hartman, D. (2014). *Skills and competency checklists*. Retrieved from http://www.ehow.com/info_8376523_skills-competency-checklists.html

Hunter, K. M. (2011). *Implementation of an electronic medication administration record and bedside verification system online journal of nursing informatics*. Retrieved from http://ojni.org/issues

Inspiration software. (2014). *Introduction to concept mapping*. Retrieved from http://www.inspiration.com/visual-learning/concept-mapping

Joliet Junior College. (2014). *Blank adjunct faculty contract.* Retrieved from http://www.jjc.edu/about/college-info/adjunct-faculty/Pages/blank-contract.aspx

Kaufman, D. (2014). *Interpretation of arterial blood gases (ABGs).* Retrieved from http://www.thoracic.org/clinical/critical-care/clinical-education/abgs.php

Lab Tests Online. (2014). *Lab tests.* Retrieved from http://www.labtestsonline.org

LearnAlberta.Ca. (2008). *Assessment strategies and tools: Anecdotal notes.* Retrieved from http://www.learnalberta.ca/content/mewa/html/assessment/anecdotalnotes.html

Lewis, S. M., Heitkemper, M., & Dirksen, S. (2010). *Medical-surgical nursing* (6th ed.). St. Louis, MO: Mosby.

Massachusetts Department of Elementary and Secondary Education. (2014). *Educator evaluation.* Retrieved from http://www.doe.mass.edu/edeval/resources/evalforms

Mayer, S. (2014). *Nursing + counseling nursing students success.* Retrieved from mcli.maricopa.edu

Merck Manual. (2011). *Home health handbook.* Retrieved from http://www.merckmanuals.com/home/index.html

Moore, M. (2005). *Nutritional assessment and care* (5th ed.). St. Louis, MO: Mosby.

National Institute on Aging. (2014). *End of life.* Retrieved from http://www.nia.nih.gov

National Institute of Health. (2014). *Drug abuse.* Retrieved from http://www.nlm.nih.gov/medlineplus/sitemap.html

National Library of Medicine. (2014). *Autoimmune disorders.* Retrieved from www.ncbi.nlm.nih.gov

Nobel Prize.Com. (2014). *Medicine educational games.* Retrieved from http://nobel prize.org/educational_games/medicine

Nursing Link. (2014). *Physical assessment.* Retrieved from http://nursinglink.monster.com/training/articles/298-physical-assessment—chapter-1-history-and-physical-examination

Pennsylvania Department of Education. (2014). *Life skill deficiency.* Retrieved from http://www.ntuaft.com/TISE/IRS%20manual/Scope/life_skill_deficiency.htm

Potter, P., & Potter, A. (2009). *Fundamentals of nursing* (7th ed.). St. Louis, MO: Mosby.

Psychology Today. (2014). *Death and dying.* Retrieved from http://www.psychology-today.com/conditions/death-and-dying

Quan, K. (2014). *Demystifying critical thinking skills.* Retrieved from http://nursinglink.monster.com/benefits/articles/18452-demystifying-critical-thinking-skills

Quintessential Careers. (1996). *Job-seeker action verbs.* Retrieved from http://www.quintcareers.com/action_verbs.html

Registered Nurse RN.com. (2014). *Nursing care plan overview and introduction: What is a care plan in nursing?* Retrieved from http://www.registerednursern.com/nursing-care-plans-free-care-plan-examples-for-a-registered-nurses-rn-students

Rural Connection Inc. (2007). *Nurses as teachers.* Retrieved from www.nursesasteachers.org

Sherman, R. (2011). *Teaching nurses to delegate.* Retrieved from http://www.emergingrnleader.com/delegationnursing-leadership

Teleflex. (2009). *Thoracic system pathology.* Retrieved from http://www.teleflex.com/en/usa/ucd/thoracic_system_pathology.php

TNTP. (2010). *Teacher evaluation.* Retrieved from tntp.org/assets/documents/Teacher-Evaluation-Oct10F.pdf

University of Portland School of Nursing. (2014). *Student clinical performance evaluation.* Retrieved from http://nursing.up.edu

U. S. Food and Drug Administration. (2014). *Information on drugs.* Retrieved from http://www.fda.gov/Drugs/InformationOnDrugs/ucm079436.htm

Van Leeuwen, A., Kranpitz, T., & Smith, L. (2006). *Davis's comprehensive handbook of laboratory and diagnostic tests with nursing implications* (2nd ed.). Philadelphia, PA: F.A. Davis Company.

Webber, N. (2014). *Uses of remediation in nursing programs.* Retrieved from http://www.ehow.com/list_6518586_uses-remediation-nursing-programs.html

Williams, E. (2014). *Leadership styles in nursing management.* Retrieved from http://work.chron.com/leadership-styles-nursing-management-16070.html

Winningham, M.,& Preusser, B. A. (2000). *Winningham and Preusser's critical thinking in medical–surgical settings: A case study approach* (2nd ed.). St. Louis, MO: Mosby.

Zacharewicz, N. (2014). *How to write an anecdotal note.* Retrieved from http://www.ehow.com/how_8683005_write-anecdotal.html

INDEX